Back To Basics

Back To Basics

Critical Care Transport Certification Review

Orchid Lee Lopez

To order additional copies of this book, contact:
Xlibris Corporation
1-888-795-4274
www.Xlibris.com
Orders@Xlibris.com
88683

Contents

Dedication

To my husband, Gene, my children, Raquel, Corinne, Alexis, Amanda, sons-in-law, Eric, Robert II and my grandchildren, Jacob, Angelee, Gavin, Taylin, Robert III—who have always been there through hard times and whose patience, understanding, encouragement, and support have never wavered during the many hours spent working on this textbook.

Acknowledgments

This critical care transport certification review textbook is also dedicated to all the hard-working EMS educators and medical directors who have spent countless hours, training and who have made a difference in improving the quality of patient care in the prehospital ground and air medical transport environment. Thank you for all that you have done and will continue to do.

John Samson, RN, CFRN, NREMT-P, FP-C
Sheryl Williams, RN, BSN, CFRN
Robert Hesse, RN, CFRN, NREMT-P, FP-C
Barb Wood, RN, RNC
Chuck Bauer, EMT-P, FP-C
Andrew Castellana, EMT-P, FP-C
Aaron Downey, EMT-P, FP-C
Chad Boesl, RN, CFRN
Gene Lopez, NREMT-P, FP-C
Mike Breithaupt, Rotor-Wing Pilot
Steve Farber, Rotor-Wing Pilot
Richard Dobson, Rotor-Wing Pilot
Karen Bajalis, RN, RNC
Carol Pribyl, RN, RNC
LeAnn Thorpe, RN, RNC
Melinda Boyer, RRT
Mike Bei, RN, RNC
Rick McKinstry, RN, CFRN
Christopher Hall, EMT-P, FP-C
Eric Lewis, RN, CFRN
Chuck Skinner, EMT-P, FP-C
Amy Caldwell, EMT-P, FP-C
John Elliott, MD
Steve Murphey, MD
Steve Maher, MD
Dave Tellez, MD
Dave Streitwieser, MD
Glenn Waterkotte, MD
Darren Braude, MD
Stephen Donohue, MD

In Memory Of
James Alan Baker, EMT-P, FP-C
New Mexico Clinical EMS Educator

Every job is a self-portrait of the person who does it.
Autograph your work with excellence. We are what we repeatedly do.
Excellence, then, is not an act, but a habit.

—Aristotle

Preface

Back To Basics Critical Care Transport Certification Review (BCCTPC) is intended to meet the needs of prehospital care providers at all levels as they strive for ever-increasing clinical excellence when preparing to take the certification examinations. Prehospital care providers are confronted daily by a variety of clinical conditions and must have an in-depth understanding of the pathophysiology of these conditions to be able to assess and provide the medical treatment necessary.

This book in organized into ten modules, which includes fifty questions in each module, with a total of five hundred practice questions that will assist the readers in preparing for the certification examination. Each question is provided with the answer and rationale, which includes a comprehensive explanation as to why the answer is correct and why the other answers are not correct. The practice questions with rationale will provide the reader with a better conceptual basic understanding of the subject matter. The figures and tables provided illustrate pertinent concepts, thereby facilitating reading comprehension. This format also makes the text useful as a quick reference guide. Study flashcards have been provided to assist the reader in testing themselves over a variety of topics and subject areas that could be included on the certification examination.

The BCCTPC examination content outlines have been provided so that the reader has a better understanding of what topics or subject areas can be asked on the certification examination. Studying is only a part of getting good results on your exam. Preparation for your examination should begin several months prior; this includes studying, reviewing study materials on a regular basis, and if possible, attending a BCCTPC-approved sixteen-hour FP-C/CCP-C review course. Students with better study methods and strategies have a better success in passing the certification examination. Everyone is different; different methods work for different people, and tips on how to study for the exam have been provided for the purpose of improving upon your current studying techniques.

The material in this textbook contains the most current information available at the time of publication. It is the responsibility of the readers to familiarize themselves and to stay informed of any new changes or recommendations in the policies and procedures set by the federal, state, and local agencies as well as the institution or agency where the reader is employed. The author and the publisher of this textbook disclaim any liability, loss, or risk resulting directly or indirectly from the suggested procedures and theory from any undetected errors or from the reader's misunderstanding of the textbook.

All information used in advanced cardiac life support reflects the current guidelines. Issues and concerns related to geriatrics, pediatrics, obstetrics, and neonates are integrated throughout the text. The national standards for cardiopulmonary resuscitation (CPR) and emergency cardiovascular care (ECC) are reviewed and revised on a regular basis and may change after the publication of this textbook. It is important that you know the most current recommended guidelines for CPR and ECC.

The *Back to Basics Critical Care Transport Certification Review* text is an independent publication and has not been authorized, sponsored, or otherwise approved by BCCTPC Inc. Please note that this textbook is independent of the actual CCP-C, FP-C, CFRN, or CTRN certification examination administration. If you are interested in taking the FP-C or CCP-C certification examination, you can contact the Board for Critical Care Transport Paramedic Certification (BCCTPC) or visit their Web site at www.bcctpc.org. If you are interested in taking the CFRN or CTRN certification examination, you can contact the Board for Certification in Emergency Nursing (BCEN) or visit their Web site at www.ena.org.

Module 1
ECG and IABP Monitoring

1. A sixty-six-year-old man complains of chest pain for three hours. The 12-lead ECG shows the following:

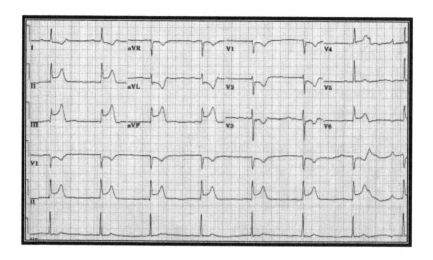

   A. Anterolateral myocardial infarction
   B. Inferior myocardial infarction
   C. Posterior myocardial infarction
   D. Lateral myocardial infarction

2. Which of the following coronary arteries supplies the majority of the circulation to the inferior portion of the heart?

   A. Left coronary
   B. Left ascending
   C. Right coronary
   D. Circumflex

3. V1-V6 chest leads are categorized as

    A. Bipolar leads
    B. Augmented leads
    C. Unipolar leads
    D. Limb leads

4. Which of the following references can be used to determine ST
    elevation, ST depression, or QRS duration on the ECG tracing?

    A. Delta wave
    B. J point
    C. Osborne wave
    D. Z point

5. Which type of myocardial infarction (MI) does the following
    12-lead ECG show?

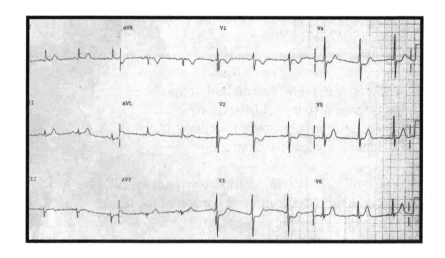

    A. Inferior
    B. Anterior
    C. Posterior
    D. Septal

6. ST elevation seen on the ECG tracing can indicate

   A. Ischemia
   B. Injury
   C. Infarction
   D. Electrolyte imbalance

7. Hyperkalemia >7.0 can exhibit which of the following changes on the ECG tracing?

   A. Inverted T waves
   B. U waves
   C. Tented or peaked T waves
   D. Flattened T waves

8. A fifty-year-old man presents with chest pain for three days. What does the following 12-lead ECG show?

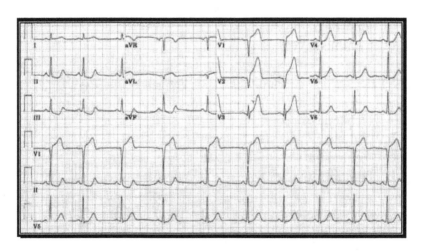

   A. Inferior MI
   B. Anterior MI
   C. Posterior MI
   D. Right ventricular MI

9. Which of the following is characteristic of the 12-lead ECG for a patient with a history of WPW?

   A. J point
   B. Delta wave
   C. Osborne wave
   D. Q wave

10. Interpret the following ECG tracing.

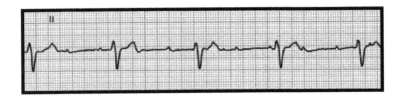

   A. Second-degree AVB, Type I
   B. Second-degree AVB, Type II
   C. First-degree AVB
   D. Complete AVB

11. ST depression can indicate all of the following, *except*

   A. Ischemia
   B. Old injury
   C. Acute injury
   D. Digitalis toxicity

12. Q waves present with ST elevation can indicate

   A. Acute ischemia
   B. Acute injury
   C. Old infarction
   D. Right ventricular MI

13. Interpret the following ECG tracing.

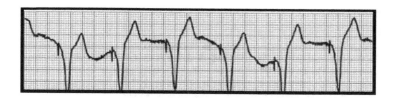

    A. 100% ventricular paced rhythm
    B. Sinus rhythm with ST elevation
    C. Atrial fibrillation with ST elevation
    D. Junctional rhythm with ST elevation

14. Your patient presents with epigastric pain, nausea, and vomiting for one hour. He describes his chest pain as "heavy in nature." What does the following 12-lead ECG show?

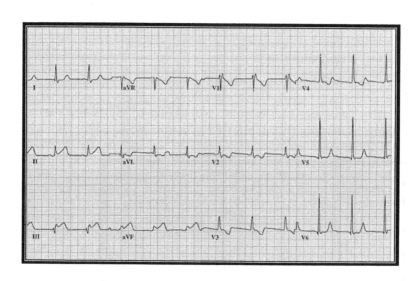

    A. Posterior MI
    B. Anterior MI
    C. Inferior MI
    D. Poor R wave progression

15. Interpret the following ECG tracing.

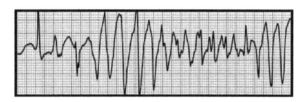

    A. Monomorphic VT
    B. Polymorphic VT
    C. Atrial fibrillation with bundle branch block
    D. Electrical alternans

16. Your patient is exhibiting ST elevation in leads II, III, and AVF. ST depression is noted in V1-V3. Which of the following may prove hazardous?

    A. Isotonic fluid bolus
    B. Heparin
    C. GII/BIIIa inhibitors
    D. Nitroglycerin

17. A fifty-five-year-old woman complains of SOB for two days. Identify what the following ECG rhythm reveals

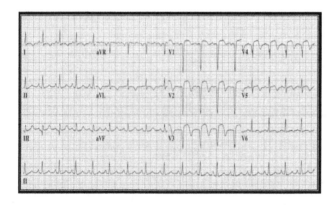

    A. Inferior MI
    B. Anteroseptal MI
    C. Lateral wall MI
    D. Poor R wave aggression

18. In which sequence does blood flow through the heart valves?

    A. Tricuspid, pulmonic, mitral, aortic
    B. Tricuspid, mitral, pulmonic, aortic
    C. Tricuspid, aortic, mitral, pulmonic
    D. Mitral, pulmonic, tricuspid, aortic

19. What condition may the following ECG indicate?

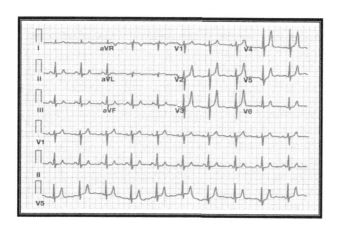

    A. Hypokalemia
    B. Hyperkalemia
    C. Hypocalcemia
    D. Hypernatremia

20. Interpret the following ECG tracing.

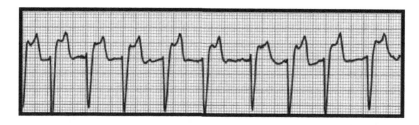

    A. Sinus rhythm with ST elevation
    B. Junctional tachycardia with ST elevation
    C. Paced 100% rhythm
    D. Atrial fibrillation with ST elevation

21. The ECG may show peaked P waves, flattened/slurred Ts, and appearance of U waves, which may indicate

    A. Hyperkalemia
    B. Hypokalemia
    C. Hypernatremia
    D. Hyperchloremia

22. Interpret the following 12-lead ECG.

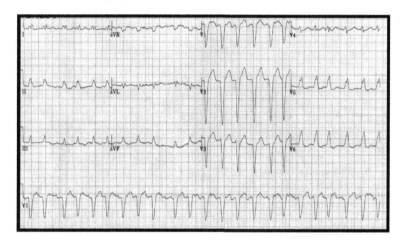

    A. Atrial flutter with bundle branch block
    B. Atrial fibrillation with bundle branch block
    C. Wide complex tachycardia
    D. Narrow complex tachycardia

23. Inferior wall MI is caused by an occlusion of which coronary artery?

    A. LAD
    B. RCA
    C. Circumflex
    D. Inferior vena cava

24. The following ECG reveals

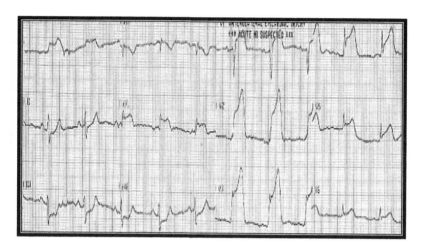

    A. Anteroseptal-lateral MI
    B. Inferior MI
    C. Posterior MI
    D. Pericarditis

25. Interpret the following ECG tracing.

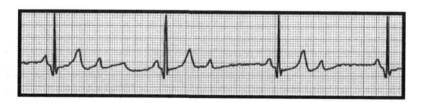

    A. Complete AVB
    B. Second-degree AVB, Mobitz I
    C. Second-degree AVB, Mobitz II
    D. AV disassociation

26. On 12-lead ECG, posterior wall MIs manifest as

    A. ST elevation in II, III, AVF
    B. ST depression in II, III, AVF
    C. ST depression in V1-V4 with abnormally tall R waves
    D. ST elevation in V1-V4 with abnormally tall R waves

27. Interpret the following 12-lead ECG.

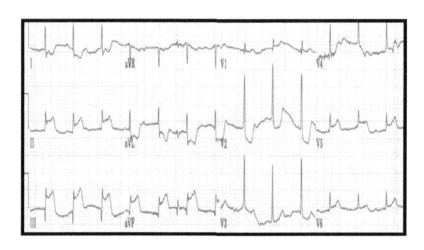

    A. Lateral wall MI
    B. Inferior-lateral wall MI
    C. Posterior wall MI
    D. Inferior wall MI

28. Interpret the following ECG tracing.

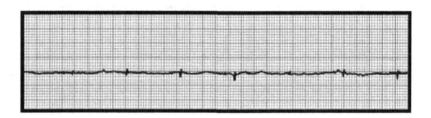

    A. Pacer spikes with failure to capture
    B. Atrial fibrillation
    C. Sinus rhythm with low QRS amplitude
    D. Sinus rhythm with electrical interference

29. Interpret the following 12-lead ECG.

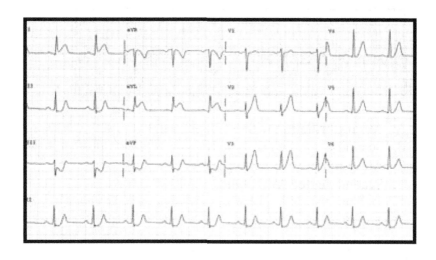

    A. Inferior MI
    B. Lateral MI
    C. Posterior MI
    D. Septal MI

30. ST elevation in leads I, aV_L, V5, and V6 are indicative of injury to which area of the heart?

    A. Inferior
    B. Lateral
    C. Anterior
    D. Posterior

31. A patient with a history of tricyclic antidepressant overdose can exhibit which of the following on the ECG tracing?

    A. Short PR interval
    B. Peaked or tented T waves
    C. Prolonged QT interval
    D. Prolonged PR interval

32. Interpret the following ECG tracing.

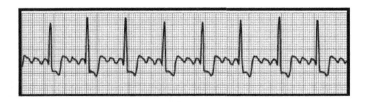

   A. Atrial fibrillation with ST depression
   B. Second-degree AVB, Type II
   C. Atrial flutter with ST depression
   D. Second-degree AVB, Type I

33. The following ECG reveals

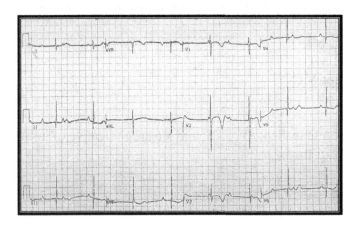

   A. First-degree AV block
   B. Second-degree AV block
   C. Sinus bradycardia
   D. Complete heart block

34. What changes in the ECG would a patient presenting with an inferior wall MI most likely have?

   A. ST depression in leads II, III, and aV_F
   B. ST elevation in leads I, aV_L, V5, and V6
   C. ST elevation in leads II, III, and aV_F
   D. ST depression in leads V1 and V2

35. Normal K⁺ lab value is

    A. 3. 0-4.0
    B. 3.5-4.5
    C. 4.0-5.0
    D. >5.5

36. Interpret the following ECG tracing.

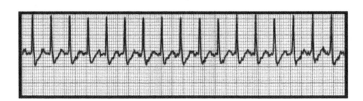

    A. Atrial fibrillation
    B. Atrial flutter
    C. Sinus tachycardia
    D. Atrial tachycardia

37. Interpret the following ECG tracing.

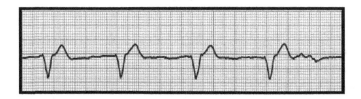

    A. Junctional bradycardia
    B. Idioventricular rhythm
    C. Complete AVB
    D. Sinus bradycardia

38. Diagnosis of a right ventricular MI includes

    A. Right-sided 12-lead ECG with ST elevation in V4
    B. Right-sided 12-lead ECG with ST depression in V2-V4
    C. Left-sided 12-lead ECG with ST elevation in V1-V4
    D. Left-sided 12-lead ECG with ST depression in V1-V2

39. Interpret the following ECG tracing.

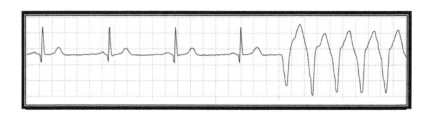

   A. Junctional bradycardia with a run of ventricular tachycardia
   B. Sinus bradycardia into ventricular tachycardia
   C. Sinus rhythm changing into 100% paced rhythm
   D. Sinus rhythm into junctional tachycardia

40. Interpret the following ECG tracing.

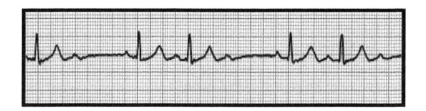

   A. Sinus rhythm with first-degree AVB
   B. Second-degree AVB, Type I
   C. Second-degree AVB, Type II
   D. Complete AVB

41. Your IABP begins to purge during ascent. The triggering mechanism for this function was initiated as a result of which gas law?

   A. Boyle's law
   B. Gay-Lussac's law
   C. Charles's law
   D. Henry's law

42. The balloon has dislodged when treating your IABP patient. Which is the most common site that will be affected?

    A. Right radial
    B. Left radial
    C. Right femoral
    D. Left femoral

43. During transport you note rust-colored "flakes" in the IABP tubing. This indicates

    A. Helium tank degredation
    B. IABP pump failure/lubricant leak
    C. Helium oxidation
    D. Balloon rupture

44. Interpret the following IABP timing strip.

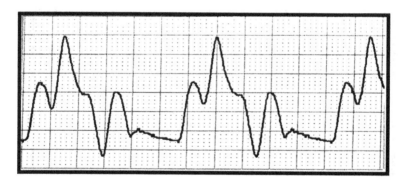

    A. Early inflation
    B. Late inflation
    C. Early deflation
    D. Late deflation

45. The primary trigger used for most IABP operations is the

    A. A-line
    B. PA catheter
    C. EKG
    D. CVP catheter

46. Inadvertent migration of the IAB may cause which of the following, *except*

    A. Loss of renal perfusion
    B. Loss of flow to subclavian artery
    C. Loss of flow to the carotid vein
    D. Loss of flow to the renal arteries

47. When timing the IABP, inflation should initiate in synchronization with

    A. ECG-P wave
    B. Anacrotic notch of the A-line
    C. Beginning systole
    D. Dicrotic notch indicated on the A-line pressure wave

48. Identify the following IABP timing strip.

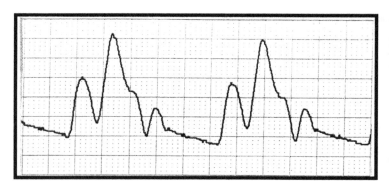

    A. Early inflation
    B. Normal timing
    C. Late inflation
    D. Late deflation

49. Which of the following is the most potentially harmful timing error?

    A. Early deflation
    B. Early inflation
    C. Late deflation
    D. None of the above is potentially harmful

50. During transport you experience a complete IABP failure. You should

A. Withdraw the IABP to 10 cm
B. Cycle the balloon manually timing with EKG visually
C. Cycle the balloon manually timing with the A-line visually
D. Cycle the balloon manually every thirty minutes regardless of timing

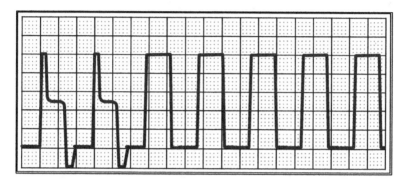

Answer Key and Rationale

1. **B:** ST elevation is present in leads II, III, and aVF. *(Review the following chart for locations of different injury, ischemia, and/or infarcted areas)*

Location	Coronary artery affected	12-lead ECG
Anterior	LAD	V3, V4
Inferior	RCA	II, III, AVF
Lateral	LCX	I, AVL, V5, V6
Septal	LAD	V1, V2
Posterior	LCX or RCA	V1-V4 ST depression, progression of tall R waves

2. **C:** The right coronary artery (RCA) supplies the majority of the inferior portion of the heart and some of the posterior portion of the heart. *(Review chart provided)*

Coronary arteries	Areas of the heart
Coronary circulation	Consists of right and left coronary arteries that arise from the coronary ostia at the aortic root
Left main coronary artery Left anterior descending (LAD) Circumflex (LCX)	LAD—supplies the anterior surface of the heart, the anterior 2/3 of the septum and part of the lateral wall LCX—primarily supplies the lateral wall of the left ventricle
Right coronary artery	Supplies the right atrium, right ventricle, and the inferior and posterior walls of the left ventricle

3. **C:** Chest leads, also known as "precordial" or unipolar leads are V1-V6 which views the heart from a horizontal plane. Traditional limb leads, also known as bipolar leads are I, II, and III, which view the heart from a vertical plane. Augmented leads are aV_R,

aV$_F$, and aV$_L$, which view the heart from a vertical plane. Most common lead used for transport is Lead II.

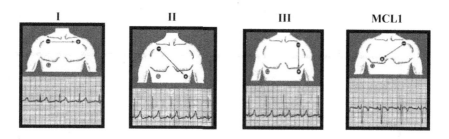

4. **B:** The junction point, also known as the J point, is known as the area where the S wave changes direction. The J point can be used to determine ST elevation, ST depression, and/or QRS duration. The delta wave is associated with WPW, the Osborne wave is associated with hypothermia, and the Z point is the reference point when measuring hemodynamic waveforms.

Junction between end of QRS and beginning of ST segment where QRS stops and makes a sudden sharp change of direction is called the J point.

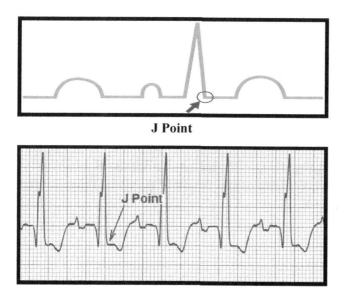

J Point

5. **C:** Posterior MI = R waves increase, ST segment depression (reciprocal changes) present in V1-V4 precordial leads. Development of tall R-waves in the right precordium should be interpreted as evidence of *posterior* MI.

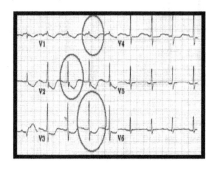 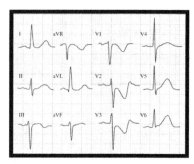

6. **B:** ST elevation is associated with myocardial injury.

ST Changes: The Three Is
- ST elevation = Injury (acute MI)
- ST depression = Ischemia
- Q waves present that measure > 25% the R wave = Infarction (necrosis)

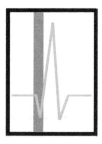

First negative deflection seen after the P wave; Q wave includes the negative downstroke and return to baseline

Are the Q Waves Significant?

- *Acute injury* = Q waves with ST elevation
- *Indeterminate* = Q waves with ST depression
- *Old infarction* = Q waves without ST changes

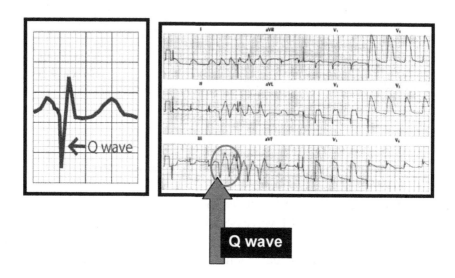

ST Measurement

Limb Leads-Bipolar

— More than 1 mm above (elevation) or below (depression) from the isoelectric line in two or more contiguous leads.

Precordial (chest) Leads-Unipolar

— More than 2 mm above (elevation) or below (depression) from the isoelectric line in two or more contiguous leads.

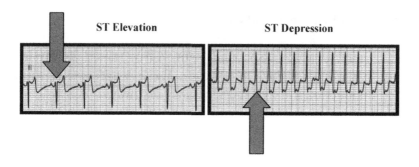

7. **C:** Tented or peaked T waves greater than 5 mm can indicate the presence of hyperkalemia.

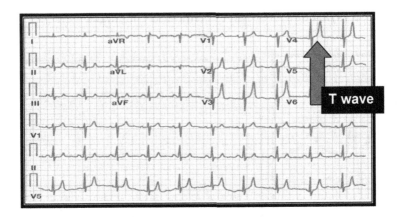

Other Changes to Look for on the ECG
- Peaked/tented T waves > 5 mm: *hyperkalemia*
- Flattened T waves/U waves present, which occur just after the T waves are usually smaller in amplitude than the T wave: *hypokalemia*

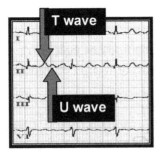

- Short PRI—may indicate WPW

- Delta wave = associated with WPW (noted bump in the beginning of the QRS wave). Delta wave is due to early conduction through the accessory pathway.

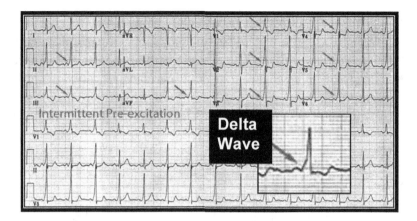

- Wide QRS: BBB present, TCA overdose

- Prolonged QT interval = TCA overdose

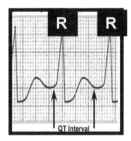

The QT Interval can be quickly assessed by using the R-R interval. QT interval measuring >½ of one R-R interval is prolonged until proven otherwise.

- Salvador Dali's Mustache = Look for the "DIG DIP," presenting as ST depression; may indicate digitalis toxicity

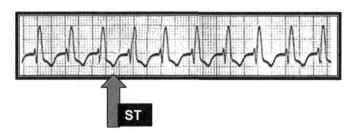

- Diffuse ST elevation across the entire ECG in conjuction with PR segment depression—suspect pericarditis/infection presenting with H/O fever or pericardial friction rub is noted
- Electrical alternans = suspect pericardial effusion/cardiac tamponde
  (amplitude of the R wave changes across the ECG "small, large, small")

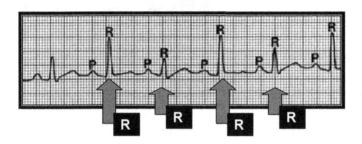

8. **B:** ST elevation present in V3, V4, Lead I, and aV$_L$ indicative of an anterior wall MI.

12-lead ECG Interpretation Review
Remember *LISA!*
- *L*ateral wall MI = I, AVL, V5, V6
- *I*nferior wall MI = II, III, AVF
- *S*eptal MI = V1, V2
- *A*nterior MI = V3, V4

9. **B:** The delta wave is due to early conduction through the accessory pathway.

10. **D:** Complete AVB, also known as AV disassociation, and third-degree heart block. ECG characteristics include no constant PRI or P wave. With every QRS, R-R interval will be regular, and the P waves will consistently march out.

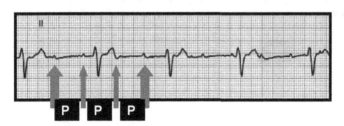

11. **C:** Acute injury is indicated by the presence of ST elevation. Ischemia, old infarction, and digitalis toxicity can present with ST depression.

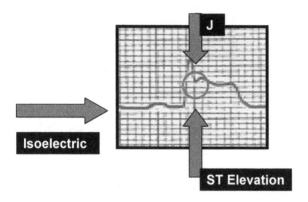

12. **B:** Q waves present with ST elevation can indicate that an acute myocardial injury is occurring.

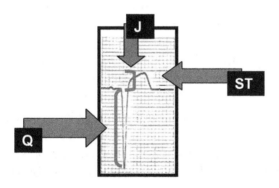

Q Wave with ST Depression or T Wave Inversion: Indeterminant

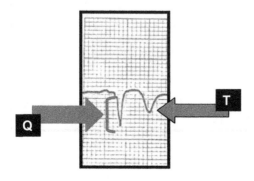

Q Wave Without ST Changes: Old Injury/Infarction

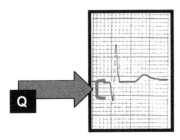

13. **A:** 100% paced rhythm with ventricular spikes present before the QRS.

14. **C:** Inferior wall MI presents with ST elevation in leads II, III, and aVF.

15. **B:** Polymorphic ventricular tachycardia, formerly known as *Torsades de pointes,* is a French word meaning "twisting of the points" and can occur with or without a pulse.

16. **D:** Patients presenting with an inferior wall MI may also have a right ventricular MI present which would affect filling pressures. Medications that decrease preload are not recommended, unless the patient has been managed with IV fluids prior to administration. Diagnosis of a right ventricular myocardial infarction (RVMI) can be done by obtaining a right-sided 12-lead ECG. The presence of ST elevation in RV4 is a highly sensitive marker for right ventricular involvement.

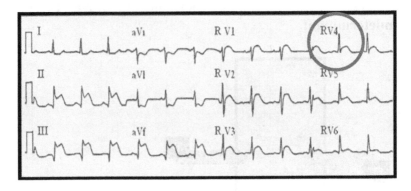

17. **B:** Anteroseptal MI presents with ST elevation in precordial leads V1-V4.

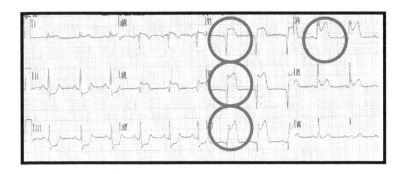

18. **A:** Remember "Toilet Paper My A_ _" for direction of blood flow through the valves. (Review chart for heart anatomy)

Anatomy of the Heart	
Area of location	Definition
Pericardium	Double-walled fibrous sac surrounding the heart
Heart chambers	Four chambers divided by septum
Heart	Contains three layers: Epicardium—thin, outermost layer Myocardium—thick, muscular middle layer Endocardium—thin, innermost layer
AV valves	Located between atria and ventricles Open as a result of lower ventricular pressures and close as a result of higher ventricular pressures Tricuspid—located between the right atrium and right ventricle Mitral (bicuspid)—located between the left atrium and left ventricle
Semilunar valves	Located between the ventricles and the great arteries Pulmonic—seperates the right ventricle from the pulmonary artery Aortic—seperates the left ventricle from the aorta
Valve order	T-P-M-A (remember *T*oilet *P*aper *My A* . . .) Tricuspid, pulmonic, mitral, aortic

19. **B:** Hyperkalemia presents with peaked or tented T waves on the ECG. Serum lab values usually greater than 7.0 when ECG changes are present.

20. **D:** Atrial fibrillation with ST elevation. R-R intervals are irregularly irregular with no obvious P waves present.

21. **B:** Hypokalemia may show peaked P waves, flattened/slurred T waves, and the presence of U waves. T wave and U wave may present as a biphasic wave.

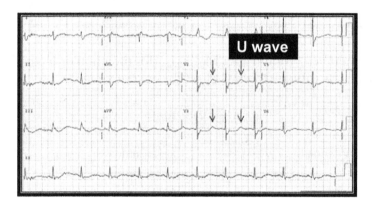

Biphasic T and Q Wave

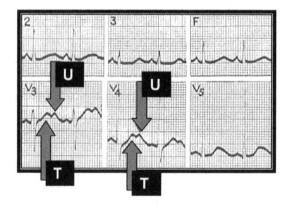

22. **B:** Atrial fibrillation with bundle branch block. R-R intervals are irregularly irregular with no discernable P waves present.

23. **B:** Right coronary artery.

24. **A:** Anteroseptal-lateral wall MI. ST elevation is present in leads I, aV_L, V5, V6 for lateral wall; V1, V2 for septal and V3, V4 for anterior wall. Reciprocal changes (ST depression) is present in the inferior leads (II, III, and aV_F).

25. **C:** Second-degree AVB, Mobitz II, also called Type II. PR interval is constant and there are more P waves present than QRS complexes. R-R interval is regular because there is a 2:1 conduction that remains constant. P waves march out.

26. **C:** Posterior wall MI. Note the progression of abnormal tall R waves and ST depression in precordial chest leads V1-V4.

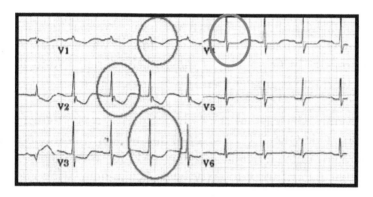

27. **B:** Inferolateral wall MI. ST elevation present in the inferior leads II, III, aV_F, and V5, V6 for the lateral leads. Reciprical changes (ST depression) present in leads I and aVL.

28. **A:** Asystole with pacer spikes present representing failure to capture.

29. **B:** Lateral wall MI. ST elevation present in lateral leads I and aV_L with reciprical changes (ST depression) in the inferior leads II, III, and aV_F.

30. **B:** Lateral wall MI

31. **C:** Prolonged Q-T interval and/or widened QRS > 0.12 seconds.

32. **C:** Atrial flutter with ST depression. Note the "flutter" waves and regular R-R intervals.

33. **D:** Complete AVB. If unable to determine rhythm, assess the continuous strip, which is usually provided at the bottom of the 12-lead ECG as lead II. The R-R interval is regular, and there is no constant PR interval and the P waves march out.

34. **C:** ST elevation (injury) in leads II, III, and aV_F.

35. **B:** Normal serum potassium range is 3.5-4.5, but it can go as high as 5.5 and can still be considered within normal range.

36. **D:** Atrial tachycardia, also known as supraventricular tachycardia (SVT). The R-R interval is regular, and the P wave, which is not visible on the ECG tracing, is most likely buried within the T wave. Heart rate is greater than 160 beats per minute.

37. **B:** Idioventricular rhythm (IVR) is defined as a ventricular rate of 20-40, wide QRS > 0.12 seconds and no P waves are present. Accelerated idioventricular rhythm (AIVR) is defined as a ventricular rate of forty to sixty beats per minute, wide QRS > 0.12 seconds and no P waves are present. The QRS duration is measured from the beginning of the QRS to the J point. Normal range is 0.04-0.12 seconds.

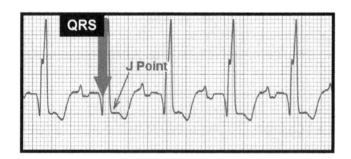

38. **A:** Highly sensitive marker for the presence of right ventricular infarction (RVI) is the presence of ST elevation in right-sided V4 lead.

39. **B:** Ventricular tachycardia (VT). The R-R interval is regular with a wide QRS constant pattern.

40. **B:** Second-degree AVB, type I, which is also known as Mobitz I or Wenckebach. The R-R interval is irregular because there is a dropped QRS complex. The P-R interval lengthens until it drops a beat.

41. **A:** Boyle's law is the expansion (ascent) or contraction (descent) of gas. Other equipment that can be affected by this law include ETT cuff, which may increase in size with ascent.

42. **B:** Left radial artery is the most common site. The distal tip of the balloon is placed in the descending aorta to displace blood both in the cephalad and distal direction to the balloon. The proximal end of the balloon is positioned just above the renal arteries.

IABP Dislodgment	
Distal displacement	Proximal displacement
Left radial artery	Renal arteries
Decrease/absent pulse	Decrease/absent urine output

43. **D:** Balloon rupture

44. **A:** Early inflation. Locate dicrotic notch (DN). Draw an imaginary line from the DN to the inflation point (IP). If the inflation point is 2 mm or more from the dicrotic notch, it indicates early inflation.

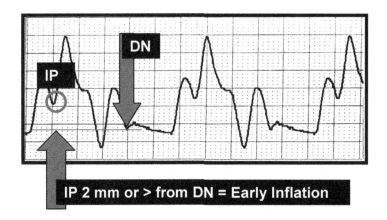

The precise timing of balloon inflation and deflation is essential to achieve the hemodynamic effects that increase coronary blood flow and decrease the workload of the heart. The arterial pressure waveform is always used to set and assess the timing. Timing is done based on the shape of the waveform and the relationship of the landmarks. Timing should always be assessed in a *1:2 assist ratio* so that a comparison of the assisted and unassisted landmarks can be made.

Review IABP Terminology

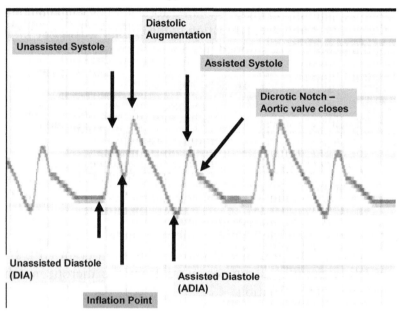

IABP terminology	
Terminology	**Definition**
PAEDP	Patient aortic end diastolic pressure—this is the patient's unassisted diastole (DIA)
PSP	Peak systolic pressure—this is the patient's unassisted systole
PDP/DA	Peak diastolic pressure or diastolic augmentation—this is the pressure generated in the aorta as the result of inflation
BAEDP	Balloon aortic end diastolic pressure—this is the lowest pressure produced by deflation of the IAB; this is assisted diastole (ADIA)
APSP	Assisted peak systolic pressure—this systole follows balloon deflation and should reflect the decrease in LV work
DN	Dicrotic notch—closure of the aortic valve

45. **C:** Inflation and deflation are synchronized with the patient's cardiac cycle. Most common is the ECG using the R wave. Mainly balloon inflation is set automatically to start in the middle of the T wave and to deflate prior to the ending QRS complex. The arterial waveform can be used when tachyarrhythmias, cardiac pacemaker function, and poor ECG signals may cause difficulties in obtaining synchronization when the ECG mode is used.

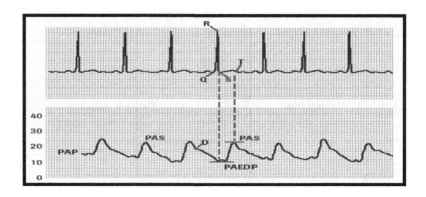

46. **C:** From the insertion site (usually the femoral artery), if the balloon is too distal to the aorta, occlusion of the brachiocephalic artery, left carotid artery, or left subclavian artery may occur. Balloon is positioned in the descending aorta, 2-4 cm below the level of the aortic arch, just distal to the left subclavian artery (radio-opaque distal tip of the balloon should be seen at the level of the second or third intercostal space on the chest x-ray). From the insertion site, if the balloon is too proximal (below the renal artery), the celiac, superior mesenteric, or renal arteries may be obstructed. Proximal end of the balloon should be positioned above the renal artery from the insertion site.

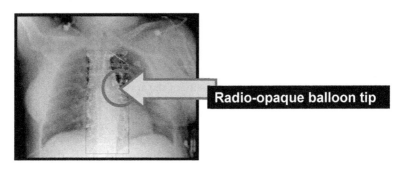

Radio-opaque balloon tip

47. **D:** It is important that the inflation of the IAB occurs at the onset of ventricular diastole, noted on the dicrotic notch on the arterial waveform. Deflation of the balloon should occur at the end of diastole just prior to the onset of ventricular systole. Balloon synchronization starts usually at a beat ratio of 1:2. This ratio facilitates comparison between the patient's own ventricular beats and augmented beats to determine ideal IABP timing.

IABP	
Balloon inflation	Balloon deflation
Inflates at the onset of ventricular diastole	Deflates just prior to the onset of ventricular systole
Increases diastolic pressure	
Increases perfusion to the coronary circulation	
Increases systemic perfusion	

48. **B:** Late deflation.

If ADIA (assisted diastole > DIA (unassisted diastole) = Late Deflation
ADIA < DIA = Normal timing

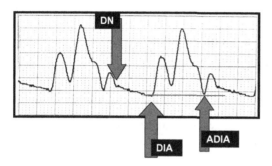

49. **C:** Late deflation. Timing errors can cause decrease in arterial pressures, decrease in cardiac output, decrease in ejection fraction, increase in heart rate, increase in pulmonary artery diastolic pressures, and increase in capillary wedge pressures.

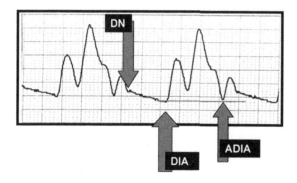

Left Ventricular Assisted Device (LVAD) Criteria
- Patient must be a heart transplant candidate
- Patient must demonstrate reversible end-stage organ disease
- Body surface area must be large enough to contain the device
- Meets the New York Heart Association Class IV hear failure criteria
- Patient has hemodynamic deterioration criteria:
    - ✓ CI < 2.0
    - ✓ Either a MAP < 65 mmHg or PAWP/PAD > 18 mmHg, or

✓ Life-threatening arrhythmias non-responsive to medical treatment, or

✓ Patient needs support of two positive inotropes, or

✓ Patient has an IABP placed

- Demonstrates the ability to manage the device or has a support person at all times

50. **D:** Cycle the balloon manually every thirty minutes regarding of timing when managing IABP failure.

Intra-Aoritc balloon pump		
Indications	Primary treatment goal	Secondary treatment goal
Acute MI Unstable angina Acute mitral valve rupture Ventricular septal defect (VSD) Left main occlusion Cardiogenic shock Postoperative CABG Bridge to heart transplantation Procedural support during coronary angiography and PTCA	Increase myocardial oxygen supply Decrease myocardial oxygen demand	Improvement of cardiac output (CO) Improvement of ejection fraction (EF) Increase of coronary perfusion pressure, systemic perfusion Decrease of heart rate, pulmonary capillary, wedge pressure, and systemic vascular resistance
Absolute contraindications	Relative contraindications	Complications
Chronic end-stage heart disease Aortic insufficiency Aortic or thoracic Aneurysm	Peripheral vascular Disease	Limb ischemia Balloon leakage Development of clots Excessive bleeding Aortic dissection
Proper IAB placement	IAB inflation/deflation	Most Lethal IABP Timing Errors
Distal end of the balloon is positioned in the descending aorta, 2-4 cm below the level of the aortic arch, just distal to the left subclavian artery *Proximal tip* should be above the renal artery from the insertion site, which is usually the femoral artery	Inflates at the onset of ventricular diastole Deflates at the onset of ventricular systole	Late deflation Early inflation

Bibliography

Antman, et al. 2004. ACC/AHA Guidelines for the management of patients with ST-elevation myocardial infarction—Executive summary. *J Am Coll Cardiol*; 44:671-719.

Association of Air Medical Services, (2004). *Guidelines for Air Medical Crew Education* Iowa, Kendall/Hunt Publishing Company.

Chelliah, YR. Ventricular arrhythmias associated with hypoglycaemia. *Anaesth Intensive Care,* 2000; 28(6):698-700.

Darovic, G. (1999). *Handbook of Hemodynamic Monitoring.* 2nd edition. Philadelphia. WB Saunders.

Oropello, JM, et al. Hemodynamic waveform detection from pulmonary artery catheters in the ICU. *J Intensive Care Med,* 1999; 14(1):46-51.

Elaine, KD. **(1990).** *Hemodynamic waveforms*, 2nd edition. St.Louis, Mosby.

Holleran, R. (1996). *Flight Nursing: Principles and Practice,* 2nd edition St. Louis, Mosby

Holleran, R. (2003). *Air and Surface Patient Transport: Principles and Practice,* 3rd edition. St. Louis, Mosby.

Holleran, Renee. (2009). *ASTNA Patient Transport: Principles and Practice,* 4th edition. St. Louis, Mosby

Krishna, M, Zacharowski, K. Principles of intra-aortic balloon pump counterpulsation. *Cont Educ Anaesth Crit Care Pain.* 2009; 9(1):24-28.

Krupa, D. (1997**)**, *Flight Nursing Core Curriculum.* Park Ridge, IL, National Flight Nurses Association.

Marino, PL. (2007). *The ICU Book,* 3rd edition. Philadelphia. Lippincott Williams & Wilkins.

Morris, F, Brady, WJ. ABC of Clinical Electrocardiography. *BMJ.* 2002; 324:831-834.

Nitasha, S, Steven MH. Cardiogenic Shock. *Hosp Pract. 2010;* 38(1):74-83.

Overwalder, PJ. Intra aortic balloon pump (IABP) Counterpulsation. *The Internet Journal of Perfusionists.* 2000; 1(1).

Overwalder, PJ. Intraaortic balloon pump (IABP) counterpulsation. *The Internet Journal of Thoracic and Cardiovascular Surgery.* 1999; 2(2).

Rippe, JM, Irwin, RS. (2003). *Irwin and Rippe's intensive care medicine*. Philadelphia, Lippincott Williams & Wilkins.

Tkachenko BI, Evlakhov VI, Poyasov IZ. Independence of changes in right atrial pressure and central venous pressure. *Bull. Exp. Biol. Med.* 2002; 134(4):318-20.

2005 American Heart Association Guidelines for Cardiopulmonary Resuscitation and Emergency Cardiovascular Care. Part 7.2: Management of Cardiac Arrest. *Circulation* 2005; 112(24 Suppl): IV 58-66.

Hirsh, J, Fuster V, Ansell J, Halperin JL. American Heart Association/ American College of Cardiology Foundation guide to warfarin therapy. *J Am Coll Cardiol.2003;* 41 (9):1633-52.

Horton, JD, Bushwick, BM. Warfarin therapy: evolving strategies in anticoagulation. *Am Fam Physician.* 1999; 59(3):635-46

Freedman. Oral anticoagulants: pharmacodynamics, clinical indications and adverse effects. *J Clin Pharmacol.* 1992; 32(3):196-209.

Gage, BF, Fihn, SD, White, RH. Management and dosing of warfarin therapy. *Am J Med. 2000;* 109(6):481-8.

Francis, CW, Kaplan, KL. (2006). Principles of antithrombotic therapy, in Lichtman MA, Beutler E, Kipps TJ, et al. *Williams Hematology* (7th edition). Chap. 21. New York. McGraw Hill Publishers Inc

Module 2
Hemodynamic Monitoring

1. Normal value for monitoring PA pressures are

   A. 2-6/8-14 mmHg
   B. 15-25/8-15 mmHg
   C. 25-35/20-30 mmHg
   D. 2.5-4.2 L/minute

2. Identify the following hemodynamic waveform tracing.

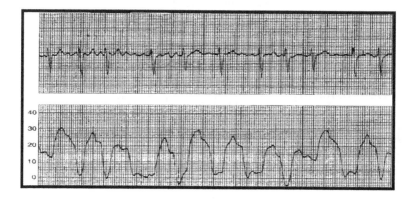

   A. pulmonary artery pressure
   B. right atrial pressure
   C. right ventricular pressure
   D. arterial pressure

3. Your initial intervention of the patient presenting with the following hemodynamic waveform tracing would be

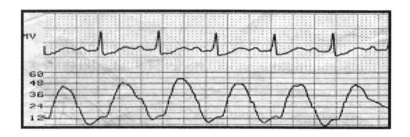

   A. synchronize cardiovert
   B. attempt to advance catheter by inflating the balloon
   C. administer precordial thump
   D. pull catheter back into the right ventricle

4. Your patient is presenting with the following hemodynamic waveform tracing

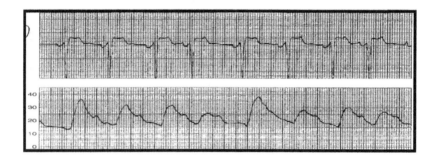

   A. CVP
   B. PA
   C. Arterial waveform
   D. RV

5. Identify the following hemodynamic waveform tracing.

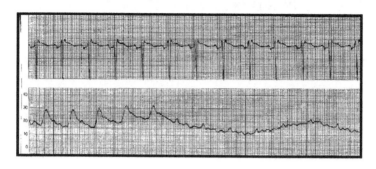

    A. RA
    B. PA
    C. RV
    D. PAWP

6. The patient's PA catheter is exhibiting a large, well defined hemodynamic waveform with an obvious "notch" on the left side of the waveform. The distal tip is most likely located in the

    A. right atrium
    B. pulmonary artery
    C. pulmonary capillary
    D. right ventricle

7. Identify what is happening with the following hemodynamic tracing.

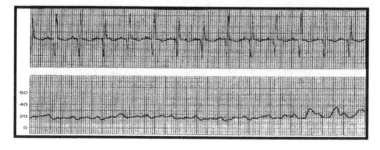

    A. CVP into RV waveform
    B. PAWP into PA waveform
    C. CVP into PA waveform
    D. PAWP into RV waveform

8. Your patient presents with the following hemodynamic parameters:
   CVP 28, CI 1.2, PA S/D 48/29, wedge 27, and SVR 2100. Identify
   the waveform tracing.

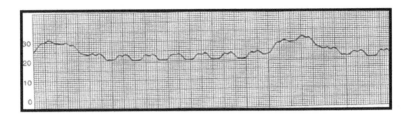

   A. CVP/RA
   B. PA
   C. Arterial
   D. PAWP

9. A common cause of elevated PA pressures is

   A. mitral valve stenosis
   B. mitral valve regurgitation
   C. left ventricular failure
   D. all of the above

10. Identify the following hemodynamic waveform tracing.

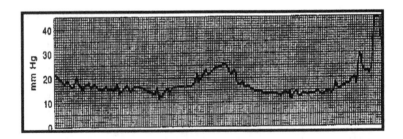

   A. CVP
   B. RV
   C. PAWP
   D. PA

11. The patient's peripheral A-line is showing a very sharp waveform with readings that appear exaggerated. This may be due to

    A. catheter embolus formation
    B. catheter whip
    C. over-dampening of the pressure system
    D. kinking of the pressure tubing

12. Your fast flush test indicates under-dampening of the system present. Which of the following may be the cause?

    A. Air in the system
    B. Low-pressure bag pressure
    C. Altitude change
    D. All of the above

13. When attempting to "wedge" a PA catheter, you should always

    A. fill the balloon with exactly 1.5 mL, no more
    B. fill the balloon with exactly 2.5 mL, no more
    C. fill the balloon with exactly 0.5 mL, no more
    D. none of the above

14. Your patient's PA waveform has suddenly changed to resemble a low-amplitude rolling waveform. This is most likely

    A. inadvertent withdrawal into the RV
    B. inadvertent withdrawal into the RA
    C. normal during inspiration
    D. inadvertent advance to wedge

15. Your patient's PA waveform is in wedge position. You would

    A. immediately withdraw the catheter to 20 cm depth
    B. have the patient cough forcefully
    C. verify chest tube drains are vented appropriately
    D. inflate the PA catheter balloon to 1.5 mL

16. Your patient presents with the following: CVP 2, CI 6.4, PA S/D 34/16, wedge 7, and SVR 400. What is your diagnosis?

    A. hypovolemic shock
    B. septic shock
    C. left ventricular failure
    D. neurogenic shock

17. Your patient presents with following parameters: CVP 20, CI 1.1, PA S/D 8/4, wedge 3, and SVR 1,800. What, is your diagnosis?

    A. hypovolemic shock
    B. right ventricular MI
    C. Congestive heart failure (CHF)/left ventricular failure
    D. sepsis

18. Identify the following hemodynamic waveform tracing.

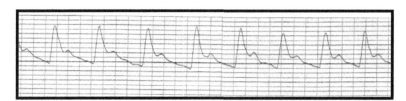

    A. PA
    B. RV
    C. arterial
    D. catheter whip

19. Central venous pressure is a reflection of

    A. right atrial pressure
    B. cardiac index
    C. left atrial pressure
    D. afterload for the right side of the heart

20. Pulmonary artery pressure reflects

    A. the filling pressure in the left ventricle
    B. the amount of blood ejected with each heart beat from the ventricles during systole
    C. right atrial pressures
    D. right- and left-sided heart pressures

21. The pulmonary artery wedge pressure evaluates

    A. the right side of the heart
    B. stroke volume
    C. the left side of the heart
    D. afterload of the left side of the heart

22. Identify what is happening in the following hemodynamic tracing.

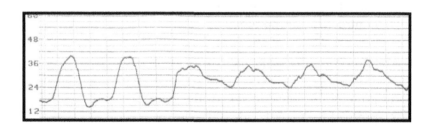

    A. PA into PAWP waveform
    B. RV into PA waveform
    C. PA into RV waveform
    D. RV into PAWP waveform

23. Normal range for cardiac output is

    A. 2-4 L/minute
    B. 4-8 L/minute
    C. 8-12 L/minute
    D. 15-20 L/minute

24. Normal range for PAWP is

    A. 2-6 mmHg
    B. 8-12 mmHg
    C. 4-8 mmHg
    D. 0-5 mmHg

25. Normal range for right atrial pressure is

    A. 2-6 mmHg
    B. 8-12 mmHg
    C. 4-8 mmHg
    D. 0-5 mmHg

26. Cardiac output is determined by

    A. blood pressure and heart rate
    B. heart rate and stroke volume
    C. cardiac index and heart rate
    D. contractility and preload

27. Systemic vascular resistance measures the

    A. preload for the right side of the heart
    B. preload for the left side of the heart
    C. afterload for the right side of the heart
    D. afterload for the left side of the heart

28. Pulmonary vascular resistance measures the

    A. preload for the right side of the heart
    B. preload for the left side of the heart
    C. afterload for the right side of the heart
    D. afterload for the left side of the heart

29. Stroke volume is

    A. measures afterload for the right side of the heart
    B. measures afterload for the left side of the heart
    C. the amount of blood ejected with each heartbeat from the ventricles during systole
    D. the amount of blood ejected with each heartbeat from the ventricle during diastole

30. The dicrotic notch signifies

    A. closure of the tricuspid valve
    B. closure of the pulmonic valve
    C. closure of the aortic valve
    D. closure of the mitral valve

31. A decrease in the patient's CVP can indicate all of the following, *except*

    A. vasodilation
    B. hypovolemia
    C. decrease in venous return
    D. right-sided heart failure

32. A decrease in the patient's SVR can indicate all of the following, *except*

    A. septic shock
    B. hypovolemic shock
    C. neurogenic shock
    D. anaphylactic shock

33. An increase in SVR can indicate all of the following, *except*

    A. cardiogenic shock
    B. right ventricular infarction
    C. septic shock
    D. hypovolemic shock

34. Medications that can decrease preload include all of the following, *except*

    A. morphine sulfate
    B. nitroglycerin
    C. vasopressin
    D. furosemide

35. Atrial waveforms are described as "filling pressures" and include which of the following?

    A. ventricular pressures
    B. right atrial and left atrial pressures
    C. right atrial pressure only
    D. left atrial pressure only

36. The PAWP tracing is an indirect measurement of

    A. right atrial pressure
    B. right ventricular pressure
    C. left atrial pressure
    D. central venous pressure

37. Arterial pressure waveforms include all of the following, *except*

    A. arterial line pressures
    B. pulmonary artery systolic pressures
    C. pulmonary artery diastole pressures
    D. ventricular pressures

38. The "a" wave seen on an atrial waveform indicates

    A. rise in atrial pressure as a result of atrial contraction
    B. decrease in atrial pressure as a result of atrial relaxation
    C. rise in ventricular pressure as result of ventricular contraction
    D. decrease in ventricular pressure as a result of ventricular relaxation

39. The "c" wave, when seen (not always visible) on an atrial waveform, indicates

    A. rise in atrial pressure when the AV valves are open
    B. rise in atrial pressure when the AV valves are closed
    C. rise in atrial pressure as it refills during ventricular contraction
    D. rise in atrial pressure as a result of atrial contraction

40. The "v" wave seen on an atrial waveform indicates

    A. rise in atrial pressure when the AV valves are open
    B. rise in atrial pressure when the AV valves are closed
    C. rise in atrial pressure as it refills during ventricular contraction
    D. rise in atrial pressure as a result of atrial contraction

41. The "a" wave, when assessing a right atrial pressure waveform, coincides with which area of the ECG cycle?

    A. mid- to late QRS
    B. at the end of the T wave
    C. in the PR interval
    D. after the QRS

42. In a right atrial waveform, if the "c" wave is present, it generally coincides with which area of the ECG cycle?

    A. mid- to late QRS
    B. immediately after the peak of the T wave
    C. in the PR interval
    D. after the QRS

43. The "v" waves, when assessing a right atrial pressure waveform, coincides with which area of the ECG cycle?

    A. mid- to late QRS
    B. immediately after the peak of the T wave
    C. in the PR interval
    D. after the QRS

44. The downslope on the "v" wave represents atrial emptying, which is called

    A. isovolumetric contraction
    B. diastasis
    C. X descent
    D. Y descent

45. The downslope of the "a" wave represents atrial relaxation, which is called

    A. isovolumetric contraction
    B. diastasis
    C. X descent
    D. Y descent

46. The period following diastole when all the four heart valves are closed is called

    A. isovolumetric contraction
    B. diastasis
    C. X descent
    D. Y descent

47. Arterial lines have which of the following pressure characteristics as compared to pulmonary artery pressures?

    A. much higher pressures
    B. much lower pressures
    C. pressures are equal
    D. none of the above

48. Positive pressure ventilation will cause cardiac pressure to

    A. rise upon inspiration
    B. rise upon expiration
    C. fall upon inspiration
    D. fall upon expiration

49. Hemodynamic pressures should be assessed and recorded at the

    A. end of exhalation
    B. beginning of exhalation
    C. end of inspiration
    D. beginning of inspiration

50. Which of the following is used as standard for measuring atrial pressures?

    A. top or peak of the "v" wave
    B. top of peak of the "a" wave
    C. identification of the "Z" point from the end of the QRS to the waveform
    D. bottom or base of the "a" wave on the right side of the downslope

Answer Key and Rationale

1. **B:** PAS 15-25 mmHg and PAD 8-15 mmHg. *(review the following chart for all hemodynamic monitoring values)*

Assessment	Normal Values
Central venous pressure (CVP Right atrial pressure (RAP)	2-6 mmHg
Right ventricular pressure (RV)—only measured when inserting catheter	SBP 15-25 mmHg DBP 0-5 mmHg
Pulmonary artery pressure (PAP)	PAS 15-25 mmHg PAD 8-12 mmHg
Pulmonary artery wedge pressure (PAWP) Pulmonary capillary wedge pressure (PCWP)	8-12
Cardiac output (CO)	4-8 L/min
Cardiac index (CI)	2.5-4.2 L/min
Stroke volume (SV)	60-135 mL
Stroke index (SI)	25-45 mL/m2
Pulmonary vascular resistance (PVR)	50-250 dyn
Systemic vascular resistance (SVR)	800-1200 dyn
Left atrial pressure (LAP)—indirect measurements of LAP can be done with measuring the PAWP	4-12 mmHg

2. **C:** Note that the anacrotic notch is seen on the left side of the waveform "looks like VT," catheter is positioned in the right ventricle. The rise in pressure begins simultaneously with ventricular depolarization (the QRS). When the right ventricle pressure is measured from a pulmonary artery catheter, the distance between the catheter tip and the transducer produces a delay between the QRS and the appearance of the rise in ventricular pressure. With a sinus rhythm, a small pressure rise in the right ventricular pressure occurs as the atrial contracts and increases the ventricular volume. Note that the wave will look taller in appearance than a PA waveform.

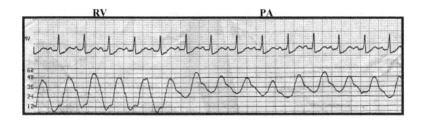

3. **B:** You must be able to recognize when the PA catheter is in the right ventricle. Initial intervention would be to attempt to float the PA catheter out of the right ventricle and into the pulmonary artery. If not successful, the PA catheter should be pulled back into the right atrium. Remember to change your lines from the proximal port to the distal port if PA catheter is repositioned in the right atrium. If the presence of the PA catheter in the right ventricle is not recognized and managed, the patient may develop PVCs and/or VT.

    What to do if catheter has been pulled back and is in the right ventricle?
    ➢ Reassess catheter centimeters at entry site
    ➢ Have the patient lay on their side
    ➢ Inflate the balloon (PAWP waveform will not be seen)
    ➢ Pull catheter back to RA position
    ➢ Change IV lines to distal port lumen if catheter has been pulled back into the right atrium

4. **B:** PA waveform, note the dicrotic notch is seen on the right side of the waveform. The pulmonary artery waveform can be correlated with the electrical activity of the right ventricle and the corresponding pressure changes occurring in the pulmonary artery. The systolic phase (PAS) reflects right ventricular contraction; therefore, the systolic pressure rise occurs after the QRS complex on the ECG.

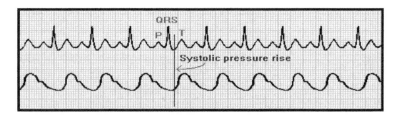

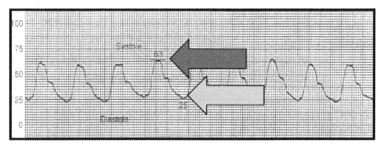

The Pulmonary Catheter
> ➢ Single thin black line equals 10 cm
> ➢ Single thick black line equals 50 cm
> ➢ Double thick black line equals 100 cm

PA Catheter Insertion Sites Commonly Used
> ➢ Right internal jugular: Shortest and straightest path to the heart
> ➢ Left subclavian: Does not require the PA catheter to enter the superior vena cava at an acute angle as compared to the right subclavian and left internal jugular
> ➢ Femoral veins: Distant sites from which passing the PA catheter into the heart may be difficult

Pulmonary Artery Catheter (PAC) Positions
> ➢ RA = 25-30 cm (proximal port/lumen)
> ➢ RV = 35-45 cm
> ➢ PA = 50-55 cm (distal port/lumen)

Proximal lumen: 25 cm from the tip of the catheter, lies in right atrium, and measures central venous pressure (CVP).

Distal lumen: at the tip of catheter (50-55 cm), lies in a branch of the pulmonary artery, and connected to a pressure transducer.

Balloon lumen: permits introduction of 1.5 mL of air into the balloon at the distal tip.

Thermistor lumen: bead situated 4 cm from the tip of the catheter and measures temperature.

Use of Pulmonary Catheter
- ➢ Assessment of volume status where CVP unreliable.
- ➢ Sampling of mixed venous blood to calculate shunt fraction.
- ➢ Measurement of cardiac output using thermodilution.
- ➢ Derivation of other cardiovascular indices, such as the pulmonary vascular resistance, oxygen delivery, and uptake.

Complications of Insertion
- ➢ Valve rupture
- ➢ Pulmonary embolism
- ➢ Pulmonary infarct
- ➢ Pulmonary artery rupture and hemorrhage
- ➢ Dysrhythmias
- ➢ Infection
- ➢ Pneumothorax
- ➢ Bleeding around site
- ➢ Labored breathing, respiratory distress
- ➢ Dampened waveform
- ➢ Balloon rupture
- ➢ Knotting of catheter in right ventricle

5. **D:** PA into "wedged" position (PAWP). The PAWP should always be lower than the mean pulmonary artery pressures (PAP). If it appears higher than mean PAP, suspect an error or that the catheter tip is not in the proper position. If it is not in the correct position, the PAWP may reflect alveolar or airway pressure and would not accurately reflect left atrial pressure. In addition to the mean PAP being higher than PAWP, pulmonary artery diastolic (PAD) pressure should be higher than PAWP. This is because the higher pressure in the pulmonary artery is needed to push the blood into the left atrium.

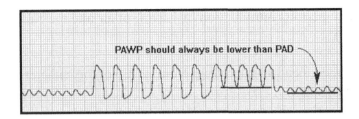

6. **D:** right ventricle *(clue: obvious notch on the left side of the waveform)* Clues that will assist in determining an RV waveform are:
   - ➢ the wave will look taller in appearance than a PA waveform
   - ➢ an RV waveform is symmetrical in shape; there is no dicrotic notch seen on the right side (downslope) of the waveform
   - ➢ the right ventricular pressure rise is closer to the QRS than with PAP waveform
   - ➢ inflation of the catheter balloon fails to produce a PAWP waveform.

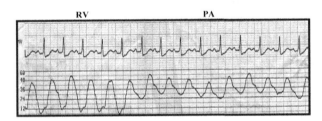

7. **B:** PAWP into PA waveform. PAWP is lower than PAD.

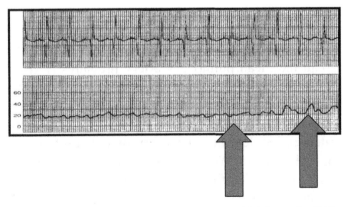

PAWP is lower than PAD

8. **A:** Atrial pressure waves are created by the pressure changes occurring in the right atrium during right atrial systole and diastole. The "a" wave is generated during atrial systole, and its height is a direct result of how much pressure is occurring in the atrium as the blood is being ejected into the ventricle.

Wave	CVP/RAP	PAWP/LAP
A	Rise in atrial pressure as a result of atrial contraction. A wave is generally seen during the PR interval before the onset of the QRS on the ECG.	Left atrial contraction "A" wave slightly later after the PR interval due to the timing delay on the ECG.
C	Not always visible, rise in the atrial pressure with closure of the AV valves (tricuspid and mitral valves) bulge upward into the atrium following valve closure. C wave generally coincides with mid- to late QRS on the ECG.	Closure of the mitral valve C wave slightly later due to the timing delay on the ECG.
V	Rise in atrial pressure as it refills during ventricular contraction. V wave is generally seen immediately after the peak of the T wave on the ECG.	Passive atrial filling. V wave slightly later due to the timing delay on the ECG.
X	Decline in right atrial pressure during atrial relaxtion ("X" in relaxation).	Left atrial relaxation (diastole).
Y	Decline in right atrial pressure: atrial emptying ("Y" in emptying).	Left atrial emptying.

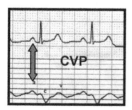

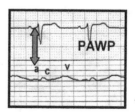

9. **D:** All of the above (Review the following chart for causes of increased and decreased hemodynamic pressures).

The hemodynamic tracing below shows a patient with severe mitral regurgitation. The pulmonary arterial (PA) pressure is severely elevated (>60 mmHg). In the distal portion of the pulmonary arterial pressure wave, a second peak is seen; this represents the V wave coincident with the ventricular contraction. V waves are usually seen in the pulmonary capillary wedge-pressure waveform; the large V wave in PA waveform signifies severe mitral regurgitation.

PA Waveform

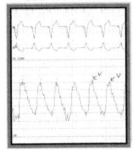

Right-heart catheterization and hemodynamic tracing of pulmonary capillary wedge-pressure (PCWP) waveform in a patient with severe mitral regurgitation. The PCWP is severely elevated (>40 mmHg). In the distal portion of the PCWP waveform, a second peak is present; this represents the V wave coincident with the ventricular contraction. A large V wave (>40 mmHg) signifies severe mitral regurgitation.

PCWP Waveform

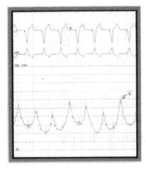

Normal parameter	Decreased pressures	Increased pressures
CVP/RAP (2-6 mmHg)	➢ Hypovolemia ➢ Vasodilation ➢ Decreased venous return (preload) ➢ Negative pressure ventilation	➢ Hypervolemia ➢ Right-sided heart failure ➢ Cardiac tamponade ➢ Positive pressure ventilation ➢ COPD ➢ Pulmonary HTN ➢ Pulmonary embolus ➢ Pulmonic stenosis ➢ Tricuspid stenosis ➢ Tricuspid regurgitation
RVP (reading only obtained when catheter is being inserted)	NA	➢ Pulmonary HTN caused by left heart failure ➢ COPD ➢ Pulmonary embolus
PAP PAS = 15-25 mmHg PAD = 8-15 mmHg	NA	➢ Fluid overload ➢ Atrial or ventricular defects ➢ Pulmonary diseases ➢ LV failure ➢ Mitral stenosis ➢ Mitral regurgitation
PAWP/PCWP (8-12 mmHg)	➢ Hypovolemia ➢ Venodilating drugs	➢ LV failure ➢ Constrictive pericarditis ➢ Mitral stenosis ➢ Mitral regurgitation ➢ Fluid overload ➢ Renal failure
PVR (50-250 dyn)	NA	➢ Pulmonary disease ➢ Hypoxia
SVR (800-1200 dyn)	➢ Septic shock ➢ Neurogenic shock ➢ Anaphylactic shock ➢ Vasodilators	➢ Hypovolemic shock ➢ Cardiogenic shock ➢ Right ventricular MI ➢ Aortic stenosis ➢ Vasoconstrictors

10. **C:** PAWP waveform *(note the "rolling" amplitude)*

What Increased PAWP Readings May Signify
- Early pulmonary congestion = 20 mmHg
- Moderate pulmonary congestion = 25 mmHg
- Severe pulmonary congestion = 30 mmHg

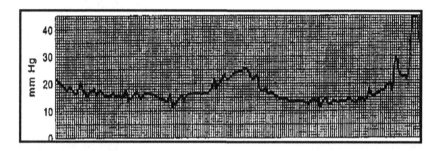

11. **B:** Catheter whip, which can be caused by hypertension. (Clue: the word "exaggerated.")

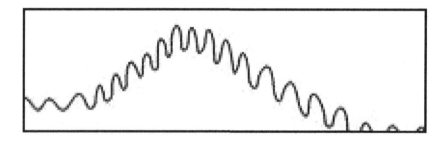

12. **D:** Properly dampened fast flush test waveform with transducer positioned properly at the phlebostatic axis. The phlebostatic axis is the point of the junction of the vena cava and the right atrium where the blood will have the lowest pressure.

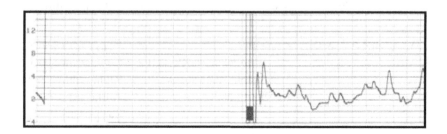

Overdampened Waveform: If the system is overdamped, then, when the fast flush is terminated, the waveform just slowly returns to baseline. This can be caused by kinking of the catheter, tip of the catheter against the wall, and increased pressure in the bag.

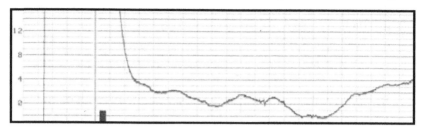

Underdampened Waveform: Shows many oscillations before returning to baseline. More than two oscillations are considered underdamped. This can be caused by air in the system, loose connections, low pressure in the bag, and altitude changes.

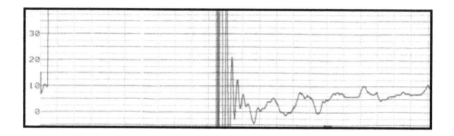

13. **D:** Balloon should only be filled until waveform is obtained but only up to no more than 1.5 mL. Balloon volumes greater than 1.5 mL can rupture the balloon.

14. **D:** Inadvertent wedge (Clue is the word *rolling* waveform)

15. **B:** Have the patient cough forcefully in an attempt to dislodge the balloon. Assure that the balloon is completely deflated, and have the patient lie on their side.

16. **B:** Know your normal and abnormal hemodyamic values

    a. CVP/RA = 2-6
    b. CI = 2.5-4.3
    c. PAS = 15-25
    d. PAD = 8-15
    e. Wedge = 8-12
    f. SVR = 800-1200

17. **B:** (Review the following types of shock and hemodynamic values.)

Type of shock or problem	CVP/RAP	Cardiac index (CI)	PAWP/PCWP (Wedge)	SVR
Hypovolemic	Low	Low	Low	High
Cardiogenic	High	Low	High	High
RVMI	High	Low	Low	High
Septic		High		Low
Neurogenic		Low (HR normal or slow)		Low
Anaphylactic		Low (HR fast)		Low

How to Assess for Type of Shock
- Afterload—Look at the SVR first
  - Right side of heart = PVR
  - Left side of heart = SVR
- SVR normal value 800-1,200
  - <800 = "Think" Distributive shock (vasodilatory shock)
    - Septic shock—look at the CI normal value, 2.5-4.3
      - CI high
    - Neurogenic shock
      - CI low
      - Heart rate slow or normal
    - Anaphylactic shock
      - CI low
      - Heart rate fast
  - >1200
    - Hypovolemia—look at the CVP/RA
      - CVP/RA low

- Cardiogenic shock
  - CVP/RA high
  - PAWP high
- RVMI
  - CVP/RA high
  - PAWP low
- Preload—look at "filling pressures" next beginning with the CVP if low hypovolemic shock is present; if high, then look at the PAWP next
  - Right side heart = CVP/RA normal value, 2-6 mmHg
    - Low < 2 mmHg—Hypovolemia
    - High > 6 mmHg—Pulmonary edema, cardiogenic shock, RVMI
  - Left side heart = PAWP normal value, 8-12 mmHg
    - Low—RVMI
    - High—Pulmonary edema
      - > 20 mmHg—Mild congestion
      - > 30 mmHg—Moderate congestion
      - > 40 mmHg—Severe congestion

18. **C:** Arterial waveform, when possible note the scale range if provided. Arterial lines and pulmonary artery pressures are categorized as arterial waveforms. The dicrotic notch is seen on the downslope of the right side of the waveform and indicates closure of the aortic valve. As pressure falls, the aortic valve closes, signaling the onset of diastole. Aortic valve closure produces a characteristic waveform known as the dicrotic notch. As diastole progresses, the pressure falls to its lowest level. The lowest point of the arterial waveform is the diastolic pressure, with a normal range of 60-90 mmHg.

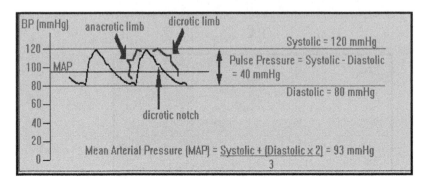

Arterial Waveforms

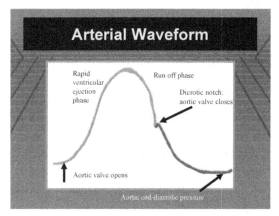

A-Line

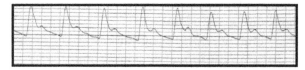

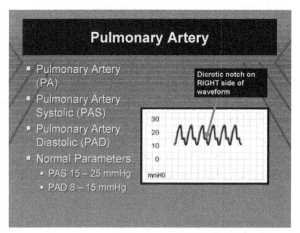

PA

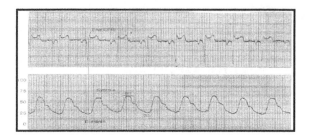

Formulas to Remember

- Coronary perfusion pressure (CPP) = DBP-PAWP (normal 50-60 mmHg)
- Mean arterial pressure (MAP) = 2 × DBP + SBP / 3 (normal 80-100 mmHg)

Arterial Lines

- Usually placed in radial or femoral arteries.
- Allen's Test (the blanching test) must be performed prior to insertion to ensure adequate radial and ulnar circulation.
- Allows for continuous BP monitoring and rapid recognition of problems requiring intervention.
- Easy access to blood gases and labs through A-line without sticking the patient.
- Slurring of the dicrotic notch occurs with aortic valve disease.

Pressure Monitoring Setup

- Purge and flush lines
- Pressurize fluid
- Place transducer at phlebostatic axis
- Attach tubing
- Close stopcock to patient
- Calibrate to ZERO
- Open to patient and fast flush

Invasive Line Transport Considerations

- Air is removed from the system to prevent air embolus and dampened waveforms.
- Tape transducer at the phlebostatic axis or on the bicep during transport.
- Limit the amount of tubing to decrease the chances of dislodgment and artifact due to aircraft vibration.
- Boyle's law will cause changes in pressure bag necessitating close attention of the flight crew members.
- Needs to be rezeroed with changes in altitude to ensure accuracy of readings.

19. **A:** evaluates preload of the right side of the heart—right atrial pressure. *(Review the following chart for hemodynamic definitions)*

Assessment	Definition
Central venous pressure (CVP Right atrial pressure (RAP)	➢ Reflection of right atrial pressure preload
Right ventricular pressure (RV)	➢ Not typically monitored but seen with insertion of the PA catheter or misplacement of catheter. ➢ Anacrotic notch appearance on left side of waveform ➢ Must recognize presence of catheter in the ventricle, PVCs or VT may occur
Pulmonary artery pressure (PAP)	➢ PA pressures reflect right—and left-sided heart pressures. ➢ Dicrotic notch is closure of the aortic valve and signals the end of systole
Pulmonary artery wedge pressure (PAWP)	➢ Evaluates pressure of the left side of the heart-preload
Cardiac output (CO)	➢ $CO = HR \times SV$
Cardiac index (CI)	➢ Is based on body surface area and is more accurate; it assesses blood flow
Stroke volume (SV)	➢ Amount of blood ejected with each heartbeat from the ventricles during systole
Stroke index (SI)	➢ Components of SV are preload, afterload, and contractility
Pulmonary vascular resistance (PVR)	➢ Measures afterload for the right heart
Systemic vascular resistance (SVR)	➢ Measures afterload for the left heart
Left atrial pressure (LAP)	➢ Reflects filling pressure in left ventricle ➢ The higher the LAP, the lower the ejection fraction from the left ventricle

20. **D:** right and left-sided heart pressures

21. **C:** evaluates preload of the left side of the heart

22. **B:** RV pressure waveform into PA pressure waveform

23. **B:** 4-8 L/minute

24. **B:** 8-12 mmHg

25. **A:** 2-6 mmHg

26. **B:** heart rate × stroke volume

27. **D:** measures afterload of the left side of the heart, whereas PVR measures afterload of the right side of the heart

28. **C:** measures afterload of the right side of the heart

29. **C:** the amount of blood ejected with each heartbeat from the ventricles during systole

30. **C:** closure of the aortic valve

31. **D:** right-sided heart failure

32. **B:** hypovolemic shock, SVR will be greater than 1,200 in shock states associated with hypovolemia, cardiogenic, and right ventricular infarction (RVI, also called right ventricular myocardial infarction-RVMI). SVR less than 800 are associated with distributive shock states, which include septic, neurogenic, and anaphylactic shock.

33. **C:** Septic shock—this is a type of distributive shock. Drug of choice recommended for a distributive shock state is *Levophed (norepinephrine), indicated in profound hypotension.* It has both alpha and beta effects, thereby increasing coronary artery blood flow. Initial adult dose is 2-12 µg/minute and titrated to desired effect.

34. **C:** Vasopressin (Pitressin) does not decrease preload

Area	Drugs that decrease	Drugs that increase
Preload	<ul><li>NTG</li><li>Morphine</li><li>Lasix</li></ul>	<ul><li>Vasoconstrictors</li><li>Fluids</li></ul>
Afterload	<ul><li>Nipride</li><li>Corlopam</li><li>Calcium-channel blockers</li><li>Dobutrex</li><li>Natrecor</li></ul>	<ul><li>Dopamine</li><li>Neosynephrine</li><li>Levophed</li><li>Epinephrine</li></ul>

35. **B:** Waveforms obtained from the right and left atria, which are CVP (right atrium; right atrial pressure) and PAWP (left atrium; left atrial pressure). More commonly, left atrial pressure waveforms are obtained through indirect measurement.

36. **C:** Left atrial pressure.

37. **D:** Right ventricular pressures are categorized under ventricular waveforms. Right ventricular waveforms are obtained during insertion of a pulmonary artery catheter or if the PA catheter dislodges backward into the right ventricle. Left ventricular waveforms are not normally observed, except during left heart catheterization.

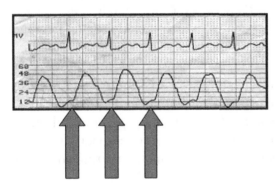

Rise in pressure "notch" seen on the downslope of left side of the waveform.

38. **A:** The "A" wave represents a rise in atrial pressure as a result of atrial contraction. (Refer to the chart for review of wave definitions provided in question answer #8.)

39. **B:** The "c" wave represents a rise in atrial pressure when the closed AV valves bulge upward into the atrium following valve closure *(refer to above chart)*.

40. **C:** The "v" wave represents a rise in the atrial pressure as it refills during ventricular contraction *(refer to above chart)*.

41. **C:** The "a" wave in a right atrial pressure waveform coincides with the PR interval on the ECG. The "a" wave begins to form as depolarization begins. The "a" wave appears slightly later after the PR interval for a left atrial pressure (PAWP) waveform *(refer to above chart)*.

42. **A:** The "c" wave in a right atrial pressure waveform coincides with mid- to late QRS on the ECG. As the pressure builds in the ventricle, the closed AV valves begin to bulge upward into the atria, producing a small rise in the pressure. This pressure rise in the atria is called the "c" wave. The "c" wave is not always visible, but when present, can be seen as a notch on the downslope of the "a" wave or as a separate wave in between the "a" wave and the "v" wave. The "c" wave in a left atrial pressure waveform will appear slightly later (after the QRS).

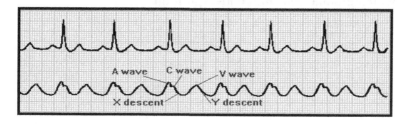

43. **B:** The "v" wave in a right atrial pressure tracing appears immediately after the peak of the T wave. It will appear slightly later in a left atrial pressure tracing.

44. **D:** The downslope of the "'v' wave, which represents a decline in the atrial pressure is referred to as the Y descent, which indicates atrial emptying.

45. **C:** The downslope of the "a" wave, which represents a decline in the atrial pressure is referred to as the X descent, which indicates atrial relaxation.

46. **A:** The closed valves prevent blood flow. The period when all four heart valves are closed is called "isovolumetric contraction," which is due to depolarization. As the pressure builds in the ventricle, the closed AV valves being to bulge upward into the atria, produces a small rise in pressure which forms the "c" wave. The "c" wave is not always visible on the tracing. Diastasis is known as middiastole and is the period when atrial and ventricular pressures are very similar, just prior to atrial depolarization.

47. **A:** Arterial lines have much higher pressures than pulmonary artery pressures.

48. **A:** Cardiac pressures rise and fall with breathing, which can be identified by increased and decreased changes in the waveform that coincide with ventilation. Positive pressure ventilation will cause cardiac pressure to rise upon inspiration. Spontaneous breathing usually produces the largest respiratory artifact, which causes a drop in vascular pressures immediately before inspiration with a gradual rise until end-expiration.

Mechanically Ventilated Patient

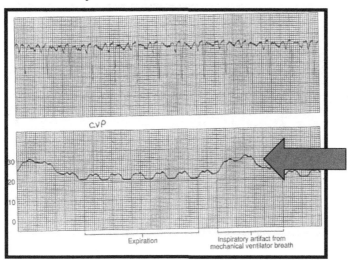

Spontaneous Breathing Patient

In a spontaneously breathing patient, inspiration is the fall in pressure and expiration is the rise in pressure. End expiration occurs just prior to the inspiratory drop in pressure.

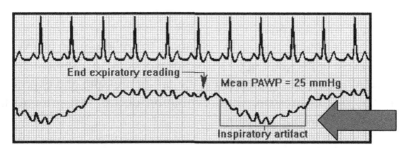

49. **A:** Record pressure measurements at the end of exhalation. For positive pressure ventilation, this will usually be at the lowest point on the waveform tracing.

Positive Pressure Ventilated Patient

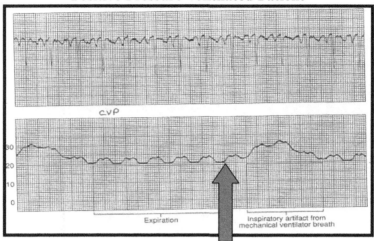

For spontaneously breathing patients, the measurement point will be just prior to the dip in respiratory artifact. Roller-coaster in appearance due to pressure changes associated with respirations. The waveform associated with end-expiration will be different for spontaneously breathing patients and mechanically ventilated patients.

In a patient on mechanical ventilation, the relationship is reversed and a rise in pressure upon inspiration occurs. In a spontaneously breathing patient, inspiration is the fall in pressure and expiration is the rise in pressure. End expiration occurs just prior to the inspiratory drop in pressure.

Spontaneously Breathing Patient

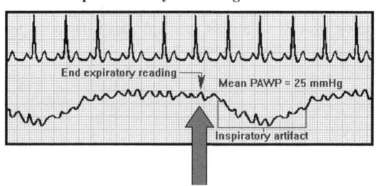

Remember that the aritifact changes seen on the waveform tracings for ventilation are reversed. Positive pressure ventilated patient will have a rise in pressure upon inspiration and spontaneous breathing patients will have a fall in pressure upon inspiration.

PAWP Waveform on a Positive Pressure Ventilated Patient

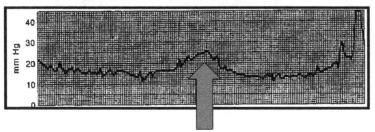

Rise in pressure upon inspiration

50. **C:** The end-diastolic pressure can be estimated by identifying the "Z" point.

Measuring Waveforms
- One way to obtain a CVP measurement is by drawing a vertical line from the end of the QRS complex through the CVP.
- We want to measure the pressure as the atria are relaxing. This occurs when the ventricles begin to contract. There are many ways to determine this, but the easiest way is to print out a strip with the ECG tracing and the CVP waveform. The end-diastolic pressure can be estimated by identifying the "Z" point. A line is drawn from the end of the QRS to the hemodynamic tracing. The point where the line intersects with the waveform is the "Z" point. The "Z" point on the PAWP tracing will be delayed by 0.08-0.12 seconds from the QRS.

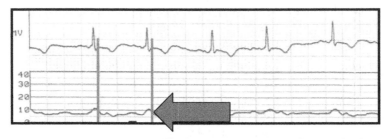

"Z" point where measurement is determined

CVP measurement		
Electrical event (ECG)	**Mechanical event**	**Right atrial pressure (RAP) 2-6 mmHg**
80-100 milliseconds after P wave	RA systole	*a* wave
	RA diastole	*x* descent
After QRS	Tricuspid valve closure	*c* wave
After peak of T wave	RA filling/tricuspid valve closed	*v* wave
	RA emptying at opening of tricuspid valve/onset of right ventricle diastole	*y* descent

Pulmonary artery pressure measurement		
Electrical event (ECG)	**Mechanical event**	**Pulmonary artery pressure (mmHg)**
T wave	Right ventricle ejection of blood into pulmonary vasculature	Systolic (PAS 15-30)
80 milliseconds after onset of QRS	Indirect indicator of LVEDP	End-diastolic (PAEDP 8-12); Mean (9-18)

PAS: pulmonary artery systolic; LVEDP: left ventricular end-diastolic pressure; PAEDP: pulmonary artery end-diastolic pressure

Pulmonary artery wedge pressure measurement		
Electrical event (ECG)	**Mechanical event**	**Pulmonary artery wedge pressure (normal PAWP is 8-12 mmHg)**
Approximately twenty milliseconds after P wave	Left atrial (LA) systole	*a* wave
	LA diastole	*x* descent
T-P interval	LA filling/mitral valve closed	*v* wave
	LA emptying at opening of mitral valve/onset of left ventricle diastole	*y* descent

Bibliography

2005 American Heart Association guidelines for cardiopulmonary resuscitation and emergency cardiovascular care. Part 7.2: Management of Cardiac Arrest. *Circulation* 2005; 112 (24 Suppl): IV 58-66.

Association of Air Medical Services. (2003) *Guidelines for Air Medical Crew Education* Iowa, Kendall/Hunt Publishing Company.

Binanay, C, Califf, RM, Hasselblad, V, et al. Evaluation study of congestive heart failure and pulmonary artery catheterization effectiveness: the ESCAPE trial. *JAMA.* 2005; 294:1625.

Darovic, G. (1999), *Handbook of Hemodynamic Monitoring.* 2nd edition. Philadelphia, W.B. Saunders

Dulak, SB. PA catheters: What the waveforms reveal. *RN.* 2003; 66:56.

Oropello, JM, et al. Hemodynamic waveform detection from pulmonary artery catheters in the ICU. *J Intensive Care Med.* 1999. 14(1):46-51.

Elaine, KD. *Hemodynamic Waveforms.* 1990. 2nd edition. St. Louis, Mosby.

Hesselvik, JF, Brodin B. Low-dose norepinephrine in patients with septic shock and oliguria. *Crit Care Med.* 1989; 17:179-180.

Holleran, R. (1996). *Flight Nursing: Principles and Practice,* 2nd edition. St Louis, Mosby.

Holleran, R. (2003). *Air and Surface Patient Transport: Principles and Practice,* 3rd edition. St. Louis, Mosby.

Holleran, R. (2009) *ASTNA Patient Transport: Principles and Practice,* 4th edition. St. Louis, Mosby.

Hotchkiss RS, Karl IE. The pathophysiology and treatment of sepsis. *N Engl J Med.* 2003; 348:138-150.

Irwin, RS.; Rippe, JM. (2003). *Intensive Care Medicine.* Philadelphia and London, Lippincott Williams & Wilkins.

Krupa, D. (1997). *Flight Nursing Core Curriculum.* Park Ridge, IL: National Flight Nurses Association.

Lough, ME, et al. (2002). *Thelan's Critical Care Nursing: Diagnosis and Management.* St. Louis, Mosby.

Lynn-McHale, D J, Carlson, K K (Eds.). (2001). *AACN procedure manual for critical care,* 4th edition. Philadelphia, W. B. Saunders.

Martin, C, et al. Effect of norepinephrine on the outcome of septic shock. *Crit Care Med* 2000; 28:2758-2765.

Nitasha, S. Steven, MH. Cardiogenic Shock. *Hosp Pract.2010;* 38(1):74-83

Pinsky, MR. Pulmonary artery occlusion pressure. *Intensive Care Med.* 2003; 29:19.

Rippe, JM, Irwin, RS. (2003). *Irwin and Rippe's intensive care medicine.* Philadelphia, Lippincott Williams & Wilkins.

Rivers E, Nguyen B, Havasted S, et al. Early goal-directed therapy in the treatment of severe sepsis and septic shock. *N Engl J Med.* 2001; 345:1368-1377.

Summerhill, EM, Baram, M. Principles of pulmonary artery catheterization in the critically ill. *Lung.* 2005; 183:209.

Tkachenko, BI, et al. Independence of changes in right atrial pressure and central venous pressure. *Bull Exp Biol Med.* 2002; 134(4):318-20.

Weed, HG. Pulmonary "capillary" wedge pressure not the pressure in the pulmonary capillaries. *Chest.* 1991; 100:1138.

Wiener, RS, Welch, HG. Trends in the use of the pulmonary artery catheter in the United States, 1993-2004. *JAMA* 2007; 298:423.

Module 3
Cardiovascular and Medical Emergencies

1. You are en-flight with a seventy-year-old male cardiac patient on 6 L of oxygen by NC. You are at 5,000 feet and the patient is becoming hypoxic. What is your initial intervention for this patient?

   A. Decrease cabin pressure
   B. Increase oxygen delivery to the patient
   C. Administer fluid bolus to increase perfusion to the heart
   D. RSI and intubate the patient

2. Which patient is not affected with altitude temperature changes?

   A. Cardiac patient
   B. Burn patient
   C. Head injured patient
   D. Spinal cord injured patient

3. Your patient presents with epigastric pain, nausea, and vomiting for the last hour. He describes his chest pain as "heavy in nature." What does the following 12-lead ECG show?

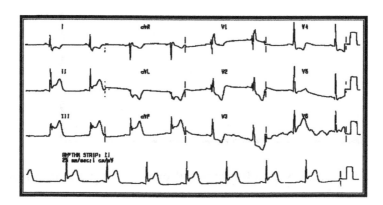

   A. Posterior MI
   B. Anterior MI
   C. Inferior MI
   D. Septal MI

4. Your patient is experiencing left ventricular diastolic failure. Therapy should be focused on

    A. Augmentation of left ventricular clearing
    B. Decreasing afterload
    C. Decreasing preload
    D. Diuretics and relief of anxiety

5. Your patient is exhibiting ST elevation in leads II, III, and AVF. ST depression is noted in V1-V3. Which of the following may prove hazardous?

    A. Isotonic fluid bolus
    B. Heparin
    C. GII/BIIIa inhibitors
    D. Nitroglycerin

6. A fifty-five-year-old woman complains of SOB for two days. Identify what the following ECG rhythm reveals.

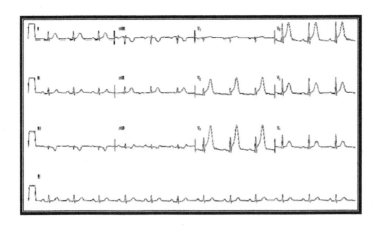

    A. Inferior wall MI with reciprocal changes in precordial leads V2-V4
    B. Anteroseptal wall MI with lateral extension and reciprocal changes in lead III and aVF
    C. Lateral wall MI with reciprocal changes in lead III and aVF
    D. Posterior wall MI with reciprocal changes in lead III and aVF

7. Electrical alternans may be caused by

   A. Pulmonary embolus
   B. Pericardial tamponade/effusion
   C. Tension pneumothorax
   D. Diaphragmatic rupture

8. Antidote for Coumadin overdose is

   A. Protamine sulfate
   B. Glucagon
   C. Vitamin K, FFP
   D. Physostigmine

9. Your patient has a chief complaint of dyspnea and weakness with the following vitals: BP 72/64, HR 112, RR 28, SpO_2 88%, temp. 99.1°F. He is on 6 L/minute of oxygen via NC. The ECG shows ST with frequent PVCs. Physical exam reveals profound vesicular rales and bronchial wheezing. Your most likely diagnosis is

   A. CHF
   B. ARDS
   C. Asthma
   D. Cardiogenic shock

10. Treatment of cardiac tamponade includes all of the following, *except*

    A. Force fluids
    B. Pericardiocentesis
    C. Rapid transport
    D. Needle thoracostomy

11. A patient presenting with Beck's triad is most likely experiencing

    A. Tension pneumothorax
    B. Increased ICP
    C. Cardiac tamponade
    D. Intra-abdominal bleeding

12. You are transporting a forty-five-year-old man with acute respiratory distress syndrome (ARDS) and MODS secondary to probable organ rejection after a heart transplant. During transport the patient becomes bradycardic with heart rate in the 30s with hypotension. Which of the following therapies will likely prove fruitless?

    A. 250-500 mL saline bolus
    B. Dopamine 5-20 µg/kg/min
    C. Transcutaneous pacing
    D. Atropine 0.5-1 mg IV push

13. Your patient presents with following parameters: CVP 20, CI 1.1, PA S/D 8/4, wedge 3, and SVR 1,800. What is your diagnosis?

    A. Hypovolemic shock
    B. RVMI
    C. CHF/LVF
    D. Sepsis

14. You are transporting a fifty-year-old man from ICU to another facility for further evaluation. The patient has been diagnosed with AMI. He has been complaining of increasing CP, SOB, and dramatic weight loss. He appears very nervous, and you note tremors. His ECG shows AF at 148. The patient may be experiencing

    A. Addison's disease
    B. Thyrotoxicosis (grave's dieases)
    C. Myxedema coma
    D. Cushing's syndrome

15. The formula to calculate MAP is

    A. 2/3 DBP × SBP
    B. 2 × DBP + SBP divided by 3
    C. 2 × SBP + DBP
    D. 2 + DBP × SBP divided by 3

16. Normal coronary perfusion pressure (CPP) is

    A. 50-60 mmHg
    B. 70-90 mmHg
    C. 80-100 mmHg
    D. <50 mmHg

17. When performing a pericardiocentesis, the insertion site is

    A. Below the subxyphoid process
    B. Just right of the subxyphoid process
    C. Just left of the subxyphoid process
    D. Above the subxyphoid process

18. You are transporting a seventy-five-year-old man with a diagnosis of inferior wall MI. During the flight you note the following rhythm. Vital signs are: 70/palp, HR 150, RR 24, SpO_2 94% on high flow oxygen with NRM at 15 L/min. He is awake and complains of chest pain and SOB. How will you manage this patient?

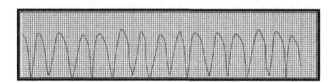

    A. Administer lidocaine and nitroglycerin
    B. Administer normal saline bolus
    C. Consider sedation and synchronize cardiovert at 100 joules
    D. Have the patient cough forcefully

19. sixty-year-old man complains of chest pain for three days with a low-grade fever. Patient complains of increased pain when lying in supine position and states that the chest pain decreases when sitting forward. What is the most likely diagnosis?

    A. Pulmonary embolism
    B. Pleurisy
    C. Pericarditis
    D. Pericardial tamponade

20. What common problem may occur with the following 12-lead presentation?

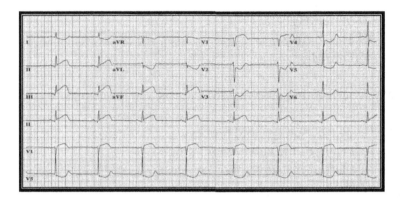

A. Ischemia
B. Right ventricular infarction
C. LAD occlusion
D. Ventricular fibrillation

21. How is the coronary perfusion pressurecalculated?

A. DBP − PCWP
B. DBP + PCWP
C. SBP − DBP
D. SBP − PCWP

22. Inferior wall MI is caused by an occlusion of which coronary artery?

A. LAD
B. RCA
C. Circumflex
D. Inferior vena cava

23. What medications would you expect to administer to a patient presenting with severe chest/abdominal pain, diaphoresis, and is restless? SBP is 170/palp and heart rate in 116. You note a difference in blood pressures when taken on each arm.

   A. Nitroglycerin and atenolol
   B. Nipride and b-blockers
   C. Lasix and nitroglycerin
   D. Bumex and Dobutrex

24. A sign of hyperventilation and hypocalcemia is

   A. Kehr's
   B. Grey Turner's
   C. Trousseau's
   D. Brudzinski's

25. All of the following are signs of cardiac tamponade, except

   A. Pulsus paradoxus
   B. Pulsus alternans
   C. Kussmual's sign
   D. Pulseless electrical activity (PEA)

26. You are transporting a sixty-year-old man complaining of severe chest pain and midscapular pain. He is short of breath and is hypertensive in the upper extremities. You auscultate a harsh systolic murmur. Your diagnosis of this patient is

   A. Cardiac tamponade
   B. Aortic rupture
   C. Myocardial rupture
   D. Tension pneumothorax

27. The MD has ordered a brain natriuretic peptide (BNP), which would evaluate the patient for

   A. Sepsis
   B. Hypovolemia
   C. Right ventricular MI
   D. CHF

28. Levine's sign relates to

   A. Meningitis; neck pain
   B. Pancreatitis; periumbilical bruising
   C. Cardiac; clenched fist over chest
   D. Splenic injury; left shoulder

29. Kussmaul's sign is a

   A. Rise in venous pressure with inspiration
   B. Crunching sound synchronized to heart beat
   C. Decrease of the SBP of > 10 mmHg with inspiration
   D. Marbled appearance of the abdomen

30. Drug of choice for treating a GI bleed is

   A. Normal saline
   B. Nipride
   C. Whole blood
   D. Sandostatin

31. You are transporting a fifty-year-old man from a rural facility. Your patient's ECG is demonstrating ST at 112 with peaked P waves. The ABG indicates pH 7.2, pCO_2 18, HCO_3 12 and pO_2 108. CMP reveals Na 130, K 2.3, Cl 95, HCO_3 10, BUN 48, creat 2.2, and glucose of 685. The most appropriate diagnosis would be

   A. Cardiogenic shock
   B. DKA
   C. Hyperglycemic, hyperosmolar nonketotic syndrome
   D. Dehydration

32. Recommended urinary output when caring for an adult patient should be

    A. 100 mL/hr
    B. 30-50 mL/hr
    C. 1-2 cc/kg/hr
    D. >200 mL/hr

33. Your patient's EKG is demonstrating ST at 130. ABG indicates pH 7.34, pCO_2 35, HCO_3 23, pO_2 104. The patient's CMP reveals: Na 132, K 2.5, Cl 97, HCO_3 22, BUN 44, creat 2.0, and glucose 1,185. The most appropriate diagnosis would be

    A. Primary hypokalemia
    B. DKA
    C. Asthma
    D. HHNK

34. A patient presenting with meningitis may exhibit which sign on assessment?

    A. Cullen's
    B. Grey Turner's
    C. Kernig's
    D. Levine's

35. Murphy's sign would indicate which of the following conditions?

    A. Splenic injury
    B. Cardiac problem
    C. Pancreatitis
    D. Gallbladder

36. A common problem seen with hepatic encephalopathy is

    A. Hyperkalemia
    B. Increased ammonia levels
    C. Low protein levels
    D. Low BUN

37. Treatment of pancreatitis would include all of the following, *except*

     A. Fluid resuscitation
     B. NPO and place OG/NG tube
     C. Morphine for pain
     D. Antibiotics for sepsis

38. The patient presenting with HHNK has a problem with

     A. Sugar
     B. Insulin
     C. Overhydration
     D. Ketoacidosis

39. The treatment of diabetes insipidus is

     A. Aggressive fluid replacement and vasopressin
     B. Restrict fluids and mannitol
     C. Aggressive fluid replacement and Dilantin
     D. Aggressive fluid replacement and octreotide

40. Adrenal insufficiency, weight loss, hypotension—the patient may be experiencing

     A. Addison's disease
     B. Thyrotoxicosis (Grave's diease)
     C. Myxedema coma
     D. Cushing's syndrome

41. Myxedema coma is also known as

     A. Thyroid storm
     B. Adrenal insufficiency
     C. Hypothyroidism
     D. Hyperaldosteronism

42. Most common presentation of a patient with hypothyroidism are all of the following, *except*

    A. Cold intolerance with coarse hair
    B. Almost exclusively over the age of sixty
    C. >90% of cases occur in the winter
    D. Primarily in men

43. Drug of choice for profound hypotension in septic shock is

    A. Isotonic crystalloid solution
    B. Levophed
    C. Nipride
    D. Dobutamine

44. You are managing a patient who has been diagnosed with hepatic encephalopathy. His ammonia levels are elevated. Your management in preparing this patient for transport is to inhibit elevated protein level by

    A. Administering whole blood
    B. Stop GI bleeding and evacuate bowel of blood
    C. Aggressive fluid resuscitation
    D. Aggressive pain control

45. Grey Turner's sign may indicate

    A. Meningitis
    B. Splenic injury
    C. Pancreatitis
    D. Gallbladder

46. Repeated doses of etomidate can cause

    A. Increased ICP
    B. Acute adrenal insufficiency
    C. AMI
    D. Pulmonary edema

47. A type of angina that can occur at rest, while sleeping, or after exercise is called

    A. Silent
    B. Prinzmetal's
    C. Stable
    D. Unstable

48. A clinical sign that indicates hypocalcemia may be present is

    A. Kehr's
    B. Grey Turner's
    C. Chvostek's
    D. Brudzinski's

49. Your patient presents upper body obesity with thin arms and legs. He has a rounded face "buffalo hump" and is complaining fatigue. He is hypertensive and hyperglycemic. What condition is he most likely presenting?

    A. Myxedema coma
    B. Thyroid storm
    C. Addison's disease
    D. Cushing's syndrome

50. Cullen's sign may indicate

    A. Meningitis
    B. Pancreatitis
    C. Gallbladder disease
    D. Cardiac problem

Answer Key and Rationale

1. **B:** Increase oxygen delivery to the patient. Hypoxic hypoxia is a deficiency in alveolar oxygen exchange. A reduction in pO_2 in inspired air or the effective gas exchange area of the lung may cause oxygen deficiency. It is also referred to as altitude hypoxia because its primary cause is exposure to low barometric pressure.

Types of hypoxia	Definition
Hypoxic hypoxia (altitude hypoxia)	Is a deficiency in the alveolar oxygen exchange, which can be caused by low barometric pressure.
Hypemic hypoxia	Is a reduction in the oxygen-carrying capacity of the blood.
Stagnant hypoxia	Occurs when conditions exist that result in reduced total cardiac output, pooling of the blood within certain regions of the body, a decreased blood flow to the tissues, or restriction of blood flow.
Histotoxic hypoxia (tissue poisoning)	Occurs when metabolic disorders or poisoning of the cytochromic oxidase enzyme results in a cell's inability to use molecular oxygen.

2. **A:** Cardiac patients are usually not affected with altitude temperature changes.

3. **C:** Inferior wall MI presents with ST elevation in leads II, III, and aVF. Reciprocal changes are present in leads I, aVL, and V1-V4.

Location	ST elevation	Reciprocal changes
Inferior wall	II, III, aVF	I, aVL, V1-V4
Anterior-septal wall	V1-V4	II, III, aVF, aVL
Lateral wall	I, aVL, V5, V6	II, III, aVF
Posterior wall	V6	V1-V4

Cardiac enzymes	Changes
CPK	onset 4-6 hours, peaks 24 hours
CPK-MB	onset 4-6 hours, peaks 12-20 hours
LDH	onset 8-12 hours, peaks 2-4 days
Troponin I normal range (most sensitive test)	0-0.1 ng/mL; onset 4-6 hours, peaks 12-24 hours, returns to normal in 4-7 days
Troponin T normal range (most sensitive test)	0-0.2 ng/mL; onset 3-4 hours, peaks 10-24 hours, returns to normal in 10-14 days

4. **D:** Diuretics and relief of anxiety. Relieving ischemia, treating atherosclerosis, and correcting renal artery stenosis are most helpful. In addition, efforts to keep patients dry, maintain a slow sinus rhythm, and control blood pressure provide a basic approach to diastolic dysfunction. When studied hemodynamically, most patients with diastolic dysfunction have normal-sized left ventricles and elevated left ventricular diastolic pressures (LVEDP) at rest when congestion is not present. This is a marker of increased stiffness. More refined hemodynamics indicates that left ventricular relaxation is slowed. Because of these changes, these patients have an inability to increase left ventricular end diastolic volume (LVEDV) without a great increase in end diastolic pressures. This inability to use the Frank-Starling mechanism of increasing LVEDV limits exercise since any increased volume markedly increases LVEDP and clinical dyspnea. A vicious cycle develops since the increased left ventricular pressure results in shortness of breath. Patients can present with marked shortness of breath, pulmonary edema, elevated BNP, peripheral edema, congestion on chest x-ray. This generates anxiety, increased sympathetic tone, an increased heart rate, and possibly an arrhythmia, such as atrial fibrillation. Ischemia, secondary to coronary stenosis, impairs relaxation further and increases LVEDP. Hypertension intensifies the impaired diastole further by enhancing concentric hypertrophy, a myocardium that is strong, but stiff. The inability to increase LVEDV compromises the ability to increase cardiac output, which, in turn, also stimulates the sympathetic and rennin angiotensin-aldosterone systems, leading to volume retention and a further increase in LVEDP.

The table below defines some of these characteristics of these two heart-failure populations:

Systolic failure	Diastolic failure
Often <65 years old	Usually >70, often >80 years old
Frequently a prior MI	More often in women
More likely ETOH use	Frequent history of hypertension
Unlikely hypertensive when congested	Frequently hypertensive when congested
More likely LBBB	More often LVH on ECG
Often an S_3 heart tone present	More likely an S_4 heart tone present
Often cardiomegaly present	Heart size not enlarged

5. **D:** Nitroglycerin. Hypotension, with distended neck veins and clear lungs occurs in patients with (RVI). This is because of occlusion of the proximal right coronary artery, the blood supply to the right ventricle. RVI patients are volume dependent because of inadequate preload to the left ventricle. The basis of therapy for a RVI is large volumes of intravenous fluids prior to administering medications that may decrease preload and inotropic support. The right ventricular involvement can be diagnosed with a predictive accuracy well above 80% by the presence of ST segment elevation of >1 mm in the right-sided precordial lead, V_{4R}, in the presence of an acute inferior or inferior-posterior MI. RVI accompanies inferior-posterior wall MIs in 30-50% of patients. Review table for management of AMI and unstable angina:

AMI/Unstable angina management goal	Treatment
Preload reduction MAP = 80-90 mmHg MAP = (2 × DBP) + SBP divided by 3	Nitrates (5-200 µg/min) Morphine (2-4 mg every 5-15 minutes) CPP = DBP-PCWP Normal CPP = 50-60
Heart rate and myocardial O_2 demand reduction	Beta-blockers Calcium-channel blockers
Clot prevention and "busting"	ASA G2BIIIA inhibitors—Reopro, Integrelin, Aggrastat Heparin Thrombolytics—Retavase, tPA, Streptokinase
Chest pain lasting less than 6 hours that is unresponsive to NTG therapy with ST segment elevation on ECG	Thrombolytics Relative contraindications: ▪ HTN, recent trauma, pregnancy Absolute contraindications: ▪ Active internal bleeding ▪ Suspected aortic dissection ▪ Known intracranial neoplasm ▪ Previous hemorrhagic stroke ▪ Stroke within the last year Complications: bleeding, intracranial hemorrhage, dysrhythmias, cardiac tamponade, pulmonary edema

6. **B:** Antero-septal wall MI with lateral extension and reciprocal changes in leads III and aVF. ST elevation > 1 mm is present in leads V2-V4 (anteroseptal) and leads I, aVL, V5, and V6 (lateral extension). The LAD supplies the anterior surface of the heart, the anterior two-thirds of the septum, and part of the lateral wall.

Type of infarct	Coronary artery involved	12-lead ECG findings
Anterior	LAD	V3, V4
Inferior	RCA	II, III, AVF
Lateral	LCX	I, AVL, V5, V6
Septal	LAD	V1, V2
Posterior	LCX or RCA	V1-V4 mirror changes, ST elevation
Wellen's syndrome	Associated with critical stenosis of the proximal LAD and impending infarct	V_2-V_3 segment turns down into a negative T at a 60-90-degree angle
Transmural MI	Extends through the full thickness of the myocardium and includes the endocardium and epicardium	
Subendocardial (nontransmural)	Necrosis is limited to the subendocardial surface	

Three Is of chest pain	Definition/Characteristics
Injury (ST elevation)	1 mm or greater in two anatomically contiguous leads in the limb leads and 2 mm or greater in two anatomically contiguous leads in the precordial leads.
Ischemia (ST depression)	Reciprocal findings from ST elevation leads.
Infarction (Q waves indicate tissue necrosis)	True Q waves are greater than 25% the height of the R wave. Pathological versus physiological: ➤ Acute—ST elevation ➤ Indeterminate—ST depression ➤ Old—No ST changes

7. **B:** Pericardial effusion leading to cardiac tamponade.

Term	Definition
Dressler's syndrome	Is a secondary form of pericarditis that occurs in the setting of injury to the heart or the pericardium, the outer lining of the heart. It is also known as post MI syndrome and postcardiotomy pericarditis. Dressler's syndrome is largely a self-limiting disease that very rarely leads to pericardial tamponade. The syndrome consists of a persistent low-grade fever, chest pain (usually pleuritic in nature), a pericardial friction rub, and /or a pericardial effusion. The symptoms tend to occur within 2-5 days post MI but can be delayed for a few weeks or even months after infarction. It tends to subside in a few days. An elevated ESR is an objective laboratory finding.
Pericardial effusion	Is the development of pericardial fluid as response to injury, acute pericarditis. Electrical alternans can be present on the ECG.
Cardiac tamponade	Consists of cardiac output being compromised by the fluid around the heart. Beck's triad can be indicative for the presence of tamponade, which includes muffled heart tones, hypotension, and jugular vein distension (JVD). Management: ABCs, intravenous fluids, and pericardiocentesis, if cardiac tamponade is present

Location of heart	Valve area
Base Right	Aortic
Base Left	Pulmonic
Left lateral sternal border	Tricuspid
Apex	Mitral

Heart Sound	Location	May indicate
S_1 A normal S_1 sound is low pitched and of longer duration than S_2.	Best heard over the mitral area at the apex which is approximately at the fifth intercostal space, midclavicular left side of the chest.	Corresponds to the closure of the mitral and tricuspid valves (atrioventricular—AV valves) at the beginning of ventricular contraction or systole.
S_2 A normal S_2 sound is higher pitched and of shorter duration than S_1	The second heart tone, or S_2, "Dub" is best heard over the aortic area which is located at the second intercostal space at the base of the heart, right sternal border. A normal S_2 sound is higher pitched and of shorter duration than S_1.	Corresponds to closure of the aortic and pulmonic valves (semilunar valves) at the end of ventricular systole.
S_3 Abnormal heart sound that may sound like the word *"Ken-tu-cky"* *in three fairly evenly spaced sounds.*	The S_3 sound is heard immediately after S_2 and is normal in children and young adolescents but usually disappears after the age of thirty.	When heard in adults, an S_3 is called a "gallop" and indicates left ventricular failure.
S_4 Abnormal heart sound that may sound like the word *"Tennessee"* where *the three syllables come quick followed by a pause.*	The S_4 sound is heard immediately before the S_1 and may be present in infants and children.	The S_4 is produced with decreased compliance of the ventricle and may indicate MI or shock.

8. **C:** Vitamin K, FFP is the antidote for Coumadin overdose. Protamine sulfate is the antidote for heparin overdose.

9. **D:** Cardiogenic shock because the patient is hypotensive. It is critical that these patients in cardiogenic shock do not receive beta-blockers as their tachycardia is functional because of their

severely limited stroke volume from an extensive MI. Perfusion to the brain and vital organs must be maintained (SBP $\geq$ 90 mmHg).

Problem	Treatment
Bradydysrhythmias with a pulse and heart rate <60 beats per minute. Assess to determine if the patient is hemodynamically compensated or decompensated.	Compensated: SBP > 90-100 mmHg without S/S of shock, good LOC, and treat the underlying cause; place combo pads as an anticipatory measure. Decompensated: SBP < 90-100 mmHg, ALOC may be present and other S/S of shock present <ul><li>F—Fluids</li><li>A—Atropine (not recommended in second-degree AVB Type II or CHB</li><li>E—External pacing</li><li>D—Dopamine drip</li><li>E—Epinephrine drip</li></ul>
Tachydysrhythmias with a pulse and heart rate > 160 beats per minute. Assess to determine if the patient is hemodynamically compensated or decompensated.	Compensated: SBP > 90-100 mmHg without S/S of shock and good LOC <ul><li>Supportive care</li><li>Vagal maneuvers—narrow complex tachycardia (SVT)</li><li>Medications</li><li>Application of combo pad as an anticipatory measure</li></ul>Decompensated: SBP < 90-100 mmHg with S/S of shock; ALOC may be present. <ul><li>Consider sedation</li><li>Synchronized cardioversion beginning at 100 joules</li><li>Medications</li></ul>

Problem	Treatment
Cardiogenic shock (hypotension present with S/S of pulmonary edema—left ventricular failure)	Inefficient pumping of the heart with hypotension ■ Dobutrex, dopamine, and Inocor to improve cardiac output ■ Vasodilators such as Nipride, NTG, and Levophed ■ IABP and LVAD therapy
CHF—beta-blockers contraindicated Right-side ventricular heart failure: ■ Back of fluid to the right side of the heart and body ■ Increased jugular venous distention (JVD) ■ Sacral edema ■ Pedal edema Left-side ventricular heart failure: ■ Back of fluid to the left side of the heart and lungs ■ Rales	Inefficient pumping of the heart without hypotension ■ Reduction of preload for relief of pulmonary edema ■ Reduction of afterload with vasodilators to enhance stroke volume and contractility ■ Natracor (neseritide)—synthetic version of BNP ■ Beta-blocker—carvidolol (Coreg) is administered PO and is a vasodilator that decrease heart rate and improve LV performance

10. **D:** Intravenous fluids, pericardiocentesis, and rapid transport are all indicated for management of a patient presenting with cardiac tamponade. Needle thoracostomy is indicated for a patient presenting with a tension pneumothorax.

11. **C:** The presence of Beck's triad is indicative of cardiac tamponade. Beck's triad includes hypotension, muffled heart tones, and jugular vein distension.

12. **D:** The administration of Atropine will not work with patients who have had a heart transplant because of denervation of the vagus nerve. Atropine works by blocking the vagus nerves, thereby increasing heart rate. Symptomatic bradycardia, second degree Type II block, high-grade AVB and CHB require placement of a pacemaker. Complications of pacing can include oversensing and failure to sense; failure to capture, myocardial penetration/perforation, and cardiac tamponade.

13. **B:** RVI because of the low PAWP. Review the following table:

Type of shock	CVP/RA 2-6	Cardiac index (CI) 2.5-4.3	PAWP/PCWP (Wedge) 8-12	SVR 800-1200
Hypovolemic	Low	Low	Low	High
Cardiogenic	High	Low	High	High
RVI	High	Low	Low	High
Septic		High		Low
Neurogenic		Low (HR slow or normal)		Low
Anaphylactic		Low (HR fast)		Low

Know your normal and abnormal hemodyamic value
- PAS = 15-25
- PAD = 8-15

To help you determine which type of shock/condition the patient is presenting with, complete the following steps in order:

1. Look at the SVR first.
2. If SVR is <800, "think" distributive shock (vasodilatory shock)
   a. Septic shock, neurogenic shock, or anaphylactic shock
   b. Next look at the cardiac index (CI)
      i. High = septic shock
      ii. Low = neurogenic shock if heart rate is within normal range or if bradycardia is present. If patient is tachycardiac, anaphylactic shock may be present. Assess for other signs and symptoms of anaphylaxis.
3. If SVR is >1200 "think" hypovolemic shock, cardiogenic shock, or right ventricular myocardial infarction (RVMI)
   c. Next look at the CVP
      i. Low = hypovolemic shock
      ii. High = cardiogenic shock or RVMI
         1. Next look at the PCWP
            a. High = cardiogenic shock
            b. Low = RVMI

14. **B:** Thyrotoxicosis, also known as Grave's disease, thyroid storm and hyperthyroidism. Avoid Aspirin because it increases T3, T4 levels and can worsen condition.

Grave's disease	Myxedema coma	Addison's disease	Cushing's disease
Hyperthyroidism	Hypothyroidism	Acute renal insufficiency	Hyperaldosteronism
Exophthalmos— "Marty Feldman" or "Betty Davis" protruding eyeballs	Infection common cause; coarse hair, deep voice, thinning or loss of the outer third of the eyebrows (Queen Ann's sign)	Hypotension is common: *caution with etomidate administration*	Hypertension
Atrial fibrillation is common	Women > 60 years; occurs in the winter months		Women have facial hair, moon-face, buffalo hump
Anxiety, tremors	Fatigue	Fatigue	Fatigue
Weight loss	Weight gain	Weight loss	Upper body obesity, thin arms and legs
Treatment: correct electrolytes and glucosteroids	Treatment: levothyroxine	Treatment: supportive care	Treatment: decrease or initiate steroids

15. **B:** (2 × DBP) + SBP divided by 3 = MAP. Normal MAP is 80-100 mmHg.

16. **A:** Normal coronary perfusion pressure is 50-60 mmHg. It can be calculated by using the following formula: DBP − PWCP. Do not confuse coronary perfusion pressure with cerebral perfusion pressure which can be calculated by using the following formula: MAP − ICP. Normal range for cerebral perfusion pressure is 70-90 mmHg. Remember that your HEAD is higher than your HEART.

17. **C:** The initial treatment of a patient with a suspected cardiac tamponade is a rapid intravenous fluid bolus. This measure improves filling pressures and temporarily improves cardiac output until pericardiocentesis can be performed. The emergent treatment of choice is pericardiocentesis. A large bore needle is placed just to the left of the patient's sub-xyphoid process

and with negative pressure applied to the syringe, it is directed toward the left scapula (shoulder) while monitoring the ECG for the presence of ventricular ectopy. The needle is placed into the pericardial sac and may withdraw as little as 15-20 mL of blood to improve the patient's condition. Pericardial blood will generally NOT CLOT because it has been defibrinated by heart motion. Pericardiocentesis is extremely challenging to perform during flight because of air turbulence and confined space.

18. **C:** Patient is hemodynamically decompensated because of the presence of hypotension. Because the patient remains conscious, sedation can be considered prior to performing synchronized cardioversion beginning at 100 joules.

19. **C:** Pericarditis is an inflammation of the pericardium which can present with chest pain radiating to the back and relieved by sitting up forward and worsened by lying down, is the classical presentation. Other symptoms of pericarditis may include dry cough, fever, fatigue, and anxiety. Pericarditis can be misdiagnosed as MI and vice versa. The classic sign of pericarditis is a friction rub. Other signs include diffuse ST-elevation and PR-depression on ECG in all leads except aVR and V1; cardiac tamponade (pulsus paradoxus with hypotension), and CHF (elevated jugular venous pressure with peripheral edema). To determine if the friction rub heard is pleuritic versus pericardial, the patient is asked to hold their breath while auscultating the chest. If the friction rub is still heard while the patient is holding their breath, it is most likely a pericardial friction rub. If the friction rub is not heard, then it is most likely a pleuritic friction rub.

20. B: RVI can be associated with inferior-posterior wall MI's in 30-50% of patients.

21. A: Coronary perfusion pressure is calculated by using the following formula:

22. **B:** Right coronary artery (RCA)

23. **B:** Nipride and Beta-blockers.

Problem	Treatment
Aortic dissection Most common site: ascending aorta Associated with Marfan's syndrome, syphilis, autoimmune diseases S/S: severe pain, originating in the back or sub-sternal region **CXR Findings:** ▪ Mediastinal widening ▪ Extension of the aortic shadow beyond the a calcified aortic wall ▪ Localized bulge on aortic arch ▪ Tracheal deviation ▪ Left pleural effusion	Debakey classification system describes three types: ▪ I = occurs in the ascending aorta and extends distally beyond the aortic arch ▪ II = process is limited to the ascending aorta (Marfan's) ▪ III = dissection distal to the origin of the left subclavian artery and extends distally to abdominal aorta **Management:** ▪ Lower SBP to 100-110 mmHg ▪ Beta-blockers blockers to slow the heart rate and decrease ejection fraction (metoprolol, esmolol), pain analgesics ▪ Fluids only if hypotensive ▪ HTN crisis: Nipride, Hyperstat to patient's normal within 30-60 min ▪ Surgery

24. **C:** Trousseau's sign is observed in patients with low calcium. This sign may be present before other manifestations of hypocalcemia such as hyperreflexia and tetany and is generally more sensitive than the Chvostek sign of hypocalcemia. To elicit Trousseau's sign, a blood pressure cuff is placed around the patient's arm and inflated to a pressure greater than the systolic blood pressure and held in place for three minutes. This will occlude the brachial artery. In the absence of blood flow, the patient's hypocalcemia and subsequent neuromuscular irritability will induce spasm of the muscles of the hand and forearm. The wrist and metacarpophalangeal joints flex, the DIP and PIP joints extend, and the fingers adduct.

25. **B:** The patient suspected of having a cardiac tamponade will exhibit signs and symptoms of decreased cardiac output such as, cool, clammy skin, altered mental sratus, tachycardia, pulsus paradoxus (a drop in systolic blood pressure > 15 mmHg during normal inspiration), distant muffled heart tones, jugular venous

distention, unless the patient is hypovolemic, hypotension, and electrical alternans.

26. **B:** Aortic rupture with 90% of patients who die at the scene. Chest x-ray findings: widening mediastinum and loss of aortic knob shadow

27. **D:** BNP is a blood test used to measure the amount of BNP hormone in the blood. BNP is produced by the heart and shows how well the heart is functioning. Normally, only a low amount of BNP is found in the heart. But if the heart has to work harder for a longer period of time, such as in heart failure, the heart releases more BNP, increasing the blood level of BNP. In some cases, this test can diagnose heart failure in a patient who does not have obvious heart failure symptoms. BNP values tend to increase with age and are higher in women than men. Lab findings—normal BNP level: 0-99 picograms per milliliter (pg/mL); Abnormal BNP level: 100 pg/mL or greater is indicative that heart failure may be present.

28. **C:** Levine's sign: patient clutching their chest, which may indicate that pain may be cardiac in origin. Review the following table for more signs and what they may indicate.

Name of sign	May indicate
Levine's	Clutching of the chest, may be cardiac in origin
Murphy's	Right upper quadrant pain, may indicate gallbladder disease
Grey Turner's	Retroperitoneal bruising, may indicate pancreatitis or trauma
Cullen's	Periumbilical bruising, may indicate pancreatitis or intra-abdominal bleeding
Halstead	Marbled appearance of the abdomen, may indicate necrosis of the pancreas
Kehr's	Shoulder pain, may indicate spleen injury on the left side or ectopic pregnancy/rupture on either side
Hamman's	Crunching sound heard with auscultation, may be synchronized with heart rate/pulse, may indicate tracheobronchial injury

29. **A:** Kussmual's sign is a rise in venous pressure with inspiration (JVD), which can be indicative of (RVI) and cardiac tamponade.

Clinical Sign/Symptom/ Term	Definition/Characteristics
S_3 heart tone	Abnormal heart sound "ventricular gallop" that is associated with CHF, mitral regurgitation, and cardiomyopathy.
S_4 heart tone	Abnormal heart sound "atrial gallop" that is associated with dilated or restrictive cardiomyopathy, aortic, and pulmonic stenosis.
Orthopnea	Increased shortness of breath in supine/lying position and is relieved by sitting and/or standing up.
Paroxysmal nocturnal dyspnea (PND)	Medical symptom, also known as *cardiac asthma*. It is defined as sudden, severe shortness of breath at night that awakens a person from sleep, often with coughing and wheezing. It is most closely associated with CHF. PND commonly occurs several hours after a person with heart failure has fallen asleep. PND is often relieved by sitting upright but not as quickly as simple orthopnea. Also unlike orthopnea, it does not develop immediately upon lying down.
Dilated cardiomyopathy	Ventricular dilation, contractile dysfunction, and symptoms of heart failure.
Hypertropic cardiomyopathy	Inappropriate LV hypertrophy (thickening of left ventricle) with preserved or enhanced contractile function. Systolic murmur can be present. Etiology unclear—IHSS (idiopathic hypertrophic subaortic stenosis).
Restrictive cardiomyopathy	Least common. Endocardial scarring of the ventricle with impaired diastolic filling.
Cardiomegaly	A medical condition wherein the heart is enlarged.

30. **D:** Sandostatin (octreotide) is a vasoactive peptide used in the management of upper gastrointestinal esophageal varices. The mechanism of action is believed to be a reduction of splanchnic blood flow. Varices are dilated veins in the distal esophagus or

proximal stomach caused by elevated pressure in the portal venous system, typically from cirrhosis. They may bleed massively but cause no other symptoms. Diagnosis is by upper endoscopy. Treatment is primarily with endoscopic banding and IV octreotide. If an acute hemorrhage episode occurs during transport, maintenance of airway and circulating volume is the first priority. As with all patient care, standard precautions should be observed. Adequate suction, IV fluids, blood, and irrigating fluid all need to be secured before transport. Adequate care must be maintained of any esophageal tubes, such as the Sengstaken-Blakemore, Linton, or Minnesota tubes, that have been placed prior to transport.

31. **B:** Diabetic ketoacidosis (DKA) is problem with insulin. Review the following tables for difference between DKA and HHNK. Treatment goal for both are aimed at administering fluids, insulin, and correcting electrolyte imbalances to control the hyperglycemia and to prevent shock and other complications.

Diabetic ketoacidosis (DKA)	Hyperglycemic hyperosmolar nonKetotic coma (HHNK)
Problem is lack of or low insulin	Problem is high sugar with high serum osmolarity
Usually can develop at any age and is most likely to occur in an insulin-dependent patient	Most patients are usually older and may have other underlying disease present. Patients may experience more sudden, severe neurologic changes than DKA
Dehydration	Severe dehydration
Acidosis present	Usually no production of ketones or presence of acidosis
Serum glucose usually < 1,000 mg/dL	Serum glucose usually > 1,000 mg/dL, (higher than DKA)

Diabetes Mellitus, often simply referred to as *diabetes*—is a condition in which a person has high blood sugar, either because the body doesn't produce enough insulin or because cells don't respond to the insulin that is produced. *This high blood sugar produces the classical symptoms of polyuria (frequent urination), polydipsia (increased thirst), and polyphagia (increased hunger).* Review the following table for the three main types of diabetes.

Type I (juvenile onset)	Type II (adult onset)	Gestational
Results from the body's failure to produce insulin and presently requires the person to inject insulin. Type 1 diabetes mellitus is characterized by loss of the *insulin-producing beta cells of the islets of Langerhans in the pancreas,* leading to insulin deficiency.	Results from insulin resistance, a condition in which cells fail to use insulin properly, sometimes combined with an absolute insulin deficiency. Type II is the common type.	Results when pregnant women, who have never had diabetes before, have a high blood glucose level during pregnancy. It may precede development of Type II diabetes. Risks to the fetus include macrosomia (high birth weight); increased fetal insulin may inhibit surfactant production. A cesarean section may be performed if there is marked fetal distress or an increased risk of injury associated with macrosomia, such as shoulder dystocia.

32. **B:** Normal adult urinary output ranges from 30-50 mL/hour. Pediatric range is from 1-2 mL/kg/hour. Expected urinary output in electrical injuries is 100 mL/hour in the adult patient and 2-4 mL/kg/hour in the pediatric patient.

33. **D:** HHNK is a problem with sugar. Review table in question no. 31.

34. **C:** *Kernig's and Brudzinski's signs* are physical examination results that are strongly suggestive of meningitis. A "stiff neck" is one of the general warning signs of meningitis, and these are some of the first steps to investigate such a finding. *Kernig's sign* is essentially a way to demonstrate that the neck is not simply "stiff" but is irritated. With the patient lying flat, the examiner flexes the hip ninety degrees and then attempts to extend the lower leg at the knee. Pain on extension is a positive sign. If positive but the straight leg raise also produces back pain, the combined sign may be due to low back muscle spasm, herniated disk, or sciatic nerve inflammation. To test for *Brudzinski's sign,* the patient lies on his or her back, and the examiner puts one hand behind the patient's head and the other on the chest. Using the hand behind the neck to raise the head but pressing on the chest with the other hand, if the hips and knees flex, the neck sign is positive.

35. **D:** Gallbladder disease may be present. Review the table in question no. 28.

36. **B:** An ammonia test measures the amount of ammonia in the blood. Most ammonia in the body forms when protein is broken down by bacteria in the intestines. The liver normally converts ammonia into urea, which is then eliminated in urine. Ammonia levels in the blood rise when the liver is not able to convert ammonia to urea. This may be caused by cirrhosis or severe hepatitis.

Hepatic encephalopathy (also known as *portosystemic encephalopathy)* is the occurrence of confusion, altered level of consciousness, and coma as a result of liver failure. In the advanced stages, it is called *hepatic coma* or *coma hepaticum.* It may ultimately lead to death. It is caused by accumulation in the bloodstream of toxic substances that are normally removed by the liver. The diagnosis of hepatic encephalopathy requires the presence of impaired liver function, and the exclusion of an alternative explanation for the symptoms. Blood tests (ammonia levels) may assist in the diagnosis. Evacuation of blood in the GI tract will decrease protein (increased protein levels in the blood can increase ammonia levels). Attacks are often precipitated by an intercurrent problem, such as infection or constipation.

Hepatic encephalopathy is reversible with treatment. This relies on suppressing the production of the toxic substances in the intestine. This is most commonly done with the laxative lactulose or with nonabsorbable antibiotics. In addition, the treatment of any underlying condition may improve the symptoms. In particular settings, such as acute liver failure, the onset of encephalopathy may indicate the need for a liver transplant. Review the following tables for other liver function tests that may be ordered to be done.

Liver function test			
Lab test name	Also known as	Normal range (µg)	Consideration
Ammonia	NH_3	Adult: 15-45 Peds: 40-80 The liver converts ammonia in the portal blood to urea for excretion by the kidneys. With impaired liver function, especially when combined with impaired portal blood flow, ammonia levels rise.	Specimen must be drawn on ice and processed immediately. Hemolysis will cause elevated levels. Excessive protein intake will cause elevated levels. Many drugs can falsely elevate or decrease levels.

Liver function test			
Lab test name	Also known as	Normal range (g/dL)	Consideration
Albumin	Alb	Adult: 3.4-5.4 Peds: 3.0-5.0 Primarily by the liver, patients with chronic liver disease accompanied with cirrhosis often have levels < 3.0 g/dL	Large amounts of IV fluids can cause inaccurate test results. Albumin levels are decreased during pregnancy. Drugs that can increase albumin measurements include anabolic steroids, androgens, growth hormone, insulin.

Liver function test			
Lab test name	Also known as	Normal range (U/L)	Consideration
Alkaline phosphatase	ALP or Alk phos	Male: 98-251 Female: 81-196 Enzyme found in the liver, the biliary tract, bone, intestines, and placenta.	Many drugs can falsely elevate or decrease levels. A hemolyzed specimen can cause falsely elevated results.

Liver function test			
Lab test name	Also known as	Normal range (mg/dL)	Consideration
Immunoglobulins	Serum Electrophoresis	IgA: 140-400 IgD: 0-8 IgG: 700-1,500 IgM: 35-375 A variety of immunoglobulins are increased in patients with chronic liver disease.	**Elevated IgA** Alcoholic liver disease, cirrhosis, hepatitis, Laennec's cirrhosis, hepatobiliary carcinoma **Elevated IgD** Chronic infections and liver diseases **Elevated IgG** Autoimmune hepatitis, hepatitis, hepatitis C, Laennec's cirrhosis **Elevated IgM** Biliary cirrhosis, hepatitis, viral infections

Liver function test			
Lab test name	Also known as	Normal range (sec)	Consideration
Prothrombin time	PT	Male: 9.6-11.8 Female: 9.5-11.3 Peds: 11-14 Neonate: 12-21 Prothrombin (PT) is a vitamin K dependent protein produced by the liver. Liver disease can lead to increased PT levels.	Many drugs can falsely elevate or decrease levels. Fibrinogen levels < 100 mg/dL can increase the PT level. Excessive agitation of sample can increase the PT level.

Liver function test			
Lab test name	Also known as	Normal range (mm^{-3})	Consideration
Platelets	PLT or Thrombocyte	Adult: 150,000-450,000 Peds: 170,000-380,000 The liver releases thrombopoietin to stimulate platelet production. Increased platelet levels can be seen with cirrhosis, and decreased platelet levels can be seen with viral infections and splenomegaly due to liver disease.	Numerous drugs can alter platelet production or counts or both. White blood cell (WBC) counts > 100,000/mm^{-3} can alter platelet counts. Handle sample gently to avoid platelet clumping.

Liver function test			
Lab test name	Also known as	Normal range	Consideration
ALT or SGPT	Alanine Aminotransferase	Male: 7-46 U/mL Female: 5-35 U/mL Peds: 3-37 U/L Enzyme produced by the liver that acts as a catalyst in amino acid production. High concentrations are found in liver cells and moderate concentrations in body fluids, heart, kidney, and skeletal muscles.	Numerous drugs including ETOH can falsely elevate levels. Uremia and Hemodialysis can falsely decrease levels. A hemolyzed specimen can cause falsely elevated levels.

Liver function test			
Lab test name	Also known as	Normal range (U/L)	Consideration
AST or SGOT	Aspartate Aminotransferase	Male: 8-26 Female: 8-20 Peds: 19-28 Enzyme that catalyzes the reversible transfer of an amino between the amino acid. High concentrations are in the liver and heart cells, with lower concentrations found in skeletal muscles, kidney, pancreas, and the brain.	Numerous drugs and vitamin A can falsely elevate levels. A hemolyzed specimen can cause falsely elevated levels.

Liver function test			
Lab test name	Also known as	Normal range (IU/L)	Consideration
GGT or GGTP	Gamma-glutamyl Transpeptidase	Male: 10-39 Female: 6-29 Peds: 0-23 Enzyme that participates in the transfer of amino acids and peptides across cellular membranes. High concentrations are found in the liver, bile ducts, and kidneys. Lower concentrations are found in the prostate gland, brain, and heart.	Numerous drugs, including ETOH can elevate levels. Oral contraceptives can lower levels. A hemolyzed specimen can cause falsely elevated results.

Liver function test			
Lab test name	Also known as	Normal range (mg/dL)	Consideration
Bilirubin	Indirect Bili and Direct Bili	Adult: Indirect Bili 0.3-1.1 Direct Bili 0.1-0.4 Bilirubin is a degradation product of the pigmented heme portion of hemoglobin. Old and abnormal red blood cells are removed from circulation by the spleen and, to some extent, by the liver.	Certain drugs can elevate bilirubin levels. A hemolyzed specimen can cause falsely elevated results. Prolonged exposure to UV or sunlight can lower bilirubin levels.

37. **C:** Morphine has been contraindicated for pain treatment in acute pancreatitis because of its presumed opioid-induced sphincter of Oddi dysfunction. Pancreatitis is the inflammation of the pancreas caused by the release of activated pancreatic enzymes. The most common triggers are biliary tract disease and chronic heavy alcohol consumption.

Pancreatitis can occur in two very different forms. Acute pancreatitis is sudden, while chronic pancreatitis is characterized by recurring or persistent abdominal pain with or without steatorrhea (presence of excess fat in the feces, foul-smelling stools that float because of high fat content) or diabetis mellitus. Severe upper abdominal pain, with radiation through to the back, is the hallmark of pancreatitis. Nausea and vomiting are prominent symptoms.

The condition ranges from mild (abdominal pain and vomiting) to severe (pancreatic necrosis and a systemic inflammatory process with shock and multiorgan failure). Findings on the physical exam will vary according to the severity of the pancreatitis, whether or not it is associated with significant internal bleeding. The blood pressure may be high (when pain is prominent) or low (if internal bleeding or dehydration has occurred).

Diagnosis is based on clinical presentation and obtaining lab tests: serum amylase and lipase. *Amylase* (the pancreatic enzyme responsible for digesting carbohydrates) is the most common blood **test** for acute **pancreatitis**. *Lipase* is more specific for pancreatitis, but both enzymes may be increased in renal failure and various abdominal conditions, such as perforated ulcer, mesenteric vascular occlusion, or intestinal obstruction. Serum amylase and lipase concentrations increase on the first day of acute pancreatitis and return to normal in three to seven days. Treatment is supportive with fluids, antiemetics, analgesics, and fasting.

38. **A:** Problem is usually higher levels of sugar (higher than DKA), high serum osmolarity, severe dehydration, lack of ketones, and acidosis. Patient with HHNK may also experience more severe and sudden neurologic changes than the patient with DKA. Review the tables in question no. 31.

39. **A:** Aggressive fluid replacement and the administration of vasopressin (Pitressin). Vasopressin is a peptide hormone which is synthesized by the hypothalamus and is stored in the pituitary gland. It controls the reabsorption of molecules in the tubules of the kidneys by affecting the tissue's permeability. Vasopressin increases peripheral vascular resistance, which in turn increases arterial blood pressure. It plays a key role in the regulation of water, glucose, and salts in the blood.

Review the following table for Diabetes insipidus (DI) and syndrome of inappropriate antidiuretic hormone (SIADH).

Diabetes insipidus (DI)	Syndrome of inappropriate antidiuretic hormone (SIADH)
A condition where the kidneys are able to conserve water; hence the phrase "peeing like a racehorse."	Occurs when excessive levels of antidiuretic hormones (arginine vasopressin, AVP) are produced, which causes the body to retain water.
Symptoms include excessive thirst and excretion of large amounts of severely diluted urine.	Symptoms include weight gain, nausea, vomiting, altered mentation, irritability, and seizures.
The most common cause is a deficiency of arginine vasopressin (AVP), also known as antidiuretic hormone (ADH)	Common causes include heart failure, diseased or injured hypothalamus, certain cancers, such as lung cancer, brain tumors.
Blood glucose, bicarbonate, calcium, and electrolyte levels need to be obtained in order to distinguish DI from other causes of excessive urination. *Hypernatremia* can develop with continued dehydration. Urinalysis demonstrates dilute urine with a low specific gravity and urine osmalarity.	Serum electrolytes need to be obtained. *Dilutional hyponatremia* is common because of water retention.
A fluid deprivation test assists in determining whether DI is caused by excessive fluid intake, a defect in ADH production, or a defect in the kidney's response to ADH.	Management can include fluid restriction, surgery, and certain medications that inhibit the secretion of ADH.

40. **A:** Acute renal insufficiency, also known as Addison's disease. Hypotension is common: *caution with etomidate administration, fatigue and weight loss.* Review the table from question no. 14 for differences of Grave's disease, myxedema coma, Cushing's disease, and Addison's disease.

41. **C:** Hypothyroidism

42. **D:** Hypothroidism occurs primarily in women, almost exclusively over the age of sixty, with 90% of the cases occurring in the winter months.

43. **B:** Levophed (norepinephrine) indication is mainly used to treat patients in vasodilatory shock states such as septic and neurogenic shock. Studies have shown a survival benefit over dopamine. Levophed functions as a peripheral vasoconstrictor (alpha-adrenergic action) and as an inotropic stimulator of the heart and dilator of coronary arteries (beta-adrenergic action).

44. **B:** Bowel cleansing is the mainstay of therapy for hepatic encephalopathy. Evacuation of gut-derived toxins (intestinal blood, bacteria) and administration of Lactulose (orally or as an enema) is one of the cornerstones of the treatment of hepatic encephalopathy. Lactulose may be given orally to acidify the ammonia in the colon and form the ammonium that can be easily excreted. It is used as a laxative for evacuating blood from intestines and for reducing ammonia production by intestinal bacteria. Gastrointestinal bleeding should also be controlled.

45. **C:** Grey Turner's sign refers to bruising of the flank areas. It can take up to twenty-four to forty-eight hours to appear, and it can predict a severe attack of acute pancreatitis. It may also be accompanied by Cullen's sign (periumbilical bruising) or Halstead's sign (marbled abdomen), which then may be indicative of pancreatic necrosis with retroperitoneal or intra-abdominal bleeding. Other causes of Grey Turner's sign can include blunt abdominal trauma, ruptured abdominal aortic aneurysm, and ruptured/hemorrhagic ectopic pregnancy.

46. **B:** Etomidate (Amidate), which is classified as a sedative-hypnotic can block the adrenal gland's production of cortisol and other steroid hormones, possibly resulting in temporary adrenal gland failure. This may cause abnormal salt and water balance, lowered blood pressure, and, ultimately, shock. Patients with known Addison's disease (acute renal insufficiency) should not be given etomidate.

47. **B:** Prinzmetal's angina. Review the following table for different types of angina.

Management of Angina

- MONA—Morphine, oxygen, nitrates, ASA
- Beta-blockers, Calcium channel blockers
- PCTA—percutaneous transluminal coronary angioplasty
- Laser therapy
- CABG—coronary artery bypass graft surgery
- IABP—intra-aortic balloon pump

Classification	Definition
Stable	Onset with physical exertion or emotional stress • Pain lasts 1-5 minutes • Pain is relieved by rest
Unstable	Stable angina that has changed in frequency, quality, duration, or intensity • Pain lasts longer than 10 minutes despite rest and NTG therapy
Variant	Spontaneous episodes of chest pain frequently noted at rest or on early rising • Circadian pattern • Relieved by NTG
Silent	Objective evidence of ischemia in asymptomatic patients
Mixed	Combination of stable and variant angina
Prinzmetal's	Can occur at rest, while sleeping, or after exercise

48. **C:** Chvostek's sign also known as the Weiss sign, is one of the signs of tetany seen in hypocalcemia. It refers to an abnormal reaction to the stimulation of the facial nerve. When the facial nerve is tapped at the angle of jaw (masseter muscle), the facial muscles on the same side of the face will contract momentarily (typically seen is twitching of the nose or lips). This sign may also be encountered in patients presenting with respiratory alkalosis, such as seen with hyperventilation, which actually causes decreased serum calcium with a normal calcium level due to shift of calcium from the blood to albumin, which has become more negative in the alkalotic state. Chvostek's sign may also be present in hypomagnesemia, frequently seen in alcoholics, patients with diarrhea, patients taking aminoglycosides or diuretics because

hypomagnesemia can cause hypocalcemia. Trousseau's sign is also often used to detect early tetany. Refer to the following table for lab values and significance.

Lab Test	Normal range	Significance
Hemoglobin	12-18	Low levels is called anemia, which can be caused by hemorrhage, lead poisoning, sickle cell anemia, suppression by chemotherapy agents and other causes. Dehydration can cause falsely high levels, which disappears once proper fluids have been administered. Other causes of high levels include living at high altitudes and smoking.
Hematacrit	36-52%	High in COPD patients and low in dehydrated or hemorrhage.
Platelets	140-400	Low levels of < 100 is called thrombocytopenia. Low levels can be caused by infection with hepatitis C, chronic liver disease, infection with HIV, pregnancy (HELLP), chemotherapy, systemic lupus, chronic lymphocytic leukemia, treatment with certain medications such as heparin and quinidine, and aplastic anemia (blood disorder that causes the body to stop making enough new blood cells).
WBC	4.5-10.5	Increases with infection and is known as leukocytosis. A decrease is called leucopenia.

Sickle-cell disease (SCD) or sickle cell anemia is a genetic blood disorder characterized by red blood cells that assume an abnormal, rigid sickle shape. The term "sickle cell crisis" is used to describe several independent acute conditions occurring in patients with sickle cell disease. Vaso-occlusive crisis (painful crisis) is managed with hydration, analgesics, and NSAIDs. Diphenhydramine is often administered for itching associated with opioid administration. A hemolytic crisis may require blood transfusions.

Lab test	Normal range	Significance
Sodium	135-145	<120 can cause seizures, managed with slow IV administration of hypertonic saline. Recommended to be maintained at 155 for head injured/bleed patient to help reduce ICP.
Potassium	3.5-5.5	>7.0 can cause ventricular dysrhythmias, peaked/tented T waves >5 mm in height on the ECG.
Calcium	8.8-10.4	Chvostek's and Trouseau's sign.
Chloride	95-112	
CO_2	24-30	<20 may indicate dehydration; assess for acidosis
BUN	6-23	May indicate blood in the gut, dehydration, or renal failure.
Creatinine	0.6-1.4	> 1.4 may indicate renal failure.
Glucose	70-110	Assess the patient's presenting condition, change in behavior, skin color, skin condition, heart rate, etc.
Serum OS	285-295	Maintain at <320 in head injured/bleed patients to reduce ICP and maintain adequate CPP. Serum OS can be decreased with the administration of mannitol, hypertonic saline, and furosemide.
Magnesium	1.5-2.5	Levels of 4-8 are indicated to prevent seizures in the pre-eclamptic pregnant patient. Levels >10 can be toxic and may require the administration of calcium.
Ammonia	Adult: 14-45 Pediatrics: 40-80	Increases in Reye's syndrome, hepatic encephalopathy.

49. **D:** Cushing's syndrome. Refer to the table in question no. 14.

50. **B:** Cullen's sign (periumbilical bruising)

Clinical Sign/Symptom/ Term	Definition/Characteristics
Hypertrophy	Increase of the size of an organ or in a select area of the tissue.
Hepatomagaly	A condition of having an enlarged liver. It is a nonspecific medical sign having many causes, which can broadly be broken down into infection, direct toxicity, hepatic tumors, or metabolic disorder. Often, hepatomegaly will present as an abdominal mass. Depending on the cause, it may sometimes be present along with jaundice.
Anasarca	Also known as "extreme generalized edema" is a medical condition characterised by widespread swelling of the skin due to effusion of fluid into the extracellular space. It is usually caused by either congestive cardiac failure, liver failure (cirrhosis of the liver), or renal failure/disease.
Ascites	Also known as *peritoneal cavity fluid, peritoneal fluid excess, hydroperitoneum* or more archaically as *abdominal dropsy,* is an accumulation of fluid in the peritoneal cavity.
Whipple's Triad	Is a collection of three criteria (called *Whipple's criteria)* that suggest a patient's symptoms result from hypoglycemia. The triad is stated in various versions, but the essential conditions are 1. Symptoms known or likely to be caused by hypoglycemia 2. A low plasma glucose measured at the time of the symptoms 3. Relief of symptoms when the glucose is raised to normal.
Wellen's syndrome	Is associated with critical stenosis of the proximal LAD and impending infarct. V_2-V_3 segment turns down into a negative T wave at a 60-96-degree angle.

Clinical Sign/Symptom/ Term	Definition/Characteristics

Acute Pericarditis	Inflammation of the pericaridium
	■ Causes: MI, infection, uremia, malignancy, drug therapy, trauma
	■ Normally 10-50 mL of pericardial fluid in the pericardial space
	■ S/S: Fever may be present, pericardial friction rub, pain decreases when patient leans forward
	   ○ Differentiating between pleuritic rub and pericardial rub: if possible, ask the patient to the hold their breath while auscultating the chest; if rub disappears—pleuritic rub (pleurisy)
	Management:
	   ○ Treat the cause
	   ○ Monitor for pericardial effusion leading to tamponade
	   ○ NSAIDS, steroids, and pain analgesia

Endocarditis	Inflammation of the endocardium
	■ Causes: bacterial infection, *streptococcus viridian* is the most common.
	■ Signs and symptoms may include the following:
	   ○ Allergy symptoms, fever, shortness of breath.
	   ○ *Janeway lesions* are nontender, small, erythematous, or hemorrhagic macules or nodules in the palms or soles, which are pathognomonic of infective endocarditis. The pathogenesis is due to septic emboli.
	   ○ *Roth's spots* are retinal hemorrhages with white or pale centers composed of coagulated fibrin.
	   ○ *Osler's nodes* are painful, red, raised lesions on the finger pulps, indicative of the heart disease subacute infective endocarditis.
	Management: treat the cause, supportive care.

Clinical sign/ Symptoms/Terms	Definition/Characteristics/Treatment

Acute arterial occlusion	Sudden interruption of blood flow
	▪ Signs and symptoms may include
	   o Pain
	   o Pallor
	   o Pulselessness—distally
	   o Parethesias—burning
	   o Cool extremity
	Management
	   o Monitor the 5 Ps
	   o Heparin
	   o Embolectomy

Venous thrombosis	*Virchow's Triad* encompasses three broad categories of factors that are thought to contribute to venous thrombosis:
	▪ Alterations in normal blood flow (stasis)
	▪ Injuries to the vascular endothelium
	▪ Alterations in the constitution of blood (hypercoagulability)
	Signs/Symptoms may include
	   o Pain
	   o Swelling
	   o Deep muscle tenderness
	Management
	   o Elevate extremity
	   o Heat
	   o Pain analgesia
	   o Anticoagulants

Hypertensive crisis	Rapid, progressive rise in BP sufficient to cause potential irreversible damage to vital organs
	▪ DBP > 130 mmHg
	▪ Organ dysfunction
	   o Hypertensive encephalopathy—true emergency
	   o Renal and cardiac damage
	Management: supportive care with a goal to decrease MAP over 30-60 minutes with Nipride, Hyperstat, and/ or labetalol

Valvular dysfunction	Definition
Mitral Stenosis	Narrowing of mitral opening. Rheumatic fever common cause.
Mitral regurgitation	Ruptured mitral valve. One leaflet ruptured, prognosis is better. S_3 and S_4 heart tones present.
Aortic stenosis	LV hypertrophy and failure.
Aortic regurgitation	Volume overloads to left ventricle, left atrial hypertension, pulmonary edema. Secondary to infective endocarditis, aortic dissection, nonpenetrating chest or upper abdominal trauma. Wide pulse pressure, diastolic murmur. IABP contraindicated.

Bibliography

Adedeji, OA, McAdam, WA. "Murphy's sign, acute cholecystitis and elderly people." *J R Coll Surg Edinb.* 1996; 41(2):88-9.

Association of Air Medical Services; (2003) *Guidelines for Air Medical Crew Education.* Iowa, Kendall/Hunt Publishing Company.

Attia, J, et al. The rational clinical examination. Does this adult patient have acute meningitis? *JAMA. 1999;* 282 (2):175-81.

Bosmann, M, et al. Coexistence of Cullen's and Grey Turner's signs in acute pancreatitis. *Am J Med.* 2009; 122(4):333-4.

Carlberg, B, et al. Atenolol in hypertension: Is it a wise choice? *Lancet.* 2004; 364(9446):1684-9.

Darovic, G. (1999), *Handbook of Hemodynamic Monitoring.* 2nd edition. Philadelphia, W.B. Saunders

Elizabeth, AH, George, EK Jr. Determining Brain Death in Adults: A Guideline for Use in Critical Care. *Crit Care Nurse.* 2004; 24: 50-56.

Goodman, DJ, et al. Effect of digoxin on atioventricular conduction. Studies in patients with and without cardiac autonomic innervation. *Circulation.* 1975; 51(2):251-256.

Francis, CW, Kaplan, KL. (2006). Principles of Antithrombotic Therapy." in Lichtman MA, Beutler E, Kipps TJ, et al. *Williams Hematology* (7th ed.). Chap. 21.

Freedman. Oral anticoagulants: pharmacodynamics, clinical indications and adverse effects. *J Clin Pharmacol.* 1992; 32(3):196-209.

Gage, BF. Fihn, SD, White, RH. Management and dosing of warfarin therapy. *Am. J. Med.* 2000; 109(6):481-8.

Ginsberg, L. Difficult and recurrent meningitis. *J Neurol Neurosurg Psychiatry.* 2004; 75 (Suppl 1): i16-21.

Hirsh, J, et al. American Heart Association/American College of Cardiology Foundation guide to warfarin therapy. *J Am Coll Cardiol. 2003;* 41(9):1633-52.

Holleran, R. (1996). *Flight Nursing: Principles and Practice, 2nd edition.* St. Louis, Mosby.

Holleran, R. (2003). *Air and Surface Patient Transport: Principles and Practice,* 3rd edition. St. Louis, Mosby.

Holleran, R. (2009). *ASTNA Patient Transport: Principles and Practice,* 4th edition. St. Louis, Mosby.

Horton, JD, Bushwick, BM. Warfarin therapy: evolving strategies in anticoagulation. *Am Fam Physician.* 1999; 59(3):635-46.

Krupa, D. (1997). *Flight Nursing Core Curriculum.* Park Ridge, IL, National Flight Nurses Association.

Law, M, Wald, NM. Lowering blood pressure to prevent myocardial infarction and stroke: a new preventive strategy. *Health Technol Assess.* 2003; 7(31):1-94.

Marik, PE, Corwin HL. Efficacy of red blood cell transfusion in the critically ill: a systematic review of the literature. *Crit Care Med.* 2008; 36:2667-2674

Packer M, Fowler MB, Roecker EB, et al. Effect of carvedilol on the morbidity of patients with severe chronic heart failure: results of the carvedilol prospective randomized cumulative survival (COPERNICUS) study. *Circulation.* 2002; 106(17):2194-9.

Rang HP, Dale MM, Ritter JM, Moore PK. (2003). Pharmacology, 5th edition. Edinburgh, Churchill Livingstone.

Sáez-Llorens, X, McCracken, GH. Bacterial meningitis in children. *Lancet.* 2003; 361(9375):2139-48.

Singer, AJet al. Correlation among clinical, laboratory, and hepatobiliary scanning findings in patients with suspected acute cholecystitis. *Ann Emerg Med.* 1996; 28(3):267-72.

Sørensen, HT, Mellemkjaer L, Blot WJ, et al. Risk of upper gastrointestinal bleeding associated with use of low-dose aspirin. *Am J Gastroenterol.* 2000; 95(9):2218-24.

Tunkel, AR, Hartman BJ, Kaplan SL, et al. Practice guidelines for the management of bacterial meningitis. *Clin Infect Dis.* 2004; 39(9):1267-84.

Van de Beek, D, de Gans J, Tunkel AR, Wijdicks EF. Community-acquired bacterial meningitis in adults. *N Engl J Med.* 2006; 354(1):44-53.

Module 4
Respiratory Emergencies

1. You are transporting a thirty-year-old man involved in a MCA from a rural area facility. The 70-kg patient is on a ventilator with the following settings: FIO_2 1.0, Vt 500, rate 16, PIP 22, and PEEP 5. The ABG results are pH 7.01, pCO_2 68, HCO_2 12, pO_2 280. Interpretation of the blood gas reveals

    A. Metabolic and respiratory acidosis
    B. Metabolic acidosis
    C. Respiratory acidosis
    D. Compensated respiratory acidosis

2. You are transporting a ten-year-old boy weighing 60 kg with diagnosis of status asthmaticus on a ventilator. $EtCO_2$ is 56 and pulse oximetry reading is 95%. Ventilator settings are at Vt 450, FIO_2 1.0, Rate 16, I:E 1:2, PEEP 5, PIP 48. How will you manage this patient?

    A. Increase tidal volume
    B. Reduce I:E ratio
    C. Increase PEEP
    D. Increase respiratory rate

3. When inserting a chest tube, correct insertion site recommended is

    A. 2nd ICS midclavicular line
    B. 4th-5th ICS anterior axillary line
    C. 4th ICS midaxillary line
    D. 5th ICS midaxillary line

4. ABG's reveal pH 7.31, pCO_2 58, Bicarb 26, pO_2 106. What is your interpretation?

    A. Metabolic acidosis
    B. Respiratory acidosis
    C. Metabolic alkalosis
    D. Respiratory alkalosis

5. A patient in early shock most probably has which acid-base imbalance?

    A. Metabolic acidosis
    B. Metabolic alkalosis
    C. Respiratory acidosis
    D. Respiratory alkalosis

6. Your patient's ABG's are: pH 7.43, pCO_2 56, HCO_3 34. You should correct the pCO_2 by

    A. Hyperventilation
    B. Ventilating at physiologic norms but greater than the patient's spontaneous rate
    C. Paralyze the patient to completely control vent rate
    D. Analyze electrolytes and replace deficiency

7. A fifty-five-year-old woman complains of SOB for 2 days. Identify what the following ECG rhythm reveals.

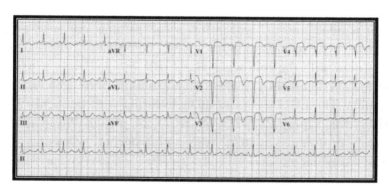

    A. Inferior MI
    B. Anteroseptal MI
    C. Lateral wall MI
    D. Posterior MI

8. Electrical alternans may be caused by

   A. Pericardial effusion
   B. Pulmonary embolus
   C. Tension pneumothorax
   D. Diaphragmatic rupture

9. You are on the scene of a thirty-year-old man involved in a single vehicle rollover accident who was reported to be ejected from the vehicle. The left chest has been decompressed with a needle. The patient is orally intubated and continues to desaturate, and you note an increase in SQ air on the left side of the chest and neck. The next intervention will be to

   A. Reneedle the left chest
   B. Insert a chest tube
   C. Advance ET tube below the level of the injury; right main stem intubation
   D. Decrease respiratory rate down to 10 per minute

10. Your patient presents with a history of asthma, coronary artery disease, hypertension, and has a chief complaint of dyspnea and weakness with the following vitals: BP 72/64, HR 112, RR 40, SpO_2 82%, temp. 99.1°F. He is on 6 L/minute of oxygen via nasal cannula. The ECG shows sinus tachycardia with frequent PVCs. ABG reveals: pH 7.28, pCO_2 68, HCO_3 24. pO_2 58. Physical exam reveals profound vesicular rales and bronchial wheezing. Your most likely diagnosis is

    A. CHF; uncompensated respiratory acidosis, hypoxemia
    B. Adult respiratory distress syndrome; compensated metabolic acidosis, hypoxemia
    C. Status asthmaticus; uncompensated metabolic acidosis, hypoxemia
    D. Cardiogenic shock; uncompensated respiratory acidosis, hypoxemia

11. You are transporting a twenty-four-year-old trauma patient from a rural facility who has just been given Anectine in preparation for endotracheal intubation. The patient's heart rate increases, muscle rigidity is present, and you observe that his end-tidal CO_2 has increased to 60 mmHg. Your next intervention would be to administer

   A. Midazolam
   B. Sodium Bicarbonate
   C. Dantrolene
   D. Glucagon

12. When performing a needle thoracostomy, which of the following is generally the preferred site?

   A. 2nd intercostal space, anterior-axillary line
   B. 5th intercostal space, anterior-midaxillary line
   C. 4th intercostal space, midclavicular line
   D. 2nd intercostal space, midclavicular line

13. Your patient presents with ABG's of pH 7.39, pCO_2 68 HCO_3 32, pO_2 82. He has history of COPD and weighs 65 kg. He presents with a history of SOB for 3 days with a RR 20 and is on 4 L/minute of oxygen by NC. He speaks in four- to five-word sentences. What acid-base disorder is present?

   A. Metabolic acidosis with partial compensation
   B. Respiratory acidosis with complete compensation
   C. Metabolic alkalosis with no compensation
   D. Respiratory alkalosis with no compensation

14. Hamman's sign may indicate which of the following?

   A. Tension pneumothorax
   B. Tracheobronchial injury
   C. Aortic rupture
   D. Cardiac tamponade

15. ABG reveals pH 7.41, pCO_2 38, HCO_3 22, pO_2 56 of a 70-kg patient on a ventilator with the following settings: Vt 700, F 14, FIO_2 0.5, I:E 1:2, PIP 46, Pplat 40, and PEEP 5. How will you manage this patient?

     A.   Increase FIO_2
     B.   Increase PEEP
     C.   Decrease Vt
     D.   All of the above

16. When managing pO_2 of <60, you would

     A.   Increase FIO_2 and apply/or increase PEEP
     B.   Increase Vt and apply/or increase PEEP
     C.   Increase FIO_2
     D.   Increase Vt

17. The patient you are transporting reveals the following ABG: pH 7.51, pCO_2 28, HCO_3 24, pO_2 110. He is a 60-kg male patient with Vt 650, F14, FIO_2 0.21, I:E 1:2, PIP 46, Pplat 42, and PEEP 0. What is your ABG interpretation, and how will you correct it?

     A.   Respiratory acidosis; increase respiratory rate (F)
     B.   Respiratory alkalosis; decrease Vt
     C.   Metabolic alkalosis; increase FIO_2
     D.   Respiratory alkalosis; increase PEEP

18. Minute ventilation is

     A.   RR × weight in kg
     B.   RR × SPO_2
     C.   Vt × weight in kg
     D.   Vt × RR

19. High-pressure alarms can be caused by all of the following, *except*

    A. Hypovolemia
    B. Connections
    C. Pneumothorax
    D. Obstructions

20. Low-pressure alarms can be caused by all of the following, *except*

    A. Hypovolemia
    B. Leaks in ventilator tubing
    C. Pneumothorax
    D. Connections

21. Vt is calculated at

    A. 3-5 mL/kg
    B. 5-8 mL/kg
    C. 6-10 mL/kg
    D. 10-15 mL/kg

22. The test most often used to diagnose a pulmonary embolism is

    A. Chest x-ray
    B. V/Q lung scan
    C. 12-lead ECG
    D. ABG

23. Acute respiratory failure is defined as

    A. pO_2 <60 mmHg and pCO_2 >50
    B. pO_2 <80 mmHg and pCO_2 >60
    C. pO_2 <60 mmHg and pCO_2 >30
    D. pO_2 <90 mmHg and pCO_2 >50

24. Situations that involve a left shift in the oxygen-hemoglobin dissociation curve are all of the following, *except*

    A. Alkalosis
    B. Hypocapnia
    C. Hypothermia
    D. Increased levels of 2,3-DPG

25. Situations that involve a right shift in the oxygen-hemoglobin dissociation curve are all of the following, *except*

    A. Alkalosis
    B. Hypercapnia
    C. Hyperthermia
    D. Increased level of 2,3-DPG

26. Repeated doses of etomidate can cause

    A. Increased ICP
    B. Acute adrenal insufficiency
    C. AMI
    D. Pulmonary edema

27. Interpret the following blood gas: pH 7.39, HCO_3 18, pCO_2 31.

    A. Respiratory alkalosis; completely compensated
    B. Respiratory acidosis; partially compensated
    C. Metabolic acidosis; partially compensated
    D. Metabolic acidosis; completely compensated

28. You are transporting a forty-year-old man from a rural ICU. The CXR reveals a ground glass appearance. The patient is on a ventilator with settings at: Vt 900 mL, rate of 16, FIO_2 0.8 with a PEEP of 5. ABG's reveal: pH 7.34, pO_2 76, pCO_2 38 and HCO_3 of 24. What pulmonary condition do you suspect?

    A. Pneumothorax
    B. Pulmonary edema
    C. ARDS
    D. Cor pulmonale

29. You would manage the above patient by

    A. Increasing the rate
    B. Increasing PEEP
    C. Performing a rapid needle decompression
    D. Administering Lasix

30. The MD has ordered a BNP, which would evaluate the patient for

    A. Sepsis
    B. Hypovolemia
    C. Right ventricular MI
    D. CHF

31. Which of the following paralytics stimulates motor end plate acetylcholine receptors causing persistent depolarization?

    A. Succinylcholine
    B. Rocuronium
    C. Vecuronium
    D. Pancuronium

32. When administering a defasciculating neuromuscular blockade, the dose recommended is

    A. 5% normal RSI dosage of NMBA
    B. 10% normal RSI dosage of NMBA
    C. 15% normal RSI dosage of NMBA
    D. 20% normal RSI dosage of NMBA

33. You are transporting a twenty-five-year-old woman with a history of suspected overdose. The following ABGs were obtained prior to your arrival at the sending facility: pH 7.52, pCO_2 27, HCO_3 24, pO_2 110. You would most likely suspect

    A. Narcotic overdose
    B. TCA overdose
    C. Early salicylate poisoning
    D. Insulin overdose

34. If the PIP does not change on a ventilator patient with respiratory acidosis, always

    A. Increase Vt before rate
    B. Decrease Vt before rate
    C. Increase rate before Vt
    D. Decrease rate before Vt

35. Trouble-shooting high-pressure alarms on the ventilator can be caused by all of the following, *except*

    A. Secretions
    B. Obstructions
    C. ET tube main-stem placement
    D. Leak in ventilator tubing

36. An elevated anion gap can indicate the presence of which of the following?

    A. Respiratory acidosis
    B. Respiratory alkalosis
    C. Metabolic acidosis
    D. Metabolic alkalosis

37. The average endotracheal tube size that should be utilized in an adult male patient is

    A. 6.0
    B. 7.0
    C. 8.0
    D. 9.0

38. The administration of Succinylcholine is contraindicated in which of the following?

    A. Hypoglycemia
    B. Hyperkalemia
    C. Hypercalemia
    D. Hypernatremia

39. Midazolam is classified as a

    A. Narcotic analgesic
    B. Hallucinogen
    C. Benzodiazepine
    D. Nondepolarizing paralytic

40. Ketamine administration is considered the drug of choice for a patient presenting with which of the following?

    A. Head injury
    B. Seizure
    C. Asthma
    D. Burns

41. Management of an intubated patient presenting with a diagnosis of ARDS would include

    A. Application of positive end-expiratory pressure
    B. Application of higher than normal tidal volumes
    C. Decreasing ventilation rate
    D. Administration of Magnesium Sulfate

42. Excess of mucous secretions and chronic inflammation of the bronchi, leading to obstruction of airflow, hypoxemia, and hypercapnea best describes which of the following conditions?

    A. Emphysema
    B. Chronic bronchitis
    C. Asthma
    D. Pneumonia

43. A chronic obstructive pulmonary disease (COPD) patient would most likely present with which of the following x-ray findings?

    A. Hyperinflation of the lungs, narrow and elongated heart shadow, increased anterior-posterior diameter of the chest
    B. Widespread pulmonary infiltrates, ground-glassy appearance
    C. Lobar infiltrates and consolidation
    D. Cardiomegaly and pulmonary vascular congestion

44. The diagnosis of ARDS would most likely present with which of the following x-ray findings?

    A. Hyperinflation of the lungs, narrow and elongated heart shadow, increased anterior-posterior diameter of the chest
    B. Widespread pulmonary infiltrates, ground-glassy appearance
    C. Lobar infiltrates and consolidation
    D. Cardiomegaly and pulmonary vascular congestion

45. An ominous sign of impending acute respiratory failure in the asthma patient would most likely be which of the following?

    A. Increased respiratory rate
    B. Increased bronchoconstriction
    C. Decreased or absence of bronchoconstriction
    D. Increased intercostal retractions

46. Signs and symptoms for a patient presenting with a tension pneumothorax would include all of the following, *except*

    A. Tachycardia
    B. Increased work of breathing
    C. Narrowing pulse pressure
    D. Widening pulse pressure

47. The normal range for pCO_2 when evaluating an arterial blood gas is

    A. 30-40 mmHg
    B. 35-45 mmHg
    C. 40-50 mmHg
    D. 50-60 mmHg

48. The normal range for pH when evaluating an arterial blood gas is

    A. 7.15-7.25
    B. 7.25-7.35
    C. 7.35-7.45
    D. 7.45-7.55

49. The normal range for HCO_3 when evaluating an arterial blood gas is

   A. 16-20 mEq/L
   B. 19-22 mEq/L
   C. 22-26 mEq/L
   D. 25-30 mEq/L

50. The most likely causes of metabolic alkalosis can include all of the following, *except*

   A. Vomiting
   B. NG suctioning
   C. Diarrhea
   D. Diuretics

Answer Key and Rationale

1. **A:** Metabolic and respiratory acidosis. The pCO_2 is high, resulting in a respiratory acidosis, and the pH and HCO_3 are low, resulting in a metabolic acidosis. Review the following table for ABG normal ranges.

ABG	Normal range
pH	7.35-7.45
pCO_2	35-45
HCO_3	22-26
pO_2	80-100

The five simple rules to ABG interpretation. Follow the rules, and you will always be right!
1. Evaluate pH. Is it normal?
2. Evaluate the pCO_2. Is it acute or chronic for respiratory disorder?
3. Evaluate the HCO_3 and calculate the anion gap for metabolic disorder or delta gap. Check if metabolic acidosis is present.
4. Identify the primary disorder.
5. Determine if compensation is present and the degree of compensation using Winter's formula. Is there more than one disorder?

Rule 1: Evaluate the pH. Is it normal?

pH		
<7.35	7.35-7.45	>7.45
Acidosis	Normal or compensated	Alkalosis

Rule 2: Evaluate the pCO_2. Is it acute or chronic for respiratory disorder?

pCO_2		
<35	35-45	>45
Alkalosis	Normal or compensated	Acidosis
Causes high pH		Causes low pH

Determine if acute or chronic respiratory disorder. Has the kidney had enough time to partially compensate?

Acute versus chronic respiratory acidosis			
Disorder	pCO_2	pH	HCO_3
Acute respiratory acidosis	For every increase of 10	There is a decrease by 0.08	And/or an increase by 1
Chronic respiratory acidosis	For every increase of 10	There is a decrease by 0.03	And/or an increase by 3

Acute versus chronic respiratory alkalosis			
Disorder	pCO_2	pH	HCO_3
Acute respiratory alkalosis	For every decrease of 10	There is a increase by 0.08	And/or a decrease by 2
Chronic respiratory alkalosis	For every decrease of 10	There is a increase by 0.03	And/or a decrease by 5

Rule 3: Evaluate the HCO_3 and calculate anion gap (AG) for primary metabolic disorder and/or delta gap if metabolic acidosis is present

HCO_3		
<22	22-26	>26
Acidosis	Normal or compensated	Alkalosis
Causes low pH		Causes high pH

Anion gap (AG)		
Formula	Normal range	Abnormal range
$AG = Na - (Cl + HCO_3)$	12 ± 4	>16
Calculate AG when primary metabolic disturbance is present	Helps narrow differential with a anion gap or nonanion gap metabolic acidosis	Nonanion gap metabolic acidosis is determined by delta gap formula

Non-anion gap		
Formula	Corrected HCO$_3$	Corrected HCO$_3$
Corrected HCO$_3$ = Measured HCO$_3$ + (AG-12).	>24, then a metabolic alkalosis coexists.	<24, then a non-anion gap metabolic acidosis coexists.
Determine if other metabolic disturbances coexist with AG metabolic acidosis.	Delta gap—accounts for increase in anion gap and shows any variation in HCO$_3$	If no other disorder is present, then the calculation should be 24

Anion gap metabolic acidosis causes	
M	Methanol
U	Uremia
D	DKA
P	Paraldahyde, propylene glycol
I	Isoniazide, iron
L	Lactic acidosis
E	Ethylene glycol. Ethanol
R	Renal failure, rhabdomyolosis
S	Salicylates, starvation ketoacidosis

Non-anion metabolic acidosis causes	
H	Hyperalimentation
A	Acetozolamide
R	Renal tubular acidosis (RTA)
D	Diarrhea
U	Rectosigmoidostomy
P	Pancreatic fistula
S	Spironolactone

Rule 4: Identify the primary acid-base disorder

Primary disorder	Primary abnormality	Compensatory response
Respiratory acidosis	Low pH and high pCO_2	High HCO_3
Respiratory alkalosis	High pH and low pCO_2	Low HCO_3
Metabolic acidosis	Low pH and low HCO_3	Low pCO_2
Metabolic alkalosis	High pH and high HCO_3	High pCO_2

Rule 5: A. Determine if compensation is present

The pCO_2 and HCO_3 are abnormal in opposite directions if compensation is present. If there is no compensation present, one component, either pCO_2 or HCO_3 is abnormal and the other is normal.

Winter's formula		
Formula	If measured pCO_2 is:	If measured pCO_2 is:
Expected pCO_2 = (1.5 × HCO_3) + 8 within ±2 of sum.	< expected pCO_2, then a coexisting respiratory alkalosis is present.	>expected pCO_2, then a coexisting respiratory acidosis is present.
Assesses appropriate respiratory compensation for metabolic disorder.	Respiratory compensation is fast.	Respiratory compensation is fast.

B. Determine degree of compensation, if present.

Partial Compensation
Evidence of compensation, but pH is still *abnormal.*

Complete Compensation
Evidence of compensation and pH is *normal.*

Respiratory acidosis		
	Uncompensated	Compensated
pH	⬇	Normal
pCO$_2$	⬆	⬆
HCO$_3$	Normal	⬆

Respiratory alkalosis		
	Uncompensated	Compensated
pH	⬆	Normal
pCO$_2$	⬇	⬇
HCO$_3$	Normal	⬇

Metabolic acidosis		
	Uncompensated	Compensated
pH	⬇	Normal
pCO$_2$	Normal	⬇
HCO$_3$	⬇	⬇

Metabolic alkalosis		
	Uncompensated	Compensated
pH	⬆	Normal
pCO$_2$	Normal	⬆
HCO$_3$	⬆	⬆

2. **B:** The normal inspiration-to-expiration (I:E) ratio to start is 1:2. This is reduced to 1:4 or greater in the presence of obstructive airway disease (asthma, COPD) in order to avoid air-trapping (breath stacking) and auto-PEEP or intrinsic PEEP (iPEEP).

Indications for mechanical ventilation		
Diagnostic criteria	Clinical criteria	Other criteria
ABGs $pO_2 < 60$ mmHg $pCO_2 > 50$ mmHg pH < 7.25 Pulmonary Function Tests Vital capacity < 10 mL/kg Negative inspiratory force <25 cmH_2O FEV1 < 10 mL/kg	Hypoventilation, apnea, respiratory distress with altered mentation, increased work of breathing unrelieved by other interventions, altered level of consciousness and need for airway protection	Controlled ventilation, such as with traumatic brain-injured patients, severe circulatory shock

Effects of Mechanical ventilation on organs		
Pulmonary	Cardiac	Renal/Hepatic/GI
Barotrauma may result in pulmonary interstitial emphysema, pneumomediastinum, pneumoperitoneum, pneumothorax, and/or tension pneumothorax. High peak inflation pressures > 40 cm H_2O are associated with an increased incidence of barotrauma.	The heart, great vessels, and pulmonary vasculature lie within the chest cavity and are subject to the increased intrathoracic pressures associated with mechanical ventilation. The result is a decrease in cardiac output due to decreased venous return to the right heart (dominant), right ventricular dysfunction, and altered left ventricular distensibility.	Positive-pressure ventilation is responsible for an overall decline in renal function with decreased urine volume and sodium excretion. Hepatic function is adversely affected by decreased cardiac output, increased hepatic vascular resistance, and elevated bile duct pressure. Mucosal ischemia and secondary bleeding may result from decreased cardiac output and increased gastric venous pressure.

Modes of mechanical ventilation	
Volume-cycled	Inhalation proceeds until a set tidal volume (TV) is delivered and is followed by passive exhalation. A feature of this mode is that gas is delivered, with a constant inspiratory flow pattern, resulting in peak pressures applied to the airways higher than that required for lung distension (plateau pressure). Since the volume delivered is constant, applied airway pressures vary with changing pulmonary compliance (plateau pressure) and airway resistance (peak pressure).
Pressure-cycled	A set peak inspiratory pressure (PIP) is applied, and the pressure difference between the ventilator and the lungs results in inflation until the peak pressure is attained and passive exhalation follows. The delivered volume with each respiration is dependent on the pulmonary and thoracic compliance.
High-frequency oscillatory support	In this ventilatory strategy, ultra-high respiratory rates (180-900 breaths per minute) are coupled with tiny tidal volumes and high airway pressures. This is a commonly accepted ventilatory setting for premature infants and has now also been used in small critical care unit studies on patients with ARDS, with reports of improving oxygenation and lung recruitment

Types of ventilatory support	
Control mode	The ventilator delivers the preset tidal volume once it is triggered regardless of patient effort. If the patient is apneic or possesses limited respiratory drive, control mode can ensure delivery of appropriate minute ventilation.
Support mode	The ventilator provides inspiratory assistance through the use of an assist pressure. The ventilator detects inspiration by the patient and supplies an assist pressure during inspiration. It terminates the assist pressure upon detecting onset of the expiratory phase. Support mode requires an adequate respiratory drive. The amount of assist pressure can be dialed in.

Methods of ventilatory support	
Continuous mandatory ventilation (CMV)	Breaths are delivered at preset intervals, regardless of patient effort. This mode is used most often in the paralyzed or apneic patient because it can increase the work of breathing if respiratory effort is present. Continuous mandatory ventilation (CMV) has given way to assist-control (A/C) mode. Many ventilators do not have a true CMV mode and offer A/C instead.
Assist-control ventilation (A/C)	The ventilator delivers preset breaths in coordination with the respiratory effort of the patient. With each inspiratory effort, the ventilator delivers a full assisted tidal volume. Spontaneous breathing, independent of the ventilator between A/C breaths is not allowed. This mode is better tolerated than CMV in patients with intact respiratory effort. A potential drawback of A/C ventilation in the patient, with obstructive airway disease, is worsening of air trapping and breath stacking.
Intermittent mandatory ventilation (IMV)	With intermittent mandatory ventilation (IMV), breaths are delivered at a preset interval and spontaneous breathing is allowed between ventilator-administered breaths. Spontaneous breathing occurs against the resistance of the airway tubing and ventilator valves, which may be formidable. This mode has given way to synchronous intermittent mandatory ventilation (SIMV).
Synchronous intermittent mandatory ventilation (SIMV)	The ventilator delivers preset breaths in coordination with the respiratory effort of the patient. Spontaneous breathing is allowed between breaths. Synchronization attempts to limit barotrauma that may occur with IMV when a preset breath is delivered to a patient who is already maximally inhaled (breath stacking) or is forcefully exhaling.
Pressure support ventilation (PSV)	For the spontaneously breathing patient, pressure support ventilation (PSV) has been advocated to limit barotrauma and to decrease the work of breathing. Pressure support differs from A/C and IMV in that a level of support pressure is set (not TV) to assist every spontaneous effort. Airway pressure support is maintained until the patient's inspiratory flow falls below a certain cutoff (e.g., 25% of peak flow).
Non-invasive positive pressure ventilation (NIPPV)	The application of mechanical ventilatory support through a mask in place of endotracheal intubation is becoming increasingly accepted and used in the emergency department. It is most commonly applied as continuous positive airway pressure (CPAP) and biphasic positive airway pressure (BiPAP). BiPAP is a form of CPAP that alternates between high and low positive airway pressures, permitting inspiration (and expiration) throughout.

Mechanical ventilator settings		
Mode of ventilation	Tailored to meet patient needs	SIMV and A/C are versatile modes that can be used for initial settings. In patients with a good respiratory drive and mild-to-moderate respiratory failure, PSV is a good initial choice.
Tidal volume (TV)	Initial 5-8 mL/kg	Is generally indicated, with the lowest values recommended in the presence of obstructive airway disease and ARDS. The goal is to adjust the TV so that plateau pressures are less than 35 cm H_2O.
Respiratory rate	8-12 breaths per minute	High rates allow less time for exhalation, increase mean airway pressure, and cause air trapping in patients with obstructive airway disease. The initial rate may be as low as 5-6 breaths per minute in asthmatic patients when using a permissive hypercapnic technique.
FIO_2	Tailored to meet patient needs	The lowest FIO_2 that produces an arterial oxygen saturation (SaO_2) greater than 90% and a $PaO_2 > 60$ mmHg is recommended.
Inspiration/ Expiration ratio (I/E)	Normal 1:2 ratio Obstructive lung disease 1: 4 or greater	The normal inspiration/expiration (I/E) ratio to start is 1:2. This is reduced to 1:4 or greater in the presence of obstructive airway disease in order to avoid air-trapping (breath stacking) and auto-PEEP or intrinsic PEEP (iPEEP). Use of inverse I/E may be appropriate in certain patients with complex compliance problems in the setting of ARDS.
Inspiratory flow rates	60 mL/ minute	Inspiratory flow rates are a function of the TV, I/E ratio, and RR and may be controlled internally by the ventilator via these other settings. If flow rates are set explicitly, 60 L/minute is typically used. This may be increased to 100 L/minute to deliver TVs quickly and allow for prolonged expiration in the presence of obstructive airway disease.
Positive end-expiratory pressure (PEEP	Physiologic PEEP 3-5 cm/H_2O	Is common to prevent decreases in functional residual capacity in those with normal lungs. The reasoning for increasing levels of PEEP in critically ill patients is to provide acceptable oxygenation and to reduce the $FIiO_2$ to nontoxic levels ($FIO_2 < 0.5$). The level of PEEP must be balanced such that excessive intrathoracic pressure does not occur (preventing barotrauma/decreased venous return).
Sensitivity	-1 to -2 cm H_2O	With assisted ventilation, the sensitivity typically is set at -1 to -2 cm H_2O. The development of iPEEP increases the difficulty in generating a negative inspiratory force sufficient to overcome iPEEP and the set sensitivity. Newer ventilators offer the ability to sense by inspiratory flow instead of negative force.

Diseases/conditions and mechanical ventilation		
Disease/ Condition	Problem	Intervention
Obstructive lung disease: Asthma and COPD	Hypoxia can generally be corrected through a high $FIiO_2$, but patients with airway obstruction are at risk of high airway pressures, breath stacking leading to intrinsic PEEP, barotrauma, and volutrauma	To minimize intrinsic PEEP, it is recommended that expiratory flow time be increased as much as possible. Permissive hypercapnia enables a low respiratory rate of 6-8 breaths per minute to be used, as well as an increased I:E ratio of 1:1.5 or 1:2. PEEP may benefit some asthmatic patients by reducing the work of breathing and maintaining open airways during expiration, but its effects are difficult to predict and must be carefully monitored.
Acute respiratory distress syndrome (ARDS)	ARDS lungs are typically irregularly inflamed and highly vulnerable to atelectasis as well as barotrauma and volutrauma. Their compliance is typically reduced, and their dead space is increased.	Initiating ventilation of patients with ARDS with A/C ventilation at a tidal volume of 6 mL/kg, with a PEEP of 5 and initial ventilatory rate of 12, titrated up to maintain a pH > 7.25. Target plateau pressure of < 30 cm H_2O.
Congestive heart failure (CHF)	Cardiac output can be dependent on preload and such patients may easily develop post-intubation hypotension.	CHF responds very well to positive-pressure ventilation, which serves the dual role of opening alveoli and reducing preload. Many patients with CHF benefit from a trial of noninvasive CPAP or BiPAP. PEEP can be increased as tolerated to improve oxygenation and reduce preload.
Traumatic brain injury (TBI)	Hyperventilation has demonstrated poor outcomes thought to be secondary to excessive cerebral vasoconstriction and reduced cerebral perfusion	PCO_2 should be maintained between 35 and 45 mmHg.

3. **B:** The chest tube is inserted in the area called the "safe zone," a region bordered by the lateral border of the pectoralis major, a horizonatal line inferior to the axilla, the anterior border of latissimus dorsi, and a horizonatal line superior to the nipple, which defines the fifth intercostal space of the anterior midaxillary line. Indications for chest tube placement may include drainage of hemothorax or large pleural effusion of any cause, drainage of large pneumothorax (greater than 25%); prophylactic placement of chest tubes in a patient, with suspected chest trauma before transport to specialized trauma center and flail chest segment requiring ventilator support and severe pulmonary contusion with effusion

4. **B:** Respiratory acidosis. The pH is low and the pCO_2 is high, indicating acidosis, so the primary disorder is respiratory acidosis. There is no indication of metabolic compensation.

Respiratory acidosis		
	Uncompensated	Compensated
pH	⬇	Normal
pCO_2	⬆	⬆
HCO_3	Normal	⬆

5. **D:** Respiratory alkalosis can be present initially as evidenced by an increase in respiratory rate in early shock as the body attempts to compensate for blood/volume loss in the compensatory stage. Other early signs of shock in the compensatory stage can include increase in heart rate, narrowing pulse pressure, and thirst.

Stages of shock			
Grades/ Class	Stages	Loss of blood volume	Results in
I	Early, reversible, compensatory	<15% (<750 mLl)	Mild increase in HR and RR
II	Early, reversible, compensatory	15-30% (750-1,500 mL)	Moderate tachycardia and begins to narrow the pulse pressure, increasing RR and delayed capillary refill time.
III	Intermediate, progressive, decompensated shock	30-40% (1,500-2,000 mL)	Compensatory mechanisms begin to fail and hypotension, tachycardia, and low urine output (<0.5 mL/kg/hr in adults) are seen. Body switches to anaerobic metabolism and lactic acids are produced.
IV	Irreversible, refractory	>40% (2,000-2,500 mL)	Profound hypotension, DIC, end-organ damage (MODS), and death.

6. **D:** The pH is normal and the HCO_3 is high, indicating a metabolic alkalosis. The pCO_2 is high, indicating compensatory response. Since the pH is normal, the patient is completely compensated.

Metabolic alkalosis		
	Uncompensated	Compensated
pH	⬆	Normal
pCO_2	Normal	⬆
HCO_3	⬆	⬆

Metabolic alkalosis is usually the result of decreased hydrogen ion concentration, leading to increased bicarbonate concentration. Loss of chloride and hydrogen ions by the alimentary tract (vomiting) or via the kidneys is usually accompanied by volume depletion. With chloride loss and volume depletion (hypochloremic alkalosis), the kidneys reabsorb sodium and HCO_3^- instead of chloride, perpetuating the metabolic alkalosis. Chronic administration of alkali also may result in transient metabolic alkalosis. Shift of hydrogen ion into the intracellular space is seen with hypokalemia. Due to a low extracellular potassium concentration, potassium shifts out of the cells. In order to maintain electrical neutrality, hydrogen shifts into the cells, raising blood pH. Compensation for metabolic alkalosis occurs mainly in the lungs, which retain carbon dioxide through hypoventilation. Management would include analyzing electrolytes frequently and replacing deficiency.

7. **B:** Antero-septal MI as evidenced by ST elevation of >2 mm in two more contiguous leads in V1-V4.

8. **A:** Pericardial effusion. Electrical alternans is an ECG alteration of the QRS complex amplitude or axis between heart beats. It is thought to be associated to changes in the ventricular axis due to fluid in the pericardium. Pericardial effusion can lead to cardiac tamponade.

9. **C:** A pneumothorax with a persistent air leak or failure of a lung to re-expand after needle thorocostomy and/or chest tube has been placed should lead the transport team to suspect a tracheobronchial injury. A tension pneumothorax may be the first visible sign of the problem. Other signs/symptoms can include hemoptysis, respiratory distress, subcutaneous, and/or mediastinal emphysema. Tracheobronchial injuries occur most often from blunt trauma. Penetrating thoracic trauma is a less common cause. If tracheobronchial injury is suspected, immediate endotracheal intubation is performed with placement of the endotracheal tube below the level of the injury.

10. **D:** Cardiogenic shock with uncompensated respiratory acidosis and hypoxemia. The hypotension indicates cardiogenic shock secondary to pump failure, leading to left ventricular heart failure

(vesicular rales and hypoxia). The pH is low and the pCO_2 is high, resulting in respiratory acidosis. The HCO_3 is normal, indicating that no compensatory response has occurred. Acute respiratory failure is defined as a $pO_2 < 60$ mmHg and a $pCO_2 > 50$ mmHg. Normal pO_2 is 80-100 mmHg.

Respiratory acidosis		
	Uncompensated	Compensated
pH	⬇	Normal
pCO_2	⬆	⬆
HCO_3	Normal	⬆

11. **C:** Malignant hyperthermia is a rare life-threatening condition that is triggered by certain medications administered during general anesthesia (gas agents) and the neuromuscular blocking agent succinylcholine (anectine). The mechanism of the condition is caused by drastic increases in intracellular calcium levels and muscle contraction, which is due to a mutation of the ryanodine receptor located in the sarcoplasmic reticulum within the skeletal muscles. Characteristic early signs of malignant hyperthermia include hypercapnea (rise in CO_2, usually assessed with capnography), tachycardia, and muscle rigidity. A late sign is the increase in body temperature up to 108°F or greater and rhabdomyolosis (muscle breakdown). Treatment with dantrolene sodium (dantrium) is usually initiated. Dantrolene sodium is classified as a muscle relaxant and is the only specific and effective treatment of malignant hyperthermia.

12. **D:** To release intrapleural pressure (tension pneumothorax), a large-bore needle should be placed into the pleural space. The second intercostal space, midclavicular approach is generally preferred. The second rib articulates with the sternomanubrial

joint (angle of Louis). The second intercostal space lies below the second rib. The needle should be placed superior to the rib margin (above the rib) to avoid the intercostal artery. An alternate site approach is the fourth or fifth intercostal anterior midaxillary line. The anterior site is used to avoid the internal mammary vessels.

13. **B:** Respiratory acidosis with complete compensation. The pCO_2 is elevated, which is the primary disorder, and the compensatory response is the increased HCO_3. The pH is normal, so there is complete compensation.

Respiratory acidosis		
	Uncompensated	Compensated
pH	⬇	Normal
pCO_2	⬆	⬆
HCO_3	Normal	⬆

14. **B:** Hamman's sign is a crunching sound heard with auscultation and may be synchronized with the patient's heart beat. This sign is associated with tracheobronchial injury.

15. **A:** The pCO_2 is < 60 mmHg, indicating hypoxemia. Treatment includes increasing the FIO_2. Increasing levels of PEEP in critically ill patients may also provide acceptable oxygenation and can reduce the FIO_2 to nontoxic levels (FIO_2 < 0.5). The level of PEEP must be balanced such that excessive intrathoracic pressure does not occur (preventing barotrauma/decreased venous return).

16. **A:** The FIO_2 can be increased and/or application of/or increasing PEEP can also provide acceptable oxygenation levels.

17. **B:** The pCO_2 is decreased and the pH is increased, indicating a respiratory alkalosis. The HCO_3 is normal, indicating there is no compensation.

Respiratory Alkalosis		
	Uncompensated	Compensated
pH	⬆	Normal
pCO_2	⬇	⬇
HCO_3	Normal	⬇

18. **D:** Tidal volume times the respiratory rate equal minute ventilation. Minute ventilation is defined as the total volume of air (gas) moved into and out of the lungs each minute. The formula is known as $VE = Vt \times f$. VE signifies minute ventilation; Vt signifies tidal volume and f signifies respiratory rate. Alveolar minute volume is the amount of gas that reaches the alveoli for gas exchange in one minute. The formula is *VAmin = (VT-VD) × Respiratory Rate.*

Lung volumes (Distinct measurements)	
Tidal volume	Volume of air inspired or expired with each normal breath. Amount 500 mL, which is approximately 5-8 mL/kg.
Inspiratory reserve volume	Extra volume of air that can be inspired above normal tidal volume. Amount 3 liters.
Expiratory reserve volume	Extra volume of air that can be expired by forceful expiration after the end of a normal tidal expiration. Amount 1,100 mL.
Residual volume	Volume of air remaining in the lungs at the end of maximum expiration. Amount 1,200 mL in a 70-kg patient.
Dead-space volume	The amount of gas in the tidal volume that remains in the air passageways unavailable for gas exchange. Anatomic dead space includes the trachea and bronchi. Physiologic dead space from COPD, obstruction, or atelactesis. Amount 150 mL.

Lung capacities (Combination of lung volumes)	
Inspiratory capacity	Tidal volume plus inspiratory reserve volume. The amount of air a person can breathe beginning at the normal expiratory level and distending the lungs to maximum capacity
Functional residual capacity (FRC)	Expiratory reserve volume plus the residual volume. The amount of air that remains in the lungs at the end of normal expiration
Vital capacity	Inspiratory reserve volume plus the tidal volume. The amount of air a person can expel from the lungs after first filling the lungs to their maximum extent and then expiring to the maximum extent.
Total lung capacity	Vital capacity plus residual volume. The maximum volume to which the lungs can be expanded with the greatest possible inspiratory effort.

19. **A**: Mechanical ventilatory complications most commonly encountered in the emergency department and during transport include hypoxia, hypotension, high-pressure alarms, and low exhaled volume alarms. Refer to the table for review.

Mechanical ventilator troubleshooting alarms			
Problem	Cause	Patient should be evaluated for	Intervention
High-pressure alarms	Are triggered when resistance to ventilation is high. This may occur secondary to reduced lung elasticity or airway obstruction or extrinsic compression.	Pneumothorax, bronchospasm, elevated abdominal pressure, mainstem intubation, tube plugs or kinks, tube biting, dynamic hyperinflation/ air trapping, psychomotor agitation, worsening pulmonary compliance, and hypovolemia.	Tube suctioning and adequate patient sedation are recommended after other causes of obstruction are ruled out.

20. **C:** Pneumothorax can trigger high-pressure alarms when resistance to ventilation is too high. Refer to the tables for review.

Mechanical ventilator troubleshooting alarms			
Problem	Cause	Patient should be evaluated for	Intervention
Low-exhaled volume alarms	Are triggered by air leaks. These are most frequently secondary to ventilatory tubing disconnection from the patient's tracheal tube but can also occur in the event of balloon deflation or tracheal tube dislodgement.	Oxygen saturation, bradycardia (especially in neonates and pediatric patients), and skin color.	Tube placement, balloon inflation, amount of oxygen in tank and connection to the ventilator should be carefully verified.

Mechanical ventilator complications		
Problem	Cause/s	Intervention
Hypoxia	May occur secondary to hypoventilation, worsening cardiac shunting, inadequate FIO_2 mainstem intubation, aspiration, tube dislodgement, or pulmonary edema	Increasing FIO_2 and adjusting ventilatory settings to increase PEEP or respiratory rate are useful first steps after excluding equipment failure and mechanical causes of hypoxia.
Hypotension	Hypotension after intubation can be caused by diminished central venous blood return to the heart secondary to elevated intrathoracic pressures. Hypotension may also be secondary to vasovagal reaction to intubation, rapid sequence induction, sedation, and tension pneumothorax.	This can be treated with fluid infusions and/or adjustment of ventilatory settings to lower intrathoracic pressure (reducing PEEP, tidal volume, and, if air trapping is suspected, respiratory rate).

21. **B:** Vt (tidal volume) of 5-8 mL/kg is generally indicated, with the lowest values recommended in the presence of obstructive airway disease and ARDS. The goal is to adjust the TV so that plateau pressures are less than 35 cm H_2O.

22. **B:** A ventilation/perfusion lung scan, also known as a V/Q lung scan, is a type of medical imaging that is used to evaluate the circulation of air and blood within the lungs. The ventilation portion of the exam assesses the ability of air to reach all sections of the lungs, and the perfusion portion evaluates how well blood circulates within the lungs. The test is commonly done to evaluate for the presence of blood clots or abnormal blood flow inside the lungs, such as a pulmonary embolism (PE).

23. **A:** Acute respiratory failure (ARF) exists when breathing fails in its ability to maintain arterial blood gases within a normal range. By definition, ARF is present when the blood gases demonstrate a pO_2 < 60 mmHg (hypoxic respiratory failure) and a pCO_2 > 50 mmHg (ventilatory respiratory failure), which is usually accompanied by fall in the pH < 7.3.

24. **D:** The oxyhemoglobin dissociation curve describes the relation between the partial pressure of oxygen and the oxygen saturation. The effectiveness of hemoglobin-oxygen binding can be affected by several factors. Refer to the table for review.

Oxyhemoglobin diassociation curve	
Right shift	Left shift
Causes a decrease in the affinity of hemoglobin to oxygen. This makes it harder for hemoglobin to bind to oxygen, but it makes it easier for hemoglobin to release bound oxygen.	Causes an increase in the affinity, making the oxygen easier for hemoglobin to pick up but harder to release.
R stands for Raised/Releases Oxygen	L stands for Low/Holds onto Oxygen
High temperature (hyperthermia)	Low temperature (hypothermia)
High 2,3-DPG levels Production increases with hypoxemia, chronic lung disease, anemia, and CHF	Low 2,3-DPG levels Production decreases with septic shock and hypophosphatemia
High pCO_2	Low pCO_2
There is no "L" in acidosis	*There is an "L" in alkalosis*

25. **A:** Alkalosis causes a left shift. Refer to table in question no. 24.

26. **B:** The use of etomidate for continued sedation of critically ill patients has been associated with increased mortality, which is due to suppression of steroid synthesis (both glucocorticoids and mineralocorticoids) in the adrenal cortex, which sometimes leads to death due to an adrenal crisis. There is no evidence that a single induction dose of etomidate has any effect on morbidity or mortality.

27. **D:** The pH is normal, HCO_3 is low (acidosis), and the pCO_2 is low (alkalosis). When both HCO_3 and pCO_2 are turned in opposite directions, the etiology is usually metabolic. The primary mechanism is a metabolic acidosis that has been fully compensated by respiratory alkalosis, making the pH within normal range.

28. **C:** ARDS, also known as respiratory distress syndrome (RDS); lungs are typically irregularly inflamed and highly vulnerable to atelectasis as well as barotrauma and volutrauma, which leads to impaired gas change, resulting in a severe oxygenation defect (hypoxemia). Their compliance is typically reduced, and their dead space increased. ARDS has gradually shifted to mean acute rather than adult. A less severe form is called acute lung injury (ALI).

ARDS was defined as the ratio of arterial partial oxygen tension (PaO_2) as fraction of inspired oxygen (FIO_2) below 200 mmHg in the presence of bilateral alveolar infiltrates on the chest x-ray. These infiltrates may appear similar to those of left ventricular failure, but the cardiac silhouette appears normal in ARDS. Also, the pulmonary capillary wedge pressure is normal (less than 18 mmHg) in ARDS but raised in left ventricular failure. A PaO_2/FIO_2 ratio less than 300 mmHg, with bilateral infiltrates indicates acute lung injury (ALI). Although formally considered different from ARDS, ALI is usually just a precursor to ARDS.

ARDS is an acute onset which is characterized by

- Bilateral infiltrates on chest radiograph sparing costophrenic angles.
- Pulmonary artery wedge pressure < 18 mmHg, if this information is available; if unavailable, then lack of clinical evidence of left ventricular failure suffices.
- If PaO_2:FIO_2 < 300 mmHg (40 kPa) acute lung injury (ALI) is considered to be present.
- If PaO_2:FIO_2 < 200 mmHg (26.7 kPa), ARDS is considered to be present.

29. **B:** Positive end-expiratory pressure (PEEP) is used in mechanically-ventilated patients with ARDS to improve oxygenation.

30. **D:** BNP is an amino acid polypeptide released by the ventricles of the heart in response to excessive stretching of the heart muscle cells. BNP is a blood test used to help in the diagnosis of CHF and is typically higher in these patients. For patients with CHF, the BNP levels will generally be >100 pg/mL. The synthetic version of BNP in medication form is Neseritide (natracor), which reduces systemic vascular resistance and cardiac output.

31. **A:** Neuromuscular blocking agents (NMBA) binds with cholinergic receptor sites of motor neurons preventing the neurotransmitter from relaying the signal. The interruption in this signal pathway is what causes paralysis. Succinylcholine (anectine) is classified as a noncompetitive depolarizing agent because it binds with the motor end-plate receptor site, causing a continuous depolarization to take place. It is this depolarization that causes the initial fasciculations (irregular muscle contractions produced by depolarization of the muscle membrane before complete cessation of muscle activity). As the acetycholinesterase enzyme breaks down the NMBA, there is a return of fasciculations.

Neuromuscular blocking agents (NMBAs)		
	Noncompetitive depolarizing	Competitive nondepolarizing
NMBA	Succinylcholine (anectine)	Rocuronium (zemuron) Vecuronium (norcuron) Pancuronium (pavulon)
Action at receptor sites	Binds with the motor-end plate and causes a continuous depolarization, which results in fasciculations.	Competitively binds with the motor-end plate and does not cause depolarization.
Result	Unresponsive to acetycholine causing paralysis	Blocks acetylcholine causing paralysis
Advantages	Short onset of action of less than 1 minute and ultra short-acting duration of 4-6 minutes	Used to extend the time of neuromuscular blockade after intubation
Disadvantages	Potential complications include hyperkalemia, bradycardia, especially in pediatric patients, bronchospasm	Longer onset of action and duration

32. **B:** The administration of a defasiculation dose of a competitivenon depolarizing NMBA, such as vecuronium (Norcuron), can prevent fasciculations that occur when succinylcholine (Anectine) is administered. Administration of 10% of the initial NMBA dose is recommended to prevent this complication, especially in trauma patients who have sustained significant skeletal fractures for the purpose of preventing further injury at the fracture site/s.

33. **C:** The ABG interpretation of a pH 7.52, pCO_2 27 and HCO_3 24 is a noncompensated respiratory alkalosis, which is present is early salicylate poisoning. The metabolic changes eventually lead to renal depletion of fluids and electrolytes, hypoglycemia, hypokalemia, and a mixed presentation of respiratory and metabolic alkalosis coupled with metabolic acidosis, which may provoke cardiac dysrhythmias, acute pulmonary edema, renal failure or neurological injury. The clinical presentation of salicylate poisoning can also include gastrointestinal bleeding and an unexplained elevated anion gap (metabolic acidosis). Salicylate levels are obtained four to six hours after ingestion.

Earlier samples may be unreliable because the pharmacokinetics is not stable before that time. The most important information in assessing severity, however is the patient's clinical condition.

Salicylate poisoning			
Severity	Clinical presentation	Plasma level in adults	Plasma level in pediatrics
Severe	Patients presenting with hallucinations, convulsions, coma, heart failure, oliguria, or renal insufficiency are *severely* toxic, no matter how high the salicylate level may be.	>75 mg/dL	>65 mg/dL in children less than 12 years of age
Moderate	When the patient presents with fever, tachypnea, loss of coordination, profuse sweating or dehydration or restlessness are *moderately* toxic.	50-70 mg/dL	40-60 mg/dL
Mild	*Mild* toxic effects are limited to burning in the mouth, lethargy, tinnitus, dizziness, nausea, or vomiting.	30-50 mg/dL	20-40 mg/dL

Since there is no specific antidote for salicylates, treatment is aimed at restoration of fluid and electrolyte, acid-base and glycemic homeostasis while preventing absorption of drug remaining in the gut and accelerating the excretion of that already absorbed.

34. **B:** Elevated peak inspiratory pressures (PIP) can be managed by decreasing the flow rate and tidal volume initially. If necessary, increasing the respiratory rate can be done to correct an underlying respiratory acidosis.

35. **D:** Leaks and/or loose connections are associated with low ventilator alarms. Refer to the tables in questions 19 and 20 for review.

36. **C:** An elevated anion gap is associated with metabolic acidosis. Refer to the table in question 1 for review of causes for elevated anion gap.

37. **C:** The average recommended ET tube for an adult male airway is 8.0-9.0 mm (size refers to the internal diameter of the tube). The average adult female airway can accommodate a 7.0-8.0-mm

tube. The balloon cuff pressure should be at minimal occluding volume of 5-10 mL. At pressures greater than 25 mmHg, mucosal ischemia begins to occur.

38. **B:** The administration of succinylcholine (Anectine) is contraindicated in patients with known and/or suspected hyperkalemia. The hyperkalemia associated with succinylcholine, which can approach or exceed life-threatening levels, is of greater consequence in patients who have a history of burns or massive muscle trauma 2 to 3 days prior, and patients may continue to be at risk for hyperkalemia for 2 to 3 months. The two absolute contraindications to use of succinylcholine are situations in which cricothyrotomy would be difficult or impossible to accomplish and the use of the medication by individuals who do not possess a thorough knowledge about the pharmacology of neuromuscular blocking agents, and they do not possess advanced airway skills or an alternative plan if they should encounter a failed airway.

39. **C:** Midazolam (versed) is classified as a benzodiazepine, schedule II controlled drug. It has potent anxiolytic, amnestic, hypnotic, anticonvulsant, skeletal muscle relaxant, and sedative properties. Major adverse effects include hypotension and respiratory depression and/or arrest. Flumazenil is a benzodiazepine antagonist that can be used to treat an overdose as well to reverse sedation.

Benzodiazepines		
Drug	Average adult dose	Average pediatric dose
Midazolam (versed)	0.1 mg/kg (2-5 mg)	0.1 mg/kg
Diazepam (valium)	2-10 mg	0.2 mg/kg
Lorazepam (ativan)	1-2 mg	0.1 mg/kg

Dexmedetomidine (precedex) is another sedative medication currently being used in the critical care unit and by anesthesiologists. It is relatively unique in its ability to provide sedation without causing respiratory depression. *Etomidate (Amidate)* is a short-acting intravenous anesthestic used for the induction of general anesthesia and sedation for short procedures. It has hypnotic and amnestic properties but no analgesic properties. Etomidate is less likely to cause hypotension and respiratory depression. Average recommended dose as an induction agent is 0.3 mg/kg, which can be repeated once if indicated. Lower doses are recommended for use of short procedures. Continued administration of etomidate can cause cortisol levels to drop, which sometimes leads to death due to adrenal crisis. Some sources advise administering a prophylactic dose of steroids, if etomidate is used.

40. **C:** *Ketamine (ketalar)* is classified as an NMDA receptor antagonist with a wide range of effects that include analgesia, anesthesia, hallucinations, elevated blood pressure, and bronchodilation. Indications include use for pediatric anesthesia and asthmatics or patients with COPD. Ketamine has been useful in managing bronchospasm because it inhibits pro-inflammatory cytokines. The accumulation of pro-inflammatory cytokines causes beta-adrenergic receptor hypofunction.

41. **A:** Application of positive end-expiratory pressure (PEEP). ARDS lungs are typically irregularly inflamed and highly vulnerable to atelectasis as well as barotrauma and volutrauma. Their compliance is typically reduced, and their dead space is increased. Initiating ventilation of patients with ARDS with A/C ventilation at a tidal volume of 6 mL/kg, with a PEEP of 5 and initial ventilatory rate of 12, titrated up to maintain a pH > 7.25. Target plateau pressure of <30 cm H_2O.

42. **B:** Chronic obstructive pulmonary disease (COPD) can be considered a continuum with asthma on one end, chronic bronchitis in the middle, and emphysema on the opposite end. It is not unusual for emphysema and chronic bronchitis to coexist in varying degrees. Physical examination may reveal pursed-lip breathing, flaring nostrils, rhonchi and/or expiratory wheezes, hyperresonant to percussion, anterior-posterior diameter of the chest is increased (barrel-chest), and tachycardia. The patient's mental status is an important component since this is the first sign showing that CO_2 level has increased beyond the patient's normal baseline level. Chronic bronchitis results in mucus-secreting cells of the bronchial walls hypersecreting copious amounts of sputum, which prevents airflow into the alveoli. The alveolar gas exchange is

normal, but the alveoli are under-ventilated because of obstruction of airflow. Refer the following tables for review of diagnostic studies, pathophysiology, and management of the COPD patient.

Chronic obstructive pulmonary disease		
COPD Triad	Problem	Management
Asthma	Airway inflammation and narrowed airway. The hypoxemia stimulates hyperventilation with a resultant decrease in PaO_2.	Ensure adequate airway, humidified oxygen, adrengeric agents, anticholinergics, corticosteroids. Intubation/mechanical ventilation is used only in severe cases.
Chronic Bronchitis (frequently referred to as "blue bloaters" because they appear edematous and cyanotic)	➢ Obstructive airflow. ➢ Hypersecretion of copious amounts of mucous, which prevents airflow into the alveoli. ➢ Hypoventilation results in hypercapnea and hypoxemia. ➢ Ventilation-perfusion (VQ) mismatch. ➢ Pulmonary hypertension and hypertrophy of the right ventricle resulting in cor pulmonale.	Humidified oxygen to thin secretions, may require endotracheal suctioning, IV fluids should be administered cautiously since there may be some degree of right-sided failure, beta agonists, methylxanthines, corticosteroids, and anticholinergics may be used.
Emphysema (frequently referred to as "pink puffers" because they markedly dyspneic with a pink skin color))	➢ Destruction of alveoli, loss of elasticity, decrease in gas exchange. Drive for respiration becomes hypoxemia. ➢ Air is trapped in the lungs, which increases residual volume. ➢ Emphysematous blebs are most often located in the apices of the lungs. ➢ Decrease elastic recoil of the lungs. Over/hyperinflation of the lungs. ➢ The expiratory phase increases as the increased resistance to airflow continues. ➢ Increased RBCs and hematacrit.	Low flow rate < 2 L/minute oxygen humidified, unless the patient is a mechanically ventilated (use cautiously since blebs may be present, which may cause a spontaneous pneumothorax to occur), pharmacologic therapy is the same treatment as chronic bronchitis.

Chronic bronchitis and emphysema diagnostic studies	
Test	Common findings
ABGs	Chronic respiratory acidosis compensated by a metabolic alkalosis in the COPD patient
Chest radiography	Hyperinflation of the lungs, narrow elongated heart shadow, increased anterior-posterior diameter, and flattened hemidiaphragms.
12-lead ECG	Low voltage may be present because of the barrel chest, large peaked P waves in the inferior leads, and a right-axis deviation as a result of elongation of the heart, signs of cor pulmonale, such as right ventricular hypertrophy.

43. **A:** Hyperinflation of the lungs, narrow elongated heart shadow, increased anterior-posterior diameter, and flattened hemidiaphragms are common findings on the chest radiography of a COPD patient. ARDS can present with widespread infilitrates, with a ground glassy appearance, pneumonia with lobar infiltrates and consolidation, and CHF with cardiomegaly and pulmonary congestion.

44. **B:** Widespread pulmonary infiltrates that is ground glassy in appearance. ARDS results from a severe alteration in pulmonary vascular permeability, which leads to a change in the lung structure and function. The outstanding characteristic is hypoxemia refractory to oxygen therapy. ARDS is most commonly seen in patients with direct or indirect acute lung injury. Because ARDS is a complication of other illnesses or injuries, the transport team must also consider the pathophysiology of the underlying problem.

45. **C:** Absence of wheezing may indicate that the patient is not able to ventilate sufficiently to produce breath sounds. The problem with a patient presenting with asthma is a prolonged expiratory phase, which can cause air trapping. These patients are not able to exhale adequately. The physical examination can reveal different degrees of respiratory distress based on the severity of their condition. The transport team should consider the situation emergent if an asthma patient presents in respiratory distress without wheezing and has difficulty in speaking. Acute respiratory failure is defined as a pO_2 < 60 mmHg and pCO_2 > 50 mmHg.

46. **D:** Perfusion becomes inadequate because of decreased venous return to the heart as a result of the increased intrapleural pressure and shift of mediastinal structures. A narrowing pulse pressure is considered a compensatory response that can occur just prior to the patient becoming hypotensive. The diastolic blood pressure becomes closer to the systolic blood pressure in a narrowing pulse pressure, whereas, the systolic blood pressure increases in a widening pulse pressure as seen with Cushing's triad (increased intracranial pressure[ICP]).

47. **B:** Normal range pCO_2 is 35-45 mmHg.

pCO_2		
<35	35-45	>45
Alkalosis	Normal or compensated	Acidosis
Causes high pH		Causes low pH

48. **C:** Normal range pH is 7.35-7.45.

pH		
<7.35	7.35-7.45	>7.45
Acidosis	Normal or compensated	Alkalosis

49. **C:** Normal range HCO_3 is 22-26.

HCO_3		
<22	22-26	>26
Acidosis	Normal or compensated	Alkalosis
Causes low pH		Causes high pH

ABG	Normal range
pH	7.35-7.45
pCO_2	35-45
HCO_3	22-26
pO_2	80-100

50. **C:** Diarrheal dehydration can cause metabolic acidosis, especially in the pediatric patient. Metabolic alkalosis can be caused by loss of hydrogen ions through the kidneys or GI tract. Vomiting or nasogastric (NG) suction generates metabolic alkalosis by the loss of gastric secretions, which are rich in hydrochloric acid (HCL). Renal losses (use of diuretics) of hydrogen ions occur when the distal delivery of sodium increases in the presence of excess aldosterone, resulting in reabsorption of sodium, leading to the secretion of hydrogen ions and potassium ions. The administration of sodium bicarbonate in amounts that exceed the capacity of the kidneys to excrete this excess bicarbonate may cause metabolic alkalosis. Shifting of hydrogen ions into the intracellular space can also occur, which is mainly seen with hypokalemia.

Acid-base imbalance		
Derangement	Problem	Common cause
Respiratory acidosis	Retention of CO_2	Hypoventilation, respiratory arrest.
Respiratory alkalosis	Blowing off CO_2	Increased respiratory rate which can be caused by different conditions.
Metabolic acidosis	Increased production of hydrogen or the inability of the body to form bicarbonate in the kidneys	Diarrhea and other main causes are best grouped by their influence on the anion gap.
Metabolic alkalosis	Loss of hydrogen ions	Vomiting, nasogastric suction, diuretics, sodium bicarbonate administration.

Bibliography

2005 American Heart Association guidelines for cardiopulmonary resuscitation and emergency cardiovascular care. Part 10.5 Near-fatal asthma. *Circulation.* 2005; 112 (Suppl 24):139.

Allen, JY. and Charles, GM. The efficacy of ketamine in pediatric emergency department patients who present with severe acute asthma. *Ann Emerg Med.* 2005; 46(1):43-50.

Association of Air Medical Services. (2003). *Guidelines for Air Medical Crew Education,* Iowa, Kendall/Hunt Publishing Company.

Breen, PH. Arterial blood gas and pH analysis. *Anesthesiol Clin North America.* 2001; (19)4:885-902.

Chipps, BE, Murphy, KR. Assessment and treatment of acute asthma in children. *J Pediatr.* 2005; 147:288.

Coleman, NJ. Evaluating arterial blood gas results. *Aust Nurs J. 1999:* (6)11 suppl 1-3.

Darovic, G. (1999). *Handbook of Hemodynamic Monitoring,* 2nd edition. Philadelphia, W.B.Saunders.

Denmark, TK et al. Ketamine to avoid mechanical ventilation in severe pediatric asthma *J Emerg Med.* 2006; 30(2):163-166.

Emergency Nursing Association. (2000). Acid-base balance. *Orientation to Emergency Nursing: Concepts, Competencies and Critical Thinking.* 1-17.

Helfaer, MA, NIchols, DG, Rogers, MC. (1996). Lower airway disease: Bronchiolitis and asthma. *In: Textbook of Pediatric Intensive Care,* 3rd edition. Rogers, MC, Nichols, DG (Eds.), Baltimore, Williams & Wilkins. p. 133.

Hills, BA. An alternative view of the role(s) of surfactant and the alveolar model. *J Appl Physiol.* 1999; 87(5):1567-1583.

Holleran, R. (1996). *Flight Nursing: Principles and Practice.* 2nd edition. St. Louis, Mosby.

Holleran, R. (2003). *Air and Surface Patient Transport: Principles and Practice,* 3rd edition. St. Louis, Mosby.

Holleran, R. (2009). *ASTNA Patient Transport: Principles and Practice,* 4th edition. St. Louis, Mosby.

Karch, AM. (2004). *Lippincott's Nursing Drug Guide.* Philadelphia, Lippincott Williams &Wilkins.

Krishnan, JA, Brower, RG. High-frequency ventilation for acute lung injury and ARDS. *Chest.* 2000; 118(3):795-807.

Krupa, D. (1997). *Flight Nursing Core Curriculum.* Park Ridge, IL, National Flight Nurses Association.

Petrillo, TM, et al. Emergency department use of ketamine in pediatric status asthmaticus. *J Asthma.* 2001; 38(8):657-664.

Rotta, AT, Asthma. (2006). *In: Pediatric Critical Care,* 3rd edition. Fuhrman, BP, Zimmerman, JJ (Eds.), Philadelphia, Mosby Elsevier. p. 589.

Schwarz, AJ, Lubinsky, PS. Acute severe asthma. (1997) *In: Essentials of Pediatric Intensive Care,* 2nd edition, Levin, DL, Morriss, FC (Eds.), Churchill Livingstone, Inc, New York. p. 130.

Tasota, FJ, Wesmiller, SW. Balancing Act: Keeping the pH in Equilibrium. *Nursing.* 1998; 98:34-40.

Venkataraman, ST, Orr, RA. (1992). Mechanical ventilation and respiratory care. *In:* Fuhrman BP, Zimmerman JJ (Eds). *Pediatric Critical Care.* St. Louis: Mosby Year Book, Chap. 48, pp. 519-543.

Wong, FW. A new approach to ABG interpretation. *AJN.* 1999; 99:34-36.

Module 5
Neurological Emergencies

1. You are preparing to transport a twenty-year-old man weighing 200 pounds with a history of a self-inflicted gunshot wound to the head. He is intubated with A/C ventilator settings of FIO_2 0.5, Vt 600, I/E 1:2, flow 5 L, RR 10, PIP 30. Vital signs are BP 100/60, HR 66, and SaO_2 94%. ICP reading of 28. His cerebral perfusion pressure is approximately

   A. 100 mmHg
   B. 70-90 mmHg
   C. 60 mmHg
   D. <50 mmHg

2. What is the initial clinical presentation that may indicate that ICP may be increasing?

   A. Hypotension
   B. Deteriorating level of consciousness
   C. Tachypnea
   D. Tachycardia

3. You are transporting an eighteen-year-old female patient with a history of being ejected from a motor vehicle accident. She is currently awake and oriented to person, place, and time; however, she is slow to respond. Vital signs are a BP of 70/42, HR 68, RR 26, SaO_2 95%, temp. 98.8°F. Hemodynamic readings are CVP 3, CI 2.0, and SVR 600. ICP reading at 6 with a urine output of 100 mL over the last two hours. Your patient is exhibiting signs and symptoms of

   A. Herniation
   B. Hypovolemic shock
   C. Spinal cord injury
   D. Diabetes insipidus

4. You are transporting a forty-year-old male diagnosed with a subarachnoid hemorrhage. Which of the following assessment findings can be associated with his diagnosis?

   A. Presence of doll's eyes reflex
   B. Positive Battle's sign
   C. Positive Brudzinski's sign
   D. Absence of ipsilateral pupillary dilation

5. You arrive on the scene to manage a fall victim. She presents with a BP 70/palp, HR 62, RR 24, Sats 96%. EMS reports brief LOC but now has a GCS of 14. You note a deformity of the right femur, and she is complaining of neck pain. The clinical presentation is most likely a diagnosis of

   A. Neurogenic shock
   B. Hypovolemic shock
   C. Epidural bleed
   D. Subdural bleed

6. Pupillary dilation in response to the oculomotor nerve insult that occurs in uncal herniation is a result of

   A. Loss of parasympathetic stimulation
   B. Loss of sympathetic stimulation
   C. Parasympathetic overstimulation
   D. Sympathetic overstimulation

7. Which formula can be used when calculating a cerebral perfusion pressure (CPP)?

   A. [(DBP × 2) + SBP] divided by 3
   B. MAP − ICP
   C. ICP − DBP
   D. [(DBP + 2) × SBP] divided by 3

8. An early sign of tentorial herniation would be

   A. Doll's eyes reflex
   B. Ataxic breathing
   C. Paralysis below the diaphragm
   D. Ipsilateral pupillary dilation

9. You have been requested to transport a thirty-two-year-old male involved in a two-car motor vehicle collision in which the right side of his head struck the "A-post." Right middle meningeal artery damage has been noted by CT with right-sided "mass effect" resulting. You would expect which of the following?

   A. Epidural hematoma
   B. Ventricular collapse
   C. Cranial midline shift to the left
   D. All of the above

10. The patient presents with a skull fracture that appears to have a central focal point with multiple fractures outward on radiography. This skull fracture would be described as

    A. Linear
    B. Linear stellate
    C. Diastatic
    D. Depressed

11. A head-injured patient would most likely experience an increased ICP as a result of which action?

    A. Hip flexion
    B. Gagging on the ETT
    C. Adduction of the arms
    D. Rotation of the head
    E. All of the above

12. You are transporting an awake multisystem trauma patient from a small rural facility with the following vital signs: BP 200/66, HR 56, RR 20-36, SaO$_2$ 97%, and temp. 99.9°F. Further assessment reveals a large laceration to the occipital area of the head, with bleeding controlled, and is moving all extremities. Pupils are reactive to light and equal at 4 mm with extraocular movements intact. The patient's clinical presentation is suggestive of which of the following?

    A. Demonstrating signs/symptoms of cushing's triad
    B. Already herniated and will likely deteriorate further
    C. Demonstrating signs/symptoms of Brown-Séquard syndrome
    D. Demonstrating signs/symptoms of hypovolemic shock

13. You are transporting a thirty-year-old female who was involved in a single vehicle rollover two hours prior to your arrival. She has a swan catheter in place with the following values: CVP 2, CI 2.0, PA S/D 12/6, wedge 7, SVR 400. Vital signs: BP 80/48, HR 46, RR 24, SaO$_2$ 90%. The patient's clinical presentation is suggestive of which diagnosis?

    A. Hypovolemic shock
    B. Septic shock
    C. Left ventricular failure
    D. Neurogenic shock

14. The expected average normal cerebral perfusion pressure range (CPP) is

    A. 80-100 mmHg
    B. 50-60 mmHg
    C. 70-90 mmHg
    D. >100 mmHg

15. The average normal ICP range is

    A. 0-10 mmHg
    B. 10-20 mmHg
    C. 20-30 mmHg
    D. >30 mmHg

16. The formula to calculate a mean arterial pressure (MAP) is

   A. 2/3 DBP × SBP
   B. [(DBP × 2) + SBP] divided by 3
   C. [(SBP × 2) + DBP] minus 3
   D. [(DBP + 2) × SBP] divided by 3

17. The patient presents with the following hemodynamic parameters: CVP 1, CI 1.7, PA S/D 12/6, wedge 6, and SVR 300. Vital signs are 78/40, HR 60, RR 16, SaO$_2$ 98%. The most likely cause is

   A. RVMI
   B. Neurogenic shock
   C. Septic shock
   D. Hypovolemic shock

18. Classic picture of neurogenic shock presents with

   A. Hypertension
   B. Absence of tachycardia
   C. Cool skin
   D. Pallor

19. You are transporting a patient with a spinal cord injury above T6 level. His baseline vital signs prior to lift off: BP 160/80, HR 62, RR 20. During transport, the patient begins to complain of a throbbing headache with nasal stuffiness. Your assessment reveals that the patient is becoming increasingly agitated. His skin color is flushed and profusely diaphoretic. Repeat vital signs are a BP 206/100, HR 52, RR 26. Your initial management of the patient would be

   A. Insert a foley catheter
   B. Administer nitroglycerin to help reduce blood pressure
   C. Hang a Nipride drip if diastolic is greater than 130 mmHg
   D. Do nothing because increased HTN is expected with altitude and spinal cord injuries

20. You have been requested to transport a forty-year-old male fall victim of approximately 25-30 feet, three hours prior to your arrival. Your assessment reveals a greater motor weakness in upper extremities than in lower extremities, with varying degrees of sensory loss. The clinical presentation may suggest which of the following spinal cord syndrome?

   A. Brown-Séquard
   B. Central cord
   C. Anterior cord syndrome
   D. Neurogenic shock

21. Hypothermia, low levels of 2,3-DPG, and hypocarbia can cause the oxyhemoglobin dissociation curve shift to go

   A. Up
   B. Down
   C. Right
   D. Left

22. In addition to glucose, which electrolyte must be maintained within normal limits when managing a head-injured patient?

   A. Calcium
   B. Magnesium
   C. Potassium
   D. Sodium

23. You are transporting a twenty-year-old male, with penetrating head and facial trauma. During transport, the patient complains of a severe headache, nausea, and vertigo. Your assessment reveals nuchal rigidity, aphasia, dysphasia, along with the patient having episodes of vomiting. What is your diagnosis?

   A. Pneumothorax
   B. Pneumocephalus
   C. Neurogenic shock
   D. Hypercapnia

24. Calculate the following patient's cerebral perfusion pressure (CPP): BP 150/75, HR 140, RR 28, SpO$_2$ 100%, CVP 2, ICP 25.

    A. 98
    B. 125
    C. 65
    D. 75

25. You are transporting a normotensive patient, who is presenting with a history of head injury and complaining of extreme thirst. Your assessment reveals he is excreting large amounts of diluted urine, sunken appearance to the eyes, dry mouth, and tachycardia is noted. The initial treatment of the patient would be?

    A. Restrict fluids
    B. Administer Sandostatin
    C. Aggressive fluid replacement and vasopressin
    D. Administer anti-thyroid medication

26. Cushing's triad includes all of the following, *except*

    A. Varying respiratory patterns
    B. Narrowing pulse pressure
    C. Widening pulse pressure
    D. Bradycardia

27. A patient presenting with an initial loss of consciousness with a period of a lucid interval, with return of a normal neurologic status, suddenly complains of a headache, with a deteriorating level of consciousness. The patient is most likely experiencing a

    A. Subdural bleed
    B. Subarachnoid bleed
    C. Intracerebral bleed
    D. Epidural bleed

28. Brudzinski's clinical sign may indicate

    A. Subarachnoid bleed or meningitis
    B. Subdural bleed or meningitis
    C. Epidural bleed or meningitis
    D. Basilar skull fracture

29. The presence of a Babinski's sign in an adult patient would exhibited by

    A. Flaccid movement of the toes
    B. Plantar flexor reflex
    C. Plantar extensor reflex
    D. Toes fanning upward

30. You have been requested to transport a thirty-two-year-old male intravenous drug user who was brought to the ED without vascular access with a history of having had a witnessed generalized tonic-clonic seizure ten minutes prior to your arrival. The patient arrived post-ictal, but responsive. No other medical history was available. On examining, the blood pressure is 130/80 mmHg, HR 88, respirations 14, and oxygen saturation of 98% on room air. The head is atraumatic, the pupils are 4 mm and reactive, cardiopulmonary exam was normal. Neurologically the patient is oriented to person only; he has no facial asymmetry, moves all four extremities, deep tendon reflexes were + 4 symmetrically, and no Babinski reflexes were present. The blood sugar is 110 mEq/dL. While looking for venous access over the patient's scarred extremities, the patient began a second generalized tonic-clonic seizure. What is the "best" first line therapy for acute seizure management?

    A. Phenytoin
    B. Phenobarbital
    C. Fosphenytoin
    D. Benzodiazepines

31. Which cranial nerve is affected with a patient presenting with Bell's Palsy?

    A. I
    B. V
    C. VII
    D. X

32. Cranial nerve III is also known as the

    A. Optic nerve
    B. Oculomotor nerve
    C. Olfactory nerve
    D. Auditory nerve

33. You are transporting a twenty-six-year-old male patient involved in a fall injury. Upon your arrival on the scene, your assessment reveals an awake patient who is not able to shrug his shoulders. Which cranial nerve is most likely affected?

    A. III
    B. VII
    C. X
    D. XI

34. A patient diagnosed with Guillan-Barre would most likely present with all of the following, *except*

    A. Descending paralysis
    B. Ascending paralysis
    C. Dysphagia
    D. Dysesthesia

35. You are transporting a twenty-five-year-old male with a history of acute alcohol intoxication who was involved in a single vehicle roll-over two hours prior to your arrival. The patient is presenting with variable loss of motor function and sensory function from the nipple line down. Which dermatome would most likely be affected and what clinical condition you do suspect?

A. C3; central cord syndrome
B. C6; Brown-séquard syndrome
C. T4; anterior cord syndrome
D. T10; anterior cord syndrome

36. You have been requested to transport a twenty-year-old male involved in a motor vehicle accident. Your assessment reveals an ethanol-like odor on his breath, GCS 15, with slurred speech, and the patient is able to grossly flex the arms at the elbow but unable to extend his arms at the elbows or wrists or flex or extend the fingers, with no sensation to the medial side of the arm and small finger. The patient was noted to have the capability of extending both lower legs at the knee, but definite weakness was present. He was able to extend and flex his ankles and toes. The clinical findings affect which dermatome and what clinical condition is suspected?

A. C5; anterior cord syndrome
B. C6; central cord syndrome
C. C8, T1; central cord syndrome
D. T4; Brown-séquard syndrome

37. The presence of a plantar extensor reflex in an adult patient can indicate

A. Damage to nerve pathways connecting the spinal cord and brain
B. Intact motor neuron function
C. Damage to the nerves in the lower extremeties
D. Increased ICP

38. Oculocephalic reflex is also known as

    A. Babinski
    B. Cold caloric
    C. Doll's eyes
    D. Consensual reflex

39. The oculovestibular reflex exam is used to assess

    A. The presence of ICP
    B. Brainstem function
    C. Spinal cord injury
    D. Pupil response

40. Mydriasis is defined as

    A. Increased salivation
    B. Pinpoint pupils
    C. Dilated pupils
    D. Fixed, midposition pupils

41. The patient presenting with Battle's and Racoon's clinical signs is most likely experiencing which of the following?

    A. Epidural bleed
    B. Basilar skull fracture
    C. Subdural bleed
    D. Increased ICP

42. Which of the following is most likely affected with a patient presenting with an epidural bleed?

    A. Middle meningeal artery
    B. Carotid artery
    C. Communicating artery
    D. Subclavian artery

43. Another term used to describe pinpoint pupils is

   A. Mydriasis
   B. Miosis
   C. Mitosis
   D. Doll's eyes

44. You would expect the normal range when measuring a mean arterial pressure (MAP) to be

   A. 50-60 mmHg
   B. 70-90 mmHg
   C. 80-100 mmHg
   D. 100-120 mmHg

45. Which clinical sign/symptom initially would indicate that a ventricular-peritoneal shunt is malfunctioning?

   A. Deteriorating level of consciousness
   B. Vomiting
   C. Hypotension
   D. Bradycardia

46. You have been requested to transport a thirty-year-old male with a history of being stabbed multiple times in the back. The patient presents with ipsilateral loss of motor function and contralateral loss of pain and temperature. The most likely diagnosis is

   A. Anterior cord syndrome
   B. Brown-Séquard syndrome
   C. Central cord syndrome
   D. Compartment syndrome

47. You are transporting a patient with a history of diving into shallow water and is presenting with complete loss of motor, pain and temperature below the injured spinal cord lesion. The patient is most likely diagnosed with

    A. Anterior cord syndrome
    B. Brown-Séquard syndrome
    C. Central cord syndrome
    D. Compartment syndrome

48. What personal protective equipment (PPE) should be worn when transporting a patient with bacterial meningitis?

    A. Mask, gloves, gown, and eye protection
    B. Gloves only
    C. Mask and gloves
    D. Gloves and eye protection

49. The patient you are transporting is exhibiting decerebrate posturing. What does this term mean?

    A. Increased tone in the extensor muscles with active tonic reflexes, resulting in all four limbs being rigidly extended and rotated internally, opisthotonos, and clenched teeth.
    B. A stooped, hyper-flexed posture, with postive Kernig's sign.
    C. Externally rotated and extended lower extremities, with upper extremities flexed at the elbows.
    D. Sustained muscular contractions, which lead to fixed contractures

50. On examining, the sixty-year-old female patient that you are preparing for transport appears awake but is unable to speak or follow commands. Vitals are: T 99, BP 168/104, HR 82, RR 18, SaO$_2$ 98% on 4 liter of oxygen by nasal cannula. She moves her left side spontaneously but has no movement of the right arm and very little movement of the right leg. The staff reports that she is right handed; radiography revealed no cranial/hip/pelvic fractures and CSF was clear, with no erythrocytes. What blood vessel do you suspect is involved?

A. Middle cerebral artery in the right hemisphere
B. Middle cerebral artery in the left hemisphere
C. Posterior cerebral artery in the parietal lobe
D. Basilar artery in the temporal lobe

Answer Key and Rationale

1. **D:** The intracranial contents have three components: cerebrospinal fluid (CSF), blood volume, and the brain. As mean systemic arterial pressure increases, cerebral arterial blood vessels constrict, preventing the increase in blood volume and flow that would normally occur. If the mean systemic arterial blood pressure decreases, the cerebral arteries dilate, increasing cerebral blood flow. A mean systolic arterial pressure of approximately 60-140 mmHg, cerebral blood flow may be maintained in a constant state. The cerebral perfusion pressure (CPP) formula equals the mean arterial pressure (MAP) minus the intracranial pressure (ICP). The mean arterial pressure (MAP) formula equals the diastolic blood pressure (DBP) × 2 and add the systolic blood pressure and then divide by 3.

Cerebral prefusion pressure	
Formula	Normal range (mmHg)
MAP = [(DBP × 2) + SBP] divided by 3	80-100
CPP = MAP − ICP	70-90
ICP	0-10

Formula answer: $60 \times 2 = 120 + 100 = 220$ divided by $3 = 73$ (MAP)

$$73 - 28 = 45 \text{ (CPP)}$$

2. **B:** All neurologic emergencies can lead to coma. During patient assessment, it is useful to use a systematic approach in evaluating the comatose patient and establishing a baseline differential diagnosis. The Glasgow Coma Scale (GCS) is widely used to measure the severity of coma in patients and is therefore and indicator of prognosis.

ALOC differential diagnosis	
A	Acidosis, AMI, alcohol
E	Epilepsy, electrolytes
I	Infection
O	Overdose, oxygen
U	Uremia
T	Trauma
I	Insulin
P	Psychosis
S	Stroke, shock

3. **C:** The patient is presenting with signs and symptoms of neurogenic shock: tachypnea, normal heart rate, and hypotension. Hemodynamic parameters to indicate the presence of neurogenic shock would include a decreased SVR < 800 and a low cardiac index (CI) < 2.5.

4. **C:** Positive Brudzinski's sign can indicate the presence of a subarachnoid hemorrhage as well as meningitis. Severe neck stiffness causes the patient's hips and knees to flex when the neck is flexed. Battle's sign consists of bruising over the mastoid process as a result of extravasation of blood along the path of the posterior auricular artery and can indicate basilar skull fracture. Doll's eye reflex also known as vestibulo-ocular reflex or oculovestibular reflex is a reflex movement during head movement by producing an eye movement in the direction opposite to head movement. The absence of the doll's eye's reflex (eyes remain in midposition when is being moved from side to side) can indicate injury to the midbrain or pons, cranial nerves III and VI. Ipsilateral (same side) pupillary dilation can indicate brain herniation.

5. **A:** Spinal cord injury can lead to neurogenic shock. The patient is presenting with tachypnea, hypotension, and a normal heart rate but can also be present with bradydysrhythmias because of loss of sympathetic tone secondary to the spinal cord injury.

Hemodynamic monitoring diagnostic criteria					
Type of shock	HR 60-100	SVR 800-1,200	CI 2.5-4.3	CVP 2-6	PCWP 8-12
Neurogenic	Normal; low	<800	Low		
Septic	High	<800	High		
Anaphylactic	High	<800	Low		
Hypovolemic	High	>1,200		Low	
Cardiogenic	High	>1,200		High	High
RVMI	High	>1,200		High	Low

6. **A:** The innermost part of the temporal lobe, the uncus, can be compressed so that it goes by the tentorium and places pressure on the brain. The uncus can compress the third cranial nerve, which can affect the parasympathetic input to the eye on the side of the affected nerve, causing the pupil on the affected side to dilate and fail to constrict in response to light as it should.

Cranial nerves		
Nerve	Name	Function and origin
I	Olfactory	Smell
II	Optic	Vision
III	Oculomotor	Eye movement; origin midbrain
IV	Trochlear	Eye movement; origin midbrain
V	Trigeminal	Mastication; origin pons
VI	Abducens	Eye movement; origin pons
VII	Facial	Facial expression; origin pons
VIII	Vestibulocochlear (auditory)	Hearing and balance
IX	Glossopharyngeal	Taste; origin medulla
X	Vagus	Swallowing; origin medulla
XI	Accessory	Sternocleidomastoid and trapezius muscles; ability to move head and shrug shoulders
XII	Hypoglossal	Muscle of tongue, speech articulation and swallowing; origin medulla

7. **B:** MAP − ICP = CPP. Refer to the table in question 1 for review.

8. **D:** Ipsilateral pupil dilation on the affected side.

9. **D:** All of the above. The middle meningeal artery runs in a groove on the inside of the cranium beneath the pterion, which is vulnerable to injury at this point, where the skull is thin. A blow or fracture of the temporal bone is often the cause of a rupture of the middle meningeal artery, which may cause an epidural hematoma (occurs between the skull and the dura). There is often significant "mass effect" with compression of the ipslateral lateral ventricle and dilatation of the opposite lateral ventricle due to obstruction of the foramen of Monro. Emergency treatment requires decompression of the hematoma, usually by craniotomy.

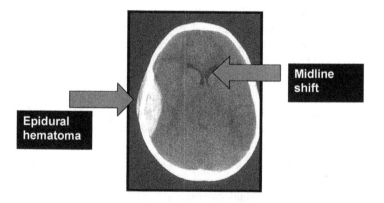

Cranial bleeds		
Type of bleed	Location of bleed	Clinical presentation
Epidural hematoma *(usually caused by tears in the artery)*	Bleeding occurs between the skull and dura mater. "Epi" meaning above the dura.	Brief loss of consciousness, lucid interval into deteriorating level of consciousness.
Subdural hematoma *(usually caused by tears in the veins)*	Bleeding occurs between the dura mater and the arachnoid mater. "Sub" meaning below the dura.	The space enlarges as the brain atrophies, so more common in the elderly patient. Can be acute or chronic. Changes in mentation can occur several weeks after injury.

10. **B:** Linear stellate is a skull fracture with multiple linear fractures radiating from the site of impact. A *growing skull fracture* (GSF) also known as a craniocerebral erosion or leptomeningeal cyst due to the usual development of a cystic mass filled with cerebral spinal fluid is a rare complication of head injury usually associated with linear skull fractures of the parietal bone in children below three years of age. There are four major types of skull fractures: linear, compressed, distatic, and basilar.

Skull fractures		
Type of fracture	Definition	Clinical manifestation
Linear	Are breaks in the bone, usually from blunt force trauma, that transverse the full thickness of the skull from the outer to inner table, are usually fairly straight and involve no displacement of the bone.	Usually of little clinical significance unless they are parallel in close proximity or transverse a suture, or they involve a venous sinus groove or vascular channel.
Compressed	Usually resulting from blunt force trauma, such as getting struck with object, getting kicked in the head.	Carry a high risk of increased pressure on the brain, crushing the delicate tissue.
Distatic	Occur when the fracture line transverses one or more sutures of the skull, causing a widening of the suture.	Usually seen in infants and children.
Basilar	Breaks in bones at the base of the skull, require more force to cause than cranial vault fractures.	Blood in the sinuses; a clear fluid called cerebrospinal fluid (CSF) leaking from the nose or ears; raccoon eyes (bruising of the orbits of the eyes that result from blood collecting there as it leaks from the fracture site); and Battle's sign (caused when blood collects behind the ears and causes bruising).

11. **E:** All of the above are considered movements/stimulators that can increase ICP. The intubated patient who is restless or who resists ventilatory support is increasing their ICP, which can be extremely critical. Seizures that develop during transport should be promptly treated because they produce hypoxia and cause increased ICP. Intravenous administration of benzodiazepines is indicated for initial seizure management. Hypotension has been found to contribute to the mortality and morbidity of head-injured patients. The patient's mean arterial pressure (MAP) should be maintained at more than 90 mmHg. Fluids and blood products should be administered to maintain blood pressure.

12. **A:** The clinical presentation of *Cushing's triad* is the triad of widening pulse pressure (rising systolic, declining diastolic), change in respiratory pattern (irregular respirations), and bradycardia. It is a sign of increased ICP, and it occurs as a result of the Cushing reflex. The normal average range for ICP is 0-10 mmHg.

13. **D:** The patient is presenting with neurogenic shock. The SVR < 800 is indicative of a distributive shock; the decreased CI < 2.5 and bradycardia narrows the type of shock to neurogenic shock. Neurogenic shock may be present in patients with cervical or high thoracic spine injury. Interruption of sympathetic outflow below the level of the injury results in loss of autoregulation, a decrease in vascular tone, and an inability of the heart to increase its intrinsic rate. With passive vasodilation and a normal bradycardic state, the patient becomes hypotensive. The sympathetic block or loss of sympathetic tone produces poikilothermy. In this state, the patient loses the ability to vasodilate and sweat in hot environments and the ability to vasoconstrict and shiver in cold environments.

14. **C:** Normal cerebral perfusion pressure range is 70-90 mmHg.

15. **A:** Normal ICP range is 0-10 mmHg, but range can go as high as 15 mmHg.

16. **B:** MAP = [(DBP × 2) + SBP] divided by 3.

17. **B:** SVR < 800, think distributive shock. Next look at the CI; is it less than 2.5? Hypotension and either a normal heart and/or bradycardia present narrows the type of distributive shock as being neurogenic shock.

18. **B:** Loss of sympathetic tone below the level of the injury results in loss of autoregulation, a decrease in vascular tone, and inability of the heart to increase its intrinisic rate. The classic picture of neurogenic shock presents with the absence of tachycardia.

19. **A:** Autonomic dysreflexia (AD), also known as "autonomic hyperreflexia or hyperreflexia," is a potentially life-threatening condition, which can be considered a medical emergency requiring immediate attention. *AD occurs most often in spinal cord-injured individuals with spinal lesions above the T6 spinal cord level.* Acute AD is a reaction of the autonomic (involuntary) nervous system to overstimulation. This condition is distinct and usually episodic, with the patient experiencing remarkably high blood pressure (often with systolic readings over 200 mmHg), intense headaches, profuse sweating, facial erythema (redness), flushing of the skin above the level of the lesion, goosebumps, nasal stuffiness, bradycardia, apprehension, anxiety, and a "feeling of doom." An elevation of 40 mmHg over baseline systolic should be suspicious for dysreflexia. Catheterization of the bladder or relief of a blocked urinary catheter tube may resolve the problem. If the noxious precipitating trigger cannot be identified, drug treatment is needed to decrease elevated ICP until further studies can identify the cause.

20. **B:** Central cord syndrome is the most common spinal cord injury (SCI) syndrome. This syndrome is unlike a complete lesion and causes loss of all sensation and movement below the level of the injury. Remember "you can dance, but you can't clap."

Spinal cord injury syndromes	
Type of syndrome	Clinical manifestation
Anterior cord	Blood supply to the anterior portion of the spinal cord is interrupted, causing a complete motor paralysis below the level of the lesion due to interruption of the corticospinal tract. Loss of pain and temperature sensation at and below the level of the lesion due to interruption of the spinothalamic tract. Retained proprioception and vibratory sensation due to intact dorsal columns. Most often occurs after hyperflexion injury.http://en.wikipedia.org/wiki/Anterior_cord_syndrome—cite_note-0#cite_note-0
Brown-Séquard	Any presentation of spinal injury that is an incomplete lesion can be called a partial Brown-Séquard or incomplete Brown-Séquard syndrome, so long as it is characterized by features of a motor loss and numbness to touch and vibration on the same side of the spinal injury and loss of pain and temperature sensation on the opposite side. Most often occurs from a penetrating injury that has damaged one side of the spinal cord.
Central cord	It is characterized by disproportionately greater motor impairment in upper compared to lower extremities and variable degree of sensory loss below the level of injury. Most often occurs after hyperextension injury.

21. **D:** A left shift causes an increase in the affinity, making the oxygen easier for the hemoglobin to pick up but harder to release. Refer to the table for review of causes.

Oxyhemoglobin diassociation curve	
Right shift	Left shift
Causes a decrease in the affinity of hemoglobin to oxygen. This makes it harder for the hemoglobin to bind to oxygen, but it makes it easier for the hemoglobin to release bound oxygen.	Causes an increase in the affinity, making the oxygen easier for the hemoglobin to pick up but harder to release.
R stands for raised/ releases oxygen	L stands for low/holds onto oxygen
High temperature (hyperthermia)	Low temperature (hypothermia)
High 2,3-DPG levelsProduction increases with hypoxemia, chronic lung disease, anemia, and CHF	Low 2,3-DPG levelsProduction decreases with septic shock and hypophosphatemia
High pCO_2	Low pCO_2
There is NO "L" in ACIDOSIS	*There is an "L" in ALKALOSIS*

22. **D:** Low serum sodium levels following traumatic brain injury (TBI) can lead to extracellular volume depletion and cerebral edema. These can all result in dangerous increases in ICP. Hypertonic saline can help avoid the negative effects of hyponatremia by increasing serum sodium levels in the acute phase of head trauma care (Johnson and Criddle, 2004; Suarez, 2004).

Maintaining serum sodium levels of 145-155 mmol/L is likely to achieve this goal. Serum sodium levels should be maintained no higher than 155 mmol/L. Higher levels are dangerous. Patients with serum sodium levels higher than 160 mmol/L are at increased risk for treatment-related renal failure, pulmonary edema, and heart failure. If serum sodium levels remain above 160 mmol/L for more than 48 hours, the risk of these problems increases even more. Furthermore, if serum sodium levels climb beyond 160 mmol/L, patients are at risk for seizures. The target serum osmolarity is less than 320 mOsmol/L. At higher levels, patients are at increased risk for treatment-related renal failure (Qureshi and Suarez, 2000; Suarez, 2004).

23. **B:** *Pneumocephalus* is the presence of air or gas within the cranial cavity. It is usually associated with disruption of the skull: after head and facial trauma, tumors of the skull base, after neurosurgery, or with scuba diving (rare). The CT scan of patients with a tension pneumocephalus typically show air that compresses the frontal lobes of the brain, which results in a tented appearance of the brain in the skull known as the *Mount Fuji sign*. The name is derived from the resemblance of the brain to Mount Fuji in Japan, a volcano known for its symmetrical cone.

The presenting symptoms of pneumocephalus vary widely, but headache is almost always present. Experience with diagnostic pneumocephalus has shown that the headache is not induced by the intracranial air alone but that the dura mater must be stretched for pain to occur. Nausea, vomiting, vertigo, nuchal rigidity, aphasia, dysphasia, hemiplegia, and obtundation have all been associated with pneumocephalus, yet all are nonspecific symptoms. Treatment options for pneumocephalus vary. In some cases, the condition resolves on its own with some watchful waiting, application of oxygen, and surgery if not resolving in a timely fashion.

24. **D:** $MAP = [(75 \times 2) + 150]$ divided by $3 = 100$. $CPP = 100-25 = 75$ mmHg

Cerebral prefusion pressure	
Formula	Normal range (mmHg)
MAP = [(DBP × 2) + SBP] divided by 3	80-100
CPP = MAP − ICP	70-90
ICP	0-10

25. **C:** Diabetes insipidus (DI) is a condition characterized by excessive thirst and excretion of large amounts of severely diluted urine, with reduction of fluid intake having no effect on the latter. There are several different types of DI, each with a different

cause. The most common type in humans is central DI, caused by a deficiency of arginine vasopressin (AVP), also known as antidiuretic hormone (ADH). The regulation of urine production occurs in the hypothalamus, which produces ADH. The hormone is stored for later release in the posterior lobe of the pituitary gland. The cause of central diabetes insipidus is usually damage to the pituitary gland or hypothalamus, most commonly due to surgery, a tumor, illness (such as meningitis), inflammation or a head injury. In some cases the cause is unknown. This damage disrupts the normal production, storage, and release of ADH.

26. **B:** Cushing's triad is defined as a widening pulse pressure (rising systolic, declining diastolic), change in respiratory pattern (irregular respirations), and bradycardia. It is sign of increased ICP, and it occurs as a result of the Cushing reflex.

The body's compensatory mechanism and response to decreased cardiac output is to stimulate the sympathetic nervous system. This will cause vasoconstriction and results in a rise in the diastolic pressure, causing a narrowed pulse pressure. A narrow pulse pressure, which is the difference between the systolic and the diastolic, is an early indication of shock. Look for hypovolemia or decreased cardiac output.

A narrowing pulse pressure in shock is consistent with hypovolemic and cardiogenic causes. Septic shock will cause a widened pulse pressure. One way to differentiate shock in your patients is to look at the pulse pressure. A narrowing pulse pressure associated with hypovolemia would be hypovolemic. A narrowing pulse pressure associated with volume overload would be cardiogenic. A widening pulse pressure associated with hypovolemia would be septic.

27. **D:** The classic symptoms include transient loss of consciousness, recovery with a lucid interval during which the patient's neurologic status returns to normal, and the secondary onset of headache and a decreasing level of consciousness. In children, bradycardia and early papilledema (optic disc swelling) may be

the only warning signs. Epidural hematomas are usually caused by tears in arteries, resulting in a buildup of blood between the dura and the skull. The dura mater also covers the spine, so epidural bleeds may also occur in the spinal column. Often due to trauma, the condition is potentially deadly because the buildup of blood may increase pressure in the intracranial space and compress delicate brain tissue. Epidural hematoma commonly results from a blow to the side of the head. The pterion region which overlies the middle meningeal artery is relatively weak and prone to injury. Epidural hematomas are classified as acute or subacute. An acute epidural hematoma that is arterial in origin generally produces symptoms within a few hours. Subacute epidural hematomas are venous in origin and take a longer time to produce symptoms. These hematomas are associated with linear skull fractures in 90% of patients. Hemorrhages commonly result from acceleration-deceleration trauma and transverse forces (10% of epidural bleeds may be venous). Venous epidural bleeds are usually due to shearing injury from rotational or linear forces, caused when tissues of different densities slide over one another.

Subdural hematoma is a collection of blood within the outermost meningeal layer, between the dura mater, which adheres to the skull, and the arachnoid mater enveloping the brain. Usually resulting from tears in veins that cross the subdural space, subdural hemorrhages may cause an increase in ICP, which can cause compression of and damage to delicate brain tissue. Subdural hematomas are classified as acute (within 24 hours), subacute (between 2-10 days), and chronic (after 2 weeks). Subdural hematomas are often life-threatening when acute, but chronic subdural hematomas are usually not deadly if treated. Elderly patients may have larger subdural hematomas, with slowly developing symptoms because they have larger potential subdural spaces as a result of cerebral atrophy. Subdural hematomas generally occur in children less than two years of age. Signs and symptoms include a bulging fontanelle and a large head (because of separation of the sutures) and retinal hemorrhages as a result of increased ICP.

28. **A:** Subarachnoid hemorrhage is bleeding into the subarachnoid space, the area between the arachnoid membrane and the pia mater surrounding the brain. This may occur spontaneously, usually from a ruptured cerebral aneurysm, or may result from head injury. Signs and symptoms can include a severe headache with a rapid onset ("thunderclap headache," which is described as the worst ever), vomiting, neck stiffness (Brudzinski's sign—severe neck stiffness causes a patient's hips and knees to flex when the neck is flexed.), confusion, or a lowered level of consciousness, and sometimes seizures (1 in 14 patients).

Intracerebral hemorrhage is a subtype of intracranial hemorrhage, which occurs within the brain tissue and not outside of it. Most intracerebral hematomas are found the frontal and temporal lobes, usually very deep, and are associated with necrosis and hemorrhage. The clinical picture may vary from no neurologic defect to deep coma. Intracerebral bleeds are the second most common cause of stroke, accounting for 30-60% of hospital admissions for stroke. High blood pressure raises the risk of spontaneous intracerebral hemorrhage by two to six times. More common in adults than in children, intraparenchymal bleeds due to trauma are usually due to penetrating head trauma but can also be due to depressed skull fractures; some may experience intense headaches. They may also go in to a coma before the bleed is noticed. A hit in the head or a fracture in the skull may also cause this bleed, acceleration-deceleration trauma, rupture of an aneurysm or arteriovenous malformation (AVM), and bleeding within a tumor.

29. **B:** The Babinski's sign can indicate upper motor neuron lesion constituting damage to the corticospinal tract (central nervous system). A normal Babinski's reflex is plantar flexor (toes curl in "claw") and an abnormal reflex is plantar extensor (toes fan out). In infants, the primitive reflexes are still present and will show an extensor reflex response. This happens because the corticospinal pathways that run from the brain down the spinal cord are not fully myelinated at this age, so the reflex is not inhibited by the cerebral cortex. The extensor response disappears and gives way to the flexor response around 12-24 months of age.

30. **D:** Seizure types are organized according to whether the source of the seizure within the brain is localized (*partial* or *focal* onset seizures) or distributed (*generalized* seizures). Partial seizures are further divided on the extent to which consciousness is affected (simple partial seizures and complex partial seizures). If consciousness is unaffected, then it is a *simple partial* seizure; otherwise, it is a *complex partial* seizure. A partial seizure may spread within the brain—a process known as *secondary generalization*. Generalized seizures are divided according to the effect on the body, but all involve loss of consciousness. These include absence, myoclonic, clonic, tonic, tonic-clonic, and atonic seizures. A *mixed seizure* is defined as the existence of both generalized and partial seizures in the same patient. Generalized epilepsy leading to status epilepticus is mostly seen in the acute state in one of the two situations: with generalized encephalopathy, including that immediately following trauma, and in patients who are known epileptics, who have reduced drug intake, and whose blood levels have fallen below therapeutic concentrations.

Use a benzodiazepine as the first-line therapy. Seizure management requires a risk benefit analysis that balances the patient's needs with the urgency of the situation. Lorazepam is the preferred first-line agent for seizure control due to its long-lasting anticonvulsant properties. Diazepam is equally effective but requires that a concomitant, long-acting antiseizure medication be administered, such as Dilantin. When the IV access is unavailable, alternate routes such as IM injections of Midazolam, rectal solutions of Diazepam, and IM Fosphenytoin should be considered; of the three, IM Midazolam is probably the fastest and easiest to use. Alternative agents that have been used to manage seizure activity include Phenobarbital, Lidocaine, etomidate, propofol, and Paraldehyde.

31. **C:** The *facial nerve* is the seventh (VII) of twelve paired cranial nerves. It emerges from the brainstem between the pons and the medulla, controls the muscles of facial expression, and functions in the conveyance of taste sensations from the anterior two-thirds of the tongue and oral cavity. It also supplies preganglionic

parasympathetic fibers to several head and neck ganglia. Patients may suffer from acute facial nerve paralysis, which is usually manifested by facial paralysis. Bell's palsy is one type of idiopathic acute facial nerve paralysis, which is more accurately described as a multiple cranial nerve ganglionitis that involves the facial nerve, and most likely results from viral infection and also sometimes as a result of Lyme disease. Voluntary facial movements, such as wrinkling the brow, showing teeth, frowning, closing the eyes tightly (inability to do so is called lagophthalmos), pursing the lips, and puffing out the cheeks, all test the facial nerve.

32. **B:** Cranial nerve III, which is the oculomotor nerve, innervates five intrinsic eye muscles: levator palpebrae superioris, superior rectus, medial rectus, inferior rectus, and inferior oblique, which collectively perform most eye movements. It also sends parasympathetic efferents (via the ciliary ganglion) to the muscles controlling pupillary constriction and accommodation. The motor fibers originate in the oculomotor nuclei of the midbrain.

33. **D:** Cranial nerve VI, which is the accessory nerve (spinal accessory nerve), originates from neurons in the medulla and in the cervical spinal cord. It has a cranial root, which joins the vagus (cranial nerve X) nerve and sends motor fibers to the muscles of the larynx, and a spinal root, which sends motor fibers to the trapezius and the sternocleidomastoid muscles. Damage to the nerve produces weakness in head rotation and shoulder elevation.

34. **A:** Guillain-Barre syndrome is an *acute inflammatory demyelinating polyneuropathy* (AIDP), an autoimmune disorder affecting the peripheral nervous system, usually triggered by an acute infectious process. It is frequently severe and usually exhibits as an ascending paralysis noted by weakness in the legs that spreads to the upper limbs and the face, along with complete loss of deep tendon reflexes. With prompt treatment by plasmapheresis or intravenous immunoglobulins and supportive care, majority of patients will regain full functional capacity.

Myasthenia gravis is an autoimmune neuromuscular disease, leading to fluctuating muscle weakness and fatiguability. It is an autoimmune disorder, in which weakness is caused by circulating antibodies that block acetylcholine receptors at the postsynaptic neuromuscular junction, inhibiting the stimulative effect of the neurotransmitter acetylcholine. Myasthenia is treated medically with cholinesterase inhibitors or immunosuppressants, and, in selected cases, thymectomy. Symptoms, which vary in type and severity, may include asymmetrical ptosis (a drooping of one or both eyelids), diplopia (double vision) due to weakness of the muscles that control eye movements, an unstable or waddling gait, weakness in arms, hands, fingers, legs, and neck, a change in facial expression, dysphagia (difficulty in swallowing), shortness of breath and dysarthria (impaired speech, often nasal due to weakness of the velar muscles). In *myasthenic crisis* a paralysis of the respiratory muscles occurs, necessitating assisted ventilation to sustain life. In patients whose respiratory muscles are already weak, crises may be triggered by infection, fever, an adverse reaction to medication, or emotional stress. Diagnostic testing is done by injecting the drug edrophonium chloride (Tensilon, Reversol) or neostigmine (Prostigmin) into a vein and watching for rapid improvement of strength, usually of eye muscles. In patients with myasthenia gravis, involving the eye muscles, Edrophonium Chloride will briefly relieve eye muscle weakness. Improvement in strength of speech may also be considered a positive test.

35. **C:** A *dermatome* is an area of skin that is mainly supplied by a single spinal nerve. There are eight cervical nerves, twelve thoracic nerves, five lumbar nerves, and five sacral nerves. Each of these nerves relays sensation (including pain) from a particular region of skin to the brain. Dermatomes are useful in neurology for finding the site of damage to the spine. Refer to the table for review of dermatomes.

Anterior Cord syndrome is a type injury that usually results from hyperflexion and is characterized by variable loss of motor and sensory function below the level of injury. However, posterior column function is maintained. Clinically this person will present with a variable degree, perhaps even complete, of motor and sensory loss below the level of injury to the spinal cord, but the capacity to perceive light touch and position sense distal to the injury is maintained.

Dermatomes	
Level of spinal cord injury	Sensory impairment area
C5	Shoulder
C6	Thumb
C7	Middle finger
C8	Small finger
T1	Medial arm
T4	Nipples
T10	Umbilicus
L1	Inguinal or groin regions
L4	Knee
L5	Great toe
S1	Little toe
S2, 3, 4	Perineum

36. **C:** Central Cord syndrome is a type of injury that usually results from hyperextension and is characterized by a disproportionally greater motor impairment of the upper than the lower extremities with variable sensory loss below the level of injury. Sacral sparing typically occurs.

Two very important determinants of an incomplete, as opposed to a complete, lesion of the spinal cord are preservation of voluntary rectal sphincter tone and perianal sensation ("sacral sparing"). To check for voluntary rectal sphincter tone, insert a gloved finger in the rectum and request the patient, if cooperative, to squeeze down as if attempting to prevent movement of the bowels. If able to do so, there is substantial indication of an incomplete, as opposed to a complete, spinal cord injury, i.e., some spinal neural pathways are intact.

37. **A:** The presence of the plantar extensor reflex (toes fan upward) in an adult patient can indicate damage to the nerve pathways connecting the spinal cord and brain. It is wrong to say that the Babinski's reflex is positive or negative; it is present (plantar extensor reflex—toes fan upward which is bad) or absent (plantar flexor response—toes curl downward which is good).

38. **C:** The absence of doll's eye sign indicates injury to the midbrain or pons, involving cranial nerves III and VI. It typically accompanies coma caused by lesions of the cerebellum and brain stem. This sign usually can't be relied upon in a conscious patient because he can control eye movements voluntarily. Absent doll's eye sign is necessary for a diagnosis of brain death. An indicator of brainstem dysfunction, the absence of the doll's eye sign is detected by rapid, gentle turning of the patient's head from side to side. The eyes remain fixed in midposition, instead of the normal response of moving laterally toward the side opposite the direction the head is turned.

39. **B:** Clinical evaluation of brain death can be performed with the application of the oculovestibular reflex (cold-caloric exam). With head on bed at 30 degrees, instill 50 mL of iced water into ear canal. A normal response (presence of oculovestibular reflex) is tonic deviation of the eyes toward the irrigated ear.

40. **C:** Mydriasis is an excessive dilation of the pupil due to disease, trauma, or the use of drugs. A *mydriatic* pupil will remain excessively large even in a bright environment and is sometimes referred to as "blown pupil." Pupillary dilation (mydriasis) indicates unopposed sympathetic activity due to impaired parasympathetic axons. This may reflect compression or distortion of the oculomotor nerve (CN III) by either primary injury or herniation. Mydriasis also may be an effect of adrenergic stimuli, such as epinephrine, anticholinergics, cocaine, PCP, and drug withdrawal. The classic fixed and dilated "blown pupil" is a unilateral phenomenon that may occur when a rapidly expanding intracranial mass, including blood from a hemorrhage, is

compressing cranial nerve III. It may also represent herniation of the uncus of the temporal lobe. The opposite, constriction of the pupil, is referred to as miosis.

41. **B:** A *basilar skull fracture* (or *basal skull fracture*) is a fracture of the base of the skull, typically involving the temporal bone, occipital bone, sphenoid bone, and/or ethmoid bone. This type of fracture is rare, occurring as the only fracture in just 4% of severe head injury patients. Such fractures can cause tears in the membranes surrounding the brain, or meninges, with resultant leakage of the cerebrospinal fluid (CSF). The leaking fluid may accumulate in the middle ear space and dribble out through a perforated eardrum (CSF otorrhea) or into the nasopharynx via the eustachian tube, causing a salty taste. CSF may also drip from the nose (CSF rhinorrhea) in fractures of the anterior skull base, yielding a halo sign. Clinical signs include Battle's sign, which is ecchymosis of the mastoid process of the temporal bone and Raccoon eyes is periorbital ecchymosis ("black eyes").

42. **A:** Epidural hematomas are usually caused by tears in arteries, resulting in a buildup of blood between the dura and the skull. The middle meningeal artery runs in a groove on the inside of the cranium beneath the pterion, which is vulnerable to injury at this point, where the skull is thin. A blow or fracture of the temporal bone is often the cause of a rupture of the middle meningeal artery, which may cause an epidural hematoma.

43. **B:** The opposite of mydriasis (dilated pupil) is constriction of the pupil and is referred to as miosis when less than or equal to two millimeters. This is a normal response to an increase in light but can also be associated with certain pathological conditions, microwave radiation exposure, and certain drugs, especially opioids.

44. **C:** Normal MAP is 80-100 mmHg.

45. **B:** The best treatment for hydrocephalus is the placement of an extracranial shunt from the ventricles to an outside absorptive surface such as ventriculoperitoneal, ventriculoatrial, or ventriculopleural. Shunts usually consist of three parts:

a. Proximal end that is radiopaque and is placed into the ventricle. This end has multiple small perforations.
b. Valve—this allows for unidirectional flow. Can adjust various opening pressures. Usually has a reservoir that allows for checking shunt pressure and sampling CSF.
c. Distal end that is placed into the peritoneum or another absorptive surface by tracking the tubing subcutaneously.

Signs and symptoms of shunt complications include headache, malaise, general unwellness, vomiting, mental status alterations, increased blood pressure, head circumference increase, Cushings triad, bulging fontanel, sixth-nerve palsy signs, Macewen's sign, changes in gait, and personality changes. There may also be an increase of seizures and a complaint of neck pain.

Macewen's sign is a sign used to help to diagnose hydrocephalus (accumulation of excess cerebrospinal fluid) and brain abscesses. Tapping (percussion) the skull near the junction of the frontal, temporal, and parietal bones will produce a stronger resonant sound when either hydrocephalus or a brain abscess is present.

46. **B:** Brown-Séquard syndrome is a type of injury that usually results from a penetrating injury which has damaged one side of the spinal cord and is characterized by motor loss on the same side and sensory loss on the opposite side of the injury. Spinal cord injury can be classified in two main forms: complete and incomplete. A complete injury is defined as one in which there is complete disruption of continuity of all spinal pathways at one or more levels of the spinal cord. The result is absent motor function, sensory and pressured (touch) sensation and position and vibratory perception to all body areas enervated by the spinal cord tissue below the level of disruption. Incomplete spinal cord injury can be defined as one in which there is a variable degree of loss of function secondary to partial disruption of the spinal cord (some pathways of neurological function are intact, some are disrupted either permanently or transiently).

47. **A:** Anterior cord syndrome is a type injury that usually results from hyperflexion and is characterized by variable loss of motor

and sensory function below the level of injury. However, posterior column function is maintained. Clinically this person will present with a variable degree, perhaps even complete, of motor and sensory loss below the level of injury to the spinal cord, but the capacity to perceive light touch and position sense distal to the injury is maintained. Refer to the table in question 20 for review of spinal cord syndromes.

48. **A:** Meningitis is inflammation of the meninges, which are the protective coverings that are present over the brain and the spinal cord. This inflammation can be either bacterial or viral in nature. Some of the common symptoms that the patient presents with include headache and neck stiffness. This is a serious and possibly fatal condition, as the inflammation of the meninges can easily spread to the brain and the spinal cord, thus, causing life-threatening complications. One of the important bacterial meningitis precautions is to see to it that the patient wears a face mask at all times. This is of paramount importance because bacterial meningitis is contagious in nature, and it is a droplet infection. *H. influenzae* and *N meningitis* may be transmitted by droplets generated during coughing, sneezing, talking, or procedures, such as intubation and bronchoscopy. Droplet precautions should therefore be used whenever there is a clinical suspicion of infection with one of these pathogens. Traditional systems of isolation precautions have relied on an understanding of the mechanisms by which disease can be spread and have focused the use of protective barrier equipment, such as gloves, gowns, masks, and protective eyewear in order to interrupt transmission and to break the chain of infection.

49. **A:** *Abnormal posturing* is an involuntary flexion or extension of the arms and legs, indicating severe brain injury. It occurs when one set of muscles becomes incapacitated, while the opposing set is not, and an external stimulus, such as pain, causes the working set of muscles to contract. Posturing can be caused by conditions that lead to large increases in ICP. Such conditions include traumatic brain injury, stroke, intracranial hemorrhage, brain tumors, and encephalopathy. Posturing due to stroke usually only occurs on one side of the body and may also be referred to as spastic hemiplegia. Progression from decorticate posturing to

decerebrate posturing is often indicative of uncal (transtentorial) or tonsilar brain herniation. Refer to the table for review of abnormal posturing.

Abnormal posturing		
Type	Location of damage	Clinical presentation
Decorticate posturing *(also known as flexor posturing)*	Cerebral hemispheres, thalamus, and midbrain	The elbows, wrists, and fingers flexed, and legs extended and rotated inward.
Decerebrate posturing *(also known as extensor posturing)*	May indicate lesion to the lower brainstem, midbrain, and cerebellum	The head is arched back (opisthotonos), the arms are extended by the sides, and the legs are extended. Both the arms and the legs are rotated internally. The body is rigid and teeth are clenched. A hallmark of decerebrate posturing is extended elbows.

50. **B:** The *middle cerebral artery* (MCA) is one of the three major paired arteries that supplies blood to the cerebrum. The left and right MCAs rise from trifurcations of the internal carotid arteries and thus are connected to the anterior cerebral arteries and the posterior communicating arteries, which connect to the posterior cerebral arteries. The MCAs are not considered a part of the Circle of Willis. Occlusion/damage of the middle cerebral artery results in middle cerebral artery syndrome, potentially showing the following: paralysis (plegia) or weakness (paresis) of the contralateral face and arm (faciobrachial); sensory loss of the contralateral face and arm; damage to the dominant hemisphere (usually the left hemisphere since most individuals are right-handed) results in aphasia (Broca's or Wernicke's); large MCA infarcts often have deviation conjugée (a gaze preference toward the side of the lesion), especially during the acute period.

Broca's Aphasia, also known as expressive asphasia, is characterized by the loss of the ability to produce language (spoken or written). Expressive aphasia differs from dysarthria, which is characterized by a patient's inability to properly move the muscles of the tongue and mouth to produce speech. *Wernicke's Aphasia,* also known as receptive or sensory aphasia, and patients may speak in long sentences that have no meaning, add unnecessary words, and even create new "words," and have great difficulty in understanding the speech of both themselves and others and are, therefore, often unaware of their mistakes.

Bibliography

2005 American Heart Association guidelines for cardiopulmonary resuscitation and emergency cardiovascular care. Part 7.2: Management of cardiac arrest. *Circulation.* 2005; 112(24 Suppl):IV58-66.

American College of Surgeons. *Atls, Advanced Trauma Life Support Program for Doctors. Bull Am Coll Surg.* 2008; p. 58.

Association of Air Medical Services. (2004). *Guidelines for Air Medical Crew Education,* Iowa, Kendall/Hunt Publishing Company.

Attia, J, Hatala, R, Cook, DJ, Wong, JG. The rational clinical examination. Does this adult patient have acute meningitis? *JAMA.* 1999; 282(2):175-81.

Carlberg, B, Samuelsson, O, Lindholm, LH. Atenolol in hypertension: is it a wise choice? *Lancet.* 2004; 364(9446):1684-9

Darovic, G. (1999). *Handbook of Hemodynamic Monitoring,* 2nd edition. Philadelphia, W. B. Saunders.

Dawodu, ST. (2007). Traumatic brain injury: Definition, epidemiology, pathophysiology. emedicine.com.

Elizabeth, A, Henneman and George, E, Karras Jr. Determining brain death in adults: A guideline for use in critical care. *Crit Care Nurse.* 2004; 24:50-56. © 2004 American Association of Critical-Care Nurses

Ginsberg, L. Difficult and recurrent meningitis. *J Neurol Neurosurg Psychiatry.* 2004; 75 (Suppl. 1): i16-21.

Holleran, R. (1996). *Flight Nursing: Principles and Practice,* 2nd edition. St. Louis, Mosby.

Holleran, R. (2003). *Air and Surface Patient Transport: Principles and Practice,* 3rd edition. St. Louis, Mosby.

Holleran, R. (2009). *ASTNA Patient Transport: Principles and Practice,* 4th edition. St. Louis, Mosby.

Krupa, D. (1997). *Flight Nursing Core Curriculum.* Park Ridge, IL, National Flight Nurses Association.

Law M, Wald N, Morris J. Lowering blood pressure to prevent myocardial infarction and stroke: a new preventive strategy. *Health Technol Assess.* 2003; 7(31):1-94.

Marx, J. (2010). *Rosen's emergency medicine: concepts and clinical practice,* 7th edition. Philadelphia, Mosby/Elsevier. P.393-396.

Smith, Jet al. (2006). *Textbook of Surgery*. Wiley-Blackwell. pp. 446.

Tunkel, AR, Hartman BJ, Kaplan SL, et al. Practice guidelines for the management of bacterial meningitis. *Clin Infect Dis.* 2004; 39(9):1267-84.

Van de Beek, D, de Gans, J, Tunkel, AR, Wijdicks, EF. Community-acquired bacterial meningitis in adults. *N Engl J Med.* 2006; 354(1):44-53.

Module 6
Trauma and Burns

1. You are on the scene where a thirty-five-year-old man having gunshot wound to the left chest. The left chest has been decompressed with a needle prior to your arrival. The patient is intubated and continues to desaturate. Your assessment reveals an increase in SQ air to the chest and neck. The next intervention would be to

   A. Reneedle the left chest
   B. Advance ET tube below the level of the injury; right main stem intubation
   C. Decrease respiratory rate down to 10 per minute
   D. Insert a chest tube

2. You are managing a burn patient who weighs 90 kg with a 65% burn surface area (BSA). How much fluid should this patient receive in the first eight hours when using the Parkland formula?

   A. 23,400 mL
   B. 11,700 mL
   C. 8,450 mL
   D. 5,850 mL

3. What does the clinical presentation of abnormal posturing generally indicate?

   A. Frontal lobe dysfunction
   B. Upper motor neuron dysfunction
   C. Severe injury/damage to the brain and brainstem
   D. Lower motor neuron dysfunction

4. Using the Consensus formula, calculate how much fluid this 70-kg patient with a 50% BSA would receive in the first 8 hours of care?

   A. 2,000-4,000 mL
   B. 7,000-14,000 mL
   C. 3,500-7,000 mL
   D. 5,000-8,000 mL

5. The most commonly abused organ orsystem is?

   A. Head
   B. Orthopedic
   C. Integumentary
   D. Genitourinary

6. You are transporting a twenty-year-old man involved in a high-speed motor vehicle accident with a history of being ejected from the vehicle two hours prior to your arrival. The patient has been intubated and remains unconscious, with abnormal posturing noted. Mechanisms of injury associated with acceleration and deceleration that occurs with high-speed motor vehicle accidents or ejection from a vehicle can cause which type of brain injury?

   A. Cerebral contusion
   B. Concussion
   C. Diffuse axonal injury
   D. Depressed skull fracture

7. When inserting a chest tube, correct insertion site recommended is

   A. 2nd ICS midclavicular
   B. 5th ICS anterior midaxillary
   C. 5th ICS midaxillary
   D. 4th ICS midaxillary

8. You are transporting a twenty-three-year-old man, with a diagnosis of left-sided hemothorax. Guidelines for tube clamping suggest that the chest tube be clamped after how many milliliters of blood have been removed in the adult patient?

    A. 100 mL
    B. 1,000 mL
    C. 1,500 mL
    D. 500 mL

9. You arrive on the scene to manage a fall victim. She presents with a BP 80/50, HR 128, RR 36, SaO$_2$ 90%. Ground EMS reports that upon their physical examination, the patient revealed decreased bowel-like breath sounds on the left side of the chest. The patient is complaining of difficulty in breathing and severe left shoulder pain. The most likely diagnosis of this patient is

    A. Diaphragmatic rupture and spleen injury
    B. Neurogenic shock and tension pneumothorax
    C. Hypovolemic shock and cardiac tamponade
    D. Hemothorax and liver injury

10. You are preparing to transport a seventy-two-kg patient presenting with second and third degree burns to his entire face, anterior torso, and complete left arm. How much fluid should the patient receive in the first eight hours using the Parkland formula?

    A. 4,600 mL
    B. 9,200 mL
    C. 3,066 mL
    D. 2,300 mL

11. A sixty-year-old male patient has been trapped under a tractor for almost six hours. Once extricated, he is most likely to experience

   A. Tension pneumothorax
   B. Massive hemothorax
   C. Rhabdomyolysis
   D. Compartment syndrome

12. Your patient was struck from behind while driving. The most common area of injury from a rear-end collision is

   A. Ankle fracture
   B. Coup Contrecoup injury pattern
   C. C2 fracture
   D. T12-L1 injuries

13. The clotting cascade can be triggered through an extrinsic pathway. The triggering mechanism is the release of

   A. Fibrinogen
   B. Prothrombin
   C. Basophils
   D. Tissue thromboplastin

14. A patient in early shock most probably would present with which of the following acid-base imbalance?

   A. Metabolic acidosis
   B. Metabolic alkalosis
   C. Respiratory acidosis
   D. Respiratory alkalosis

15. Which blood component does not require typing and crossmatching before administration?

   A. Platelets
   B. Fresh frozen plasma
   C. Cyropercipitate
   D. Albumin

16. You are transporting a twenty-five-year-old female that presents with the following 12-lead ECG. What does the following 12-lead ECG show?

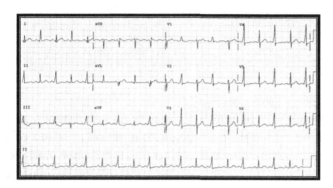

   A. U waves
   B. Electrical alternans
   C. Osborne wave
   D. Prolonged QT interval

17. Platelets are considered low at

   A. <600
   B. <450
   C. <240
   D. <150

18. Electrical alternans may be caused by a

   A. Pulmonary embolus
   B. Pericardial effusion
   C. Tension pneumothorax
   D. Diaphragmatic rupture

19. Normal K^+ value is

   A. 3.0-4.0
   B. 3.5-4.5
   C. 4.0-5.0
   D. 1.5-2.5

20. You are managing a twenty-five-year-old man with burns to the entire face, left forearm, right hand, and anterior portion of the entire left leg. His BSA would be

   A. 12%
   B. 19%
   C. 24%
   D. 30%

21. A twenty-one-year-old patient with history of stab wounds to the chest, presenting with a drop in the systolic blood pressure of 20 mmHg during inspiration, a narrowing pulse pressure, and clear equal breath sounds bilaterally would most likely be managed with all of the following, *except*

   A. Intravenous fluid bolus
   B. Pericardiocentesis
   C. Rapid transport
   D. Needle thoracostomy

22. A patient presenting with Beck's triad is most likely experiencing

   A. Tension pneumothorax
   B. Increased ICP
   C. Cardiac tamponade
   D. Intra-abdominal bleeding

23. Immediate release of intrapleural pressure should be performed where

   A. Fourth intercostal space, anterior axillary line
   B. Fifth intercostal space, anterior midaxillary line)
   C. Fourth intercostal space, midclavicular line
   D. Second intercostal space, midclavicular line

24. An object in motion will remain in motion and an object at rest will remain at rest unless acted upon by a force; this law is known as

A. Newton's first law
B. Newton's second law
C. Newton's third law
D. Ohm's law

25. Your patient was involved in a single car roll-over and is complaining of neck and left shoulder pain. You note bruising to the left chest wall. Vital signs are BP 80/48, HR 130, RR 28, SpO$_2$ 96%. The most likely cause is

A. Cardiac tamponade
B. Tension pneumothorax
C. Splenic injury
D. Intra-abdominal bleeding

26. What is a common problem associated with electrical injuries?

A. Myoglobinuria
B. Ventricular fibrillation
C. Diabetes insipidus
D. Hypokalemia

27. When managing a patient with an electrical injury that presents with hematochromagen urine, you should maintain a urine output of

A. 30-50 mL/hr
B. 50-100 mL/hr
C. 1-2 mL/kg/hr
D. A minimum 100 mL/hr

28. Normal cerebral perfusion pressure is at least?

A. 80-100 mmHg
B. 50-60 mmHg
C. 70-90 mmHg
D. >100 mmHg

29. Your patient presents with following parameters: CVP 0, CI 1, PA S/D 8/4, wedge 3, and SVR 1,800. What is your diagnosis?

    A. Hypovolemic shock
    B. Right ventricular infarction
    C. CHF
    D. Sepsis

30. Normal ICPis

    A. 0-10 mmHg
    B. 10-20 mmHg
    C. 20-30 mmHg
    D. > 30 mmHg

31. The formula used to calculate mean arterial pressure is:

    A. 2/3 DBP × SBP
    B. [(DBP × 2) + SBP] divided by 3
    C. 2 × SBP + DBP
    D. [(2 + DBP) × SBP] divided by 3

32. What is the formula used when calculating cerebral perfusion pressure?

    A. [(2 × DBP) + SBP] divided by 3
    B. MAP − ICP
    C. ICP − DBP
    D. [(2 + DBP) × SBP] divided by 3

33. Grey Turner's sign may indicate

    A. Meningitis
    B. Splenic injury
    C. Retroperitoneal bleed
    D. Gallbladder

34. Most commonly seen injuries with side impact or "lay it down" motorcycle crashes include all of the following, *except*

A. Open fracture of the femur
B. Pelvic fractures
C. Abrasions to the affected side
D. Tibia/fibula or malleolus fractures

35. Predictable injuries that can occur with falls can include all of the following, *except*

A. Calcaneus fractures
B. C2 fracture
C. T12-L1 back injuries
D. Bilateral wrist fractures

36. Dry chemicals such as lime should be

A. Brushed off before irrigation
B. Neutralized with a special agent before irrigation
C. Irrigated immediately with water or physiologic saline
D. Wrapped in a dressing and not irrigated

37. Hamman's sign may indicate the presence of

A. Tension pneumothorax
B. Tracheobronchial injury
C. Aortic rupture
D. Cardiac tamponade

38. Recommended urinary output when managing a burn patient without an electrical injury is

A. 100 mL/hr
B. 10-20 mL/hr
C. 30-50 mL/hr
D. >100 mL/hr

39. Hydrofluoric burns can be managed with copious amounts of water and

   A. Calcium gluconate
   B. Osmotic diuretics
   C. Glucagon
   D. Pyroxidine

40. The management approach for a patient experiencing brain herniation can include all of the following, *except*

   A. Serum sodium goal 155
   B. Serum osmolality less than 320
   C. Hypertonic saline, mannitol
   D. Hyperventilation to maintain $EtCO_2$ at 20-30 mmHg

41. Classic picture of neurogenic shock presents with

   A. Hypertension
   B. Absence of tachycardia
   C. Cool skin
   D. Pallor

42. Your patient presents with motor loss, numbness to touch, vibration on the same side of the spinal injury, loss of pain, and temperature sensation on the opposite side. You suspect that the most likely spinal cord syndrome present is

   A. Brown-Séquard
   B. Central cord
   C. Anterior cord syndrome
   D. Neurogenic shock

43. When should escharotomies ideally be performed?

   A. Circumferential burns are present in the chest or extremities and transport time exceeds greater than thirty minutes
   B. Circumferential burns to the extremities or digits have adequate circulatory stability
   C. Circumferential burns to the chest decrease chest wall compliance
   D. Circumferential burns are present on any pediatric patient

44. A patient presents with a further drop in MAP of 20% with an increase in fluid loss of over 1,800 mL. Vasoconstriction continues and leads to oxygen deficiency. Physiologically, the body switches to anaerobic metabolism, forming lactic acid as a waste product. The patient would most likely be in which stage of shock?

   A. Early reversible and compensated shock
   B. Late shock
   C. Intermediate or progressive and decompensated shock
   D. Refractory or irreversible shock

45. Calculate the following patient's cerebral perfusion pressure (CPP): BP 180/90, HR 120, RR 24, SpO_2 98%, CVP 2, ICP 25.

   A. 80
   B. 120
   C. 65
   D. 95

46. All of the following conditions are considered a form of obstructive shock, *except*

   A. Cardiac tamponade
   B. ICP
   C. Tension pneumothorax
   D. Massive pulmonary embolism

47. You are managing a 100-kg burned patient with 70% BSA. How much fluid will the patient receive in the first eight hours using the Consensus formula?

   A. 14,000-28,000 mL
   B. 7,000-14,000 mL
   C. 3,500-7,000 mL
   D. 28,000 mL

48. Late signs and symptoms of a tension pneumothorax can include all of the following, *except*

   A. Narrowing pulse pressure
   B. Hypotension
   C. Bradycardia
   D. Tracheal shift away from the affected side

49. The most common cause of pulseless electrical activity in a trauma patient is

   A. Hypoxia
   B. Hypovolemia
   C. Tension pneumothorax
   D. Cardiac tamponade

50. You have responded to a fire in a building with five victims. You notice that a large portion of the synthetic carpet has been burned in the room where you are treating the patients. The patients are exhibiting increasing signs of respiratory distress and coughing after high oxygen has been applied. What may be causing the patients' signs and symptoms?

   A. Cyanide
   B. Ammonia
   C. Carbon dioxide
   D. Hydrocarbon

Answer Key and Rationale

1. **B:** *Tracheobronchial injury* (TBI) is damage to the tracheobronchial tree (the structure of airways involving the trachea and bronchi). It can result from blunt or penetrating neck or chest trauma, causing a tear in the trachea or bronchus, allowing air to enter the pleural space or mediastinum. These injuries are characterized by palpable subcutaneous emphysema (in the neck, face, and thorax), dyspnea, hemoptysis (coughing up blood), and absent breath sounds to the affected side. *Hamman's sign,* which is a crunching sound auscultated to the anterior chest that is synchronized to the patient's heart beat, may also be present. A pneumothorax that reaccumulates after needle decompression has been performed or chest tube has been placed, should heighten the suspicion for tracheobronchial injury. The airways may also be injured by inhaling harmful fumes or aspirating liquids or objects. Intubation with placement of the tube distal to the injury site should be accomplished (right mainstem intubation in most cases). These patients should be closely monitored for development of a tension pneumothorax during transport.

2. **B:** Once the burning process has been stopped, the patient should be volume resuscitated according to the Parkland formula. This formula dictates the amount of Lactated Ringer's solution or Hartmann's solution to deliver in the first twenty-four hours after the time of injury. Half of this volume is given in the first eight hours with the remaining half to be administered in the subsequent sixteen hours. This formula excludes first-degree burns, so erythema (redness of the skin) alone is discounted.

Parkland Formula
[(4 mL × weight in kg) × % of TBSA] = Total fluids in twenty-four hours

Half of the total fluids calculated administered in the first eight hours and the rest in the subsequent sixteen hours.

$4 \times 90 = 360 \times 65\% = 23$; 400 mL total fluids in twenty-four hours with half of the total fluids calculated to be administered in the first eight hours. *Answer is 11,700 mL.*

Modified Brooke Formula

[(2 mL × weight in kg) × % TBSA] = Total fluids in twenty-four hours with half of the total fluids calculated administered in the first eight hours and the rest in the subsequent sixteen hours.

Consensus Formula *(Parkland and modified Brook formulas combined)*

[(2-4 mL × weight in kg) × % TBSA] = Total fluids in twenty-four hours with half of the total fluids calculated administered in the first eight hours and the rest in the subsequent sixteen hours.

3. **C:** *Abnormal posturing* is an involuntary flexion or extension of the arms and legs, indicating severe brain injury. It occurs when one set of muscles becomes incapacitated, while the opposing set is not, and an external stimulus, such as pain, causes the working set of muscles to contract. Patients with decorticate posturing present with the arms flexed, or bent inward on the chest, the hands clenched into fists, and the legs extended, and feet turned inward. Progression from decorticate posturing to decerebrate posturing is often indicative of uncal (transtentorial) or tonsilar brain herniation. In decerebrate posturing, the head is arched back, the arms are extended by the sides, and the legs are extended. A hallmark of decerebrate posturing is extended elbows. The arms and legs are extended and rotated internally. The patient is rigid, with the teeth clenched.

4. **C:** The burn formulas are a guide only and infusions must be tailored to the urine output and central venous pressure. Inadequate fluid resuscitation causes renal failure and death, but over-resuscitation also causes morbidity and mortality.

    Consensus Formula *(Parkland and modified Brook formulas combined)*
    [(2-4 mL × weight in kg) × % TBSA] = Total fluids in twenty-four hours with half of the total fluids calculated administered in the first eight hours and the rest in the subsequent sixteen hours.

    $2 \times 70 = 140 \times 50\% = 7,000$ mL, which is the low end of the range and 14,000 mL is the high end of the range. Half of this volume is given in the first eight hours with the remaining half to be administered in the subsequent sixteen hours. This formula excludes first-degree burns, so erythema (redness of the skin) alone is discounted.

Answer is 3,500-7,000 mL

5. **C:** The integumentary system is the largest organ system that protects the body from damage, comprising the skin and its appendages (including hair, scales, feathers, and nails). The integumentary system has a variety of functions; it may serve as waterproof, cushion, and protect the deeper tissues, excrete wastes, regulate temperature, and is the attachment site for sensory receptors to detect pain, sensation, pressure, and temperature. In humans, the integumentary system also provides vitamin D synthesis.

6. **C:** Diffuse axonal injury occurs when the delicate axons of the brain are stretched and damaged as a result of rapid movement of the brain, involving mechanism of injury associated with acceleration and deceleration that occurs with high-speed motor vehicle accidents or ejection from a vehicle. This type of brain injury is generally severe with a high morbidity and mortality.

7. **B:** All pneumothoraces greater than 20% or any pneumothorax present in patients requiring positive pressure ventilation should be treated with tube thoracostomy prior to transport. Treatment consists of placement of an appropriate-sized chest tube to the fifth intercostal space, at the anterior midaxillary line of the affected side. An alternate site for chest tube placement is the second intercostal space at the midclavicular line of the affected hemothorax. The anterior approach (alternate site) is inappropriate if both air and fluid are suspected in the pleural space.

8. **B:** Hemothorax occurs when blood accumulates in the pleural space. When more than 1,500 mL of blood accumulates in the pleural space, a hemothorax is deemed massive. Clinical presentation can include dyspnea, chest pain, decreased or absent breath sounds over the affected side, and dullness to percussion of the affected hemothorax. Signs of shock, which would be related to the blood loss, may be evident. Advanced Trauma Life

Support (ATLS) guidelines state the tube should be *clamped after 1,000 mL of blood is removed* in adult patients. Pediatric patients have a circulating volume of 80 mL/kg. The 1,000 mL in adults represents one fifth of the circulating volume, so a similar 20% loss in children may require thoracostomy tube clamping. It is important to remember that tube clamping is a temporizing measure until open thoracotomy can be performed.

9. **A:** Blunt injury to the diaphragm, resulting in rupture or partial tear, occurs when a tremendous force is applied to the abdomen. Diaphragmatic tears can occur without herniation of bowel into the chest cavity. If an intestinal herniation into the pleural space does occur, intestinal strangulation may develop. The left diaphragm is injured more often than the right because the liver absorbs the impact of the force on the right side. If a right-sided tear has occurred, liver injury will probably accompany it. Spleen injuries often occur with left-sided diaphragmatic trauma. Specific treatment for a known or suspected diaphgramatic tear with possible herniation should focus on airway management, oxygenation, and ventilation because of the potentially decreased lung capacity.

10. **A:** The assessment of the patient with burn injuries begins with the ABCs of the primary assessment. Burn wounds are often very dramatic in appearance and can lure the transport team's attention away from more immediate life-threatening problems. The goal of initial fluid resuscitation is to restore and maintain adequate tissue perfusion and vital organ function, in addition to preserving heat-injured but viable tissue in the zone of stasis. Refer to the table for review.

Rule of nines		
Body area	Adult	Pediatric
Head	9%	18%
Anterior torso	18%	18%
Back	18%	18%
Each arm	9%	9%
Each leg	18%	14%
Neck or genital area	1%	0%

Entire face = 4.5%, anterior torso = 18%, complete left arm = 9%, which totals to 31.5% TBSA

***Parkland Formula** [(4 mL × weight in kg) × % TBSA] = Total fluids in 24 Hours*
4 × 72 = 288 × 32 = 9,216 mL in twenty-five hours with half of the total amount of fluids calculated is administered in the first eight hours. *Answer: 4,600 mL in the first eight hours*

11. **C:** *Rhabdomyolysis* is the rapid breakdown (*lysis*) of skeletal muscle (*rhabdomyo*) due to injury to muscle tissue. The muscle damage may be caused by physical (e.g., crush injury), chemical, or biological factors. The destruction of the muscle leads to the release of the breakdown products of damaged muscle cells into the bloodstream; some of these, such as myoglobin (a protein), are harmful to the kidney and may lead to acute kidney failure. Treatment is with intravenous fluids, and dialysis or hemofiltration, if necessary. Swelling of the damaged muscle occasionally leads to compartment syndrome, the compression by swollen muscle of surrounding tissues in the same fascial compartment (such as nerves and blood vessels), leading to damage or loss of function in the part of the body, supplied by these structures. Symptoms of this complication include, decreased blood supply, decrease in sensation, or pain in the affected limb. Release of the components of muscle tissue into the bloodstream, leads to disturbances in electrolytes, causing, nausea, vomiting, confusion, coma, and cardiac arrhythmias. Furthermore, damage to the kidneys may lead to dark *(tea-colored)* urine or a marked decrease *(oliguria)* or absence *(anuria)* of urine production, usually about 12-24 hours after the initial muscle damage. Finally, disruptions in blood clotting may lead to the development of a state called disseminated intravascular coagulation (DIC). The most reliable test in the diagnosis of rhabdomyolysis is the level of creatine kinase (CK) in the blood. CPK levels greater than 20,000 are ominous and are indicative of later DIC, acute kidney failure, and potentially dangerous hyperkalemia.

http://en.wikipedia.org/wiki/Rhabdomyolysis—cite_ note-CritCare2005-0#cite_note-CritCare2005-0

12. **D:** An automobile hit from behind rapidly accelerates, causing the car to move forward under the patient. *Predictable injuries* are to the back with T12-L1 being the common area of injury, femur fractures, tibia/fibula fractures, ankle fractures, cervical strain, and C2 fractures caused by hyperextension if the head restraint is not in the proper position.

Patterns of injury	
Mechanism of injury	Predictable injuries
Head-on collision	Fractured ribs, pneumothorax, hemopneumothorax, concussion, skull fractures, patella and femur fractures, dislocated hips, acetabular fractures, ruptured spleen, lacerated liver, and ruptured/torn thoracic aorta.
Side-impact	Clavicles, ribs, femur fracture, tibia/fibula fractures, and ruptured spleens.
Rollover	Potential for multisystem injuries.
Falls	Falls from heights greater than 15-20 feet are associated with severe injuries. Calcaneus fractures, compression fractures to T 12-L1, and bilateral wrist fractures.
Motorcycle	Head-on: fractured femurs, tibias and fibulas; chest and abdominal injuries; head and neck injuries. Side impact: most commonly seen injuries are fractures of the femur, tibia/fibula, and malleolus. Laying down the motorcycle: commonly seen are abrasions to the affected side and fractures may occur if the patient hits the road hard or comes in contact with another object.

13. **D:** Thromboplastin is the combination of both phospholipids and tissue factor, both needed in the activation of the extrinsic pathway. However, partial thromboplastin is just phospholipids and not tissue factor. Tissue factor is not needed to activate the intrinsic pathway. Partial thromboplastin is used to measure the intrinsic pathway. This test is called the aPTT, or activated partial thromboplastin time.

14. **D:** Rapid and shallow respirations are seen with a shock patient, which is due to sympathetic nervous system stimulation and acidosis.

Shock	
Types of shock	Common clinical findings
Hypovolemic	Rapid, weak, thready pulse due to decreased blood flow combined with tachycardia; cool, clammy skin due to vasoconstriction and stimulation of vasoconstriction; increased thirst, altered mentation, and hypotension. *Hemodynamic readings: SVR > 1,200, CVP low*
Cardiogenic	Distended jugular veins due to increased jugular venous pressure; crackles; weak or absent distal pulses; hypotension and arrhythmias, often tachycardia. *Hemodynamic readings: SVR > 1,200, CVP high, PAWP high*
Neurogenic	Hypotension; may be accompanied by profound bradycardia due to loss of the cardiac accelerating nerve fibers from the sympathetic nervous system at T1-T4; the skin is warm and dry or a clear sweat line exists, above which the skin is diaphoretic; priapism due to peripheral nervous system stimulation. *Hemodynamic readings: SVR < 800, CI low, and heart rate is either normal or bradycardia is present.*
Septic	Pyrexia (fever) due to increased level of cytokines; systemic vasodilation resulting in hypotension; warm and sweaty skin due to vasodilation; activation of the coagulation pathways, resulting in disseminated intravascular coagulation. *Hemodynamic readings: SVR < 800, CI high*
Anaphylactic	Erythema (red skin), urticaria (hives), and pruritis (itching); localized edema, especially around the face and tongue; weak and rapid pulse; breathlessness and cough due to narrowing of airways and swelling of the throat; wheezing due to bronchoconstriction secondary to the histamine release; hypotension. *Hemodynamic readings: SVR < 800, CI low, and tachycardia*
Obstructive	Distended jugular veins due to increased jugular venous pressure; pulsus paradoxus in the presence of tamponade or tension pneumothorax. Other causes are aortic stenosis and massive pulmonary embolism.

15. **D:** A *blood product* is any component of the blood, which is collected from a donor for use in a blood transfusion. Whole blood is uncommonly used in transfusion medicine at present; most blood products consist of specific processed components, such as red blood cells, blood plasma, or platelets. Type and crossmatch refers to the complex testing that is performed prior to a blood transfusion to determine if the donor's blood is compatible with the blood of an intended recipient, or to identify matches for organ transplants.

Crossmatching is usually performed only after other less complex tests have not excluded compatibility. Blood compatibility has many aspects and is determined not only by the blood types (O, A, B, AB), but also by blood factors (Rh, Kell, etc.). Albumin is a blood protein that is mainly produced in the liver and helps maintain volume of the blood by maintaining the oncotic pressure. Albumin IV is a plasma volume expander made from pooled human venous plasma, which does require type and crossmatching. Indications of Albumin IV include hypovolemia and hypoalbuminemia, which can be caused by burns, major injury, hemorrhage, pancreatitis, infection, liver failure, or liver cirrhosis.

Blood products	
Type of blood product	**Indication for administration**
Cryoprecepitate	Is a frozen blood product prepared from plasma and each 15 mL unit typically contains 100 IU of factor VIII, and 250 mg of fibrinogen. Use for hemophilia, Von Willebrand's disease, hypofibrinogenemia (low fibrinogen levels), DIC.
Platelets	Also known as thrombocytes, play a fundamental role in hemostasis, which leads to the formation of blood clots. If the number of platelets are to low (thrombocytopenia), excessive bleeding can occur. If the number of platelets are too high, blood clots can form (thrombosis).
Packed red blood cells	PRBCs are a preparation of red blood cells that are transfused to correct low blood levels in anemic patients. This increases the amount of hemoglobin in the blood that can carry oxygen perfused from alveoli of the lungs to tissues. One unit of PRBCs typically will raise the hematocrit by 3-4% and the blood hemoglobin concentration by 1 gm/dL.
Fresh frozen plasma	Refers to the liquid portion of human blood that has been frozen and preserved quickly after a blood donation and will be used for blood transfusion. Indications for use are limited to the treatment of deficiencies of coagulation proteins for which specific factor concentrates are unavailable or undesirable; reversal of warfarin; massive blood transfusion.

16. **B:** *Electrical alternans* is an electrocardiographic phenomenon of alternation of QRS complex amplitude or axis between beats (high, low, high). Also a wandering baseline may be seen. It is

seen in cardiac tamponade and is thought to be related to changes in the ventricular electrical axis due to fluid in the pericardium.

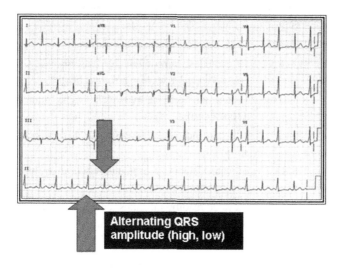

Alternating QRS amplitude (high, low)

17. **D:** In an adult, a normal count is about 150,000-400,000 (150-450) platelets per microliter of blood. If platelet levels fall below 20,000 per microliter, massive bleeding may occur and is considered a life-threatening risk.

18. **B:** *Pericardial effusion* ("fluid around the heart") is an abnormal accumulation of fluid in the pericardial cavity. Because of the limited amount of space in the pericardial cavity, fluid accumulation will lead to an increased intrapericardial pressure, and this can negatively affect heart function. When there is a pericardial effusion, with enough pressure to adversely affect heart function, this is called cardiac tamponade. Normal levels of pericardial fluid are from 15 to 50 mL. The so-called "water-bottle heart" is a radiographic sign of pericardial effusion, in which the cardiopericardial silhouette is enlarged and assumes the shape of a flask or water bottle. *Electrical alternans* is seen in cardiac tamponade and is thought to be related to changes in the ventricular electrical axis due to fluid in the pericardium.

19. **B:** Normal range of K^+ is 3.5-4.5. Some laboratories go as high as 5.5 for upper normal range.

Laboratory values		
Lab test	Normal range	Clinical manifestation
Sodium	135-145	<120 or >160 can cause seizures.
Potassium	3.5-4.5	>7 can cause ventricular dysrhythmias; ECG findings peaked/tented T wave > 5 mm in height.
Calcium	8.8-10.4	Trouseau's and Chvostek's signs can indicate hypocalcemia.
CO_2	24-30	<20 can indicate acidosis; look for cause; calculate anion gap.
BUN	6-23	Elevated BUN can indicate dehydration, blood in the gut, or renal failure.
Creatinine	0.6-1.4	Elevated reading indicates renal failure; BUN elevated.
Glucose	70-110	Assess for changes in behavior
Serum Os	285-295	Maintain <320 in the head-injured patient.
Magnesium	1.5-2.5	Levels of 4-8 are therapeutic levels in the preeclampsia obstetrical patient to prevent seizures. Levels >10 can be toxic and may require the administration of calcium.
Ammonia	Adult: 15-45 Pediatric: 40-80	Increased levels with Reye's syndrome and hepatic encepholapathy. Evacuate the bowel of any blood (blood contains protein, which increases ammonia levels).
BNP	<100	Measurable peptide used to diagnose CHF but can be nonspecific. Levels >500 CHF diagnosis.
Hemoglobin	12-18	Low indicates anemia; high many causes
Hematacrit	36-52%	Low indicates anemia; high can indicate dehydration and other conditions.
Platelets	150-400	Low platelets (thrombocytopenia), high platelets (thrombosis).
WBC	4.5-10.5	Are more elevated in the pediatric patient but is considered normal range.
CK/CPK	60-400	>20,000 are ominous and are indicative of later DIC, acute renal failure, and potentially dangerous hyperkalemia in heatstroke.

20. **B:** Entire face 4.5%, left forearm 4.5%, right hand 1%, and anterior portion of the entire left leg 9% = BSA of 19%

Rule of nines		
Body area	Adult	Pediatric
Head	9%	18%
Anterior torso	18%	18%
Back	18%	18%
Each arm	9%	9%
Each leg	18%	14%
Neck or genital area	1%	0%

21. **D:** *Cardiac tamponade* also known as *pericardial tamponade,* is an emergency condition in which fluid accumulates in the pericardium (the sac in which the heart is enclosed). If the fluid significantly elevates the pressure on the heart, it will prevent the heart's ventricles from filling properly. This, in turn, leads to a low-stroke volume. The end result is ineffective pumping of blood, shock, and often death. Clinical presentation can include; tachycardia, bradycardia, Beck's triad (muffled heart tones, hypotension, jugular venous distension), pulsus paradoxus, and the presence of electrical alternans on the ECG. Management of a cardiac tamponade in the prehospital setting includes rapid transport to the closest, most appropriate facility, intravenous fluids (this measure improves filling pressures and temporarily improves cardiac output) until pericardiocentesis can be performed. Landmark for performing a pericardiocentesis is the *infrasternal angle* or *subcostal angle,* into the apex of which the xiphoid process projects with the needle and syringe directed toward the left shoulder/scapula. A needle placed into the pericardial sac, with aspiration of as little as 15-20 mL of blood can improve the patient's condition. Pericardial blood will generally not clot because it has been defibrinated by heart motion.

22. **C:** *Beck's triad* is a collection of three medical signs associated with acute cardiac tamponade, an emergency condition wherein fluid accumulates around the heart and impairs its ability to pump blood. The result is the triad of low arterial blood pressure, jugular venous distention (unless the patient is hypovolemic), and distant, muffled heart sounds. Pulsus paradoxus, a fall in the systolic blood

pressure >15 mmHg during normal inspiration and a narrowing pulse pressure may also be observed prior to hypotension.

23. **D:** A pneumothorax can lead to severe oxygen shortage and low blood pressure, progressing to cardiac arrest unless treated; this situation is termed as *tension pneumothorax*. Clinical presentation can include dyspnea, tachycardia, altered mentation, narrowing pulse pressure, pulsus paradoxus, jugular venous distension, hypotension, diminished/absent breath sounds on the affected side, shock, and cardiac arrest. Initial treatment of a tension pneumothorax is performing a needle thoracostomy, with definitive treatment to include placement of a chest tube. To release intrapleural pressure, a large-bore needle should be placed into the second intercostal space, two-finger breadths lateral to the sternal border on the affected side. The needle should then be placed superior to the rib margin to avoid the intercostal artery. The anterior site should be used for avoidance of the internal mammary vessels.

24. **A:** *Newton's laws of motion* are three physical laws that form the basis for classical mechanics. They describe the relationship between the forces acting on a body and its motion due to those forces.

Newton's laws of motion	
Law	Definition
First law	Every body remains in a state of rest or uniform motion (constant velocity), unless it is acted upon by an external unbalanced force.
Second law	The total force applied on a body is equal to the time derivative of linear momentum of the body.
Third law	The mutual forces of action and reaction between two bodies are equal, opposite, and collinear.

25. **C:** Injury to the spleen is the most common serious complication of abdominal injury, resulting from trauma. *Kehr's sign* is the occurrence of acute pain in the tip of the shoulder due to the presence of blood or other irritants in the peritoneal cavity when a person is lying down and the legs are elevated. Kehr's sign in the left shoulder is considered a classical symptom of a ruptured spleen. It may result from diaphragmatic or peridiaphragmatic lesions, renal calculi, splenic injury, or ectopic pregnancy. Kehr's sign is a classical

example of referred pain: irritation of the diaphragm is signaled by the phrenic nerve as pain in the area above the collarbone. This is due to the fact that the supraclavicular nerves have the same cervical nerves origin as the phrenic nerve, C3 and C4.

26. **A:** *Electrical injuries* occurs upon contact of a human body with any source of voltage high enough to cause sufficient current through the skin, muscles, or hair. Voltage is defined as the force with which the electrical movement occurs. High voltage injuries (>1,000 volts) and low voltage injures (<1,000 volts) are both common, and either type can cause death. The higher the voltage, the more significant the injury. The type of current, alternating (AC) or direct (DC), can also determine the significance of the injury. Alternating current produces a tetanic contraction of muscles that "freezes" the victim to the source and has a greater potential in causing ventricular fibrillation. This is not seen with direct current. Low voltage AC can be more dangerous than a low voltage DC. Lactic acidosis is common because of the significant muscle damage caused by electrical injury. It is essential to maintain higher rates of urinary output because hemoglobinuria and myoglobinuria are common with electrical injuries.

27. **D:** The fluid resuscitation must be based on actual urine flow. A minimum of 50-100 mL/hour of urine must be maintained. If blood-colored urine is present, then the fluid volume must be sufficient enough to maintain a minimum output of 100 mL/hr.

28. **C:** *Cerebral perfusion pressure,* or *CPP,* is the net pressure gradient, causing blood flow to the brain (brain perfusion). It must be maintained within narrow limits because too little pressure could cause brain tissue to become ischemic (having inadequate blood flow) and too much could raise ICP.

Cerebral prefusion pressure	
Formula	Normal range (mmHg)
MAP = [(DBP × 2) + SBP] divided by 3	80-100
CPP = MAP − ICP	70-90
ICP	0-10

29. **A:** Careful interpretation of the CVP is important! *Central venous pressure* (CVP) describes the pressure of blood in the thoracic vena cava, near the right atrium of the heart. CVP reflects the amount of blood returning to the heart and the ability of the heart to pump the blood into the arterial system. It is a good approximation of right atrial pressure, which is a major determinant of right ventricular end-diastolic volume. The CVP should always be considered in conjunction with other cardiovascular parameters. Under normal circumstances, the right-sided heart pressures should indirectly reflect left-sided pressures, and the left-sided filling pressure may be an indicator of left ventricular function.

Preload (end-diastolic volume) is the pressure stretching the ventricle of the heart at the beginning of systole after passive filling of the ventricle and subsequent atrial contraction. *Afterload* (end-systolic volume) is the ventricular pressure at the end of systole.

Hemodynamic monitoring simplified	
Parameter	Evaluates
CVP (central venous pressure)	Preload of the right side of the heart
PCWP (pulmonary capillary wedge pressure)	Preload of the left side of the heart
PVR (pulmonary vascular resistance)	Afterload of the right side of the heart
SVR (systemic vascular resistance)	Afterload of the left side of the heart

30. **A:** ICP monitoring uses a device placed inside the head, which senses the pressure inside the skull and sends its measurements to a recording device. The intraventricular catheter is thought to be the most accurate method, but if immediate access is needed, a subarachnoid bolt is typically used. Normal value ranges may vary slightly among different laboratories (upper limits of the range can go as high as 15 mmHg).

Cerebral prefusion pressure	
Formula	Normal range (mmHg)
MAP = [(DBP × 2) + SBP] divided by 3	80-100
CPP = MAP − ICP	70-90
ICP	0-10

31. **B:** Refer to the table in question 30.

32. **B:** Refer to the table in question 30.

33. **C:** *Grey Turner's sign* refers to bruising of the flanks and can indicate retroperitoneal or intra-abdominal bleeding, which can take up to 24-48 hours to show up on assessment. It can be caused by acute pancreatitis, blunt abdominal trauma, ruptured abdominal aortic aneurysm, or ruptured/hemorrhagic ectopic pregnancy. It may be accompanied by Cullen's sign (superficial edema and bruising in the subcutaneous fatty tissue around the umbilicus), which may then be indicative of pancreatic necrosis, with retroperitoneal or intra-abdominal bleeding. Murphy's sign is useful for differentiating pain in the right upper quadrant. Typically, it is positive in cholecystitis (gallbladder disease). Kernig's and Brudzinski's signs when elicited can indicate meningitis. Kehr's sign (referred shoulder pain) can be indicative of a spleen injury or ectopic pregnancy.

34. **B:** Injuries associated with a side-impact motorcycle crash are related to the body parts crushed between the cycle and the second object. Most commonly seen injuries involve the leg and foot on the impact side. Open fracture of the femur, tibia/fibula, and malleolus are predictable. Motorcycle riders have learned the technique of laying down the bike and sliding off to the side before colliding with another object. Commonly seen are abrasions on the affected side.

35. **B:** Falls from heights greater than 15-20 feet are associated with severe injuries. Three predictable injuries are seen with falls. The forces involved are deceleration and compression. The first injury, calcaneus fractures, is caused by compression of the feet on impact. Second, as the energy dissipates after impact and the top of the body pushes down toward the point of impact, compression fractures to T12-L1 are seen. Finally, as the body moves forward and the patient puts both arms out to complete the fall, bilateral wrist fractures occur. It is important to estimate the distance fallen and what the patient landed on. A soft-landing surface (dirt or sand) will absorb much more energy than a hard surface, such as concrete.

36. **A:** Chemical burns differ from thermal burns in that the burning process continues until the agent is inactivated by reaction of tissues: neutralized or diluted with water. Dry chemicals, such as lime, should be brushed off before irrigation. Water and physiologic saline are fluids of choice for wound irrigation.

37. **B:** Tracheobronchial injuries occur when blunt or penetrating trauma causes a tear in the trachea or bronchus, allowing air to enter the pleural space or mediastinum. These injuries are characterized by palpable subcutaneous emphysema in the neck, face, and thorax. Other clinical findings include dyspnea, hemoptysis (coughing up blood), and absent breath sounds on the affected side. Hamman's sign is a crunching sound auscultated on the anterior chest wall and is synchronized to the patient's heartbeat. A pneumothorax that reaccumulates after chest tube insertion and placement to water seal drainage and suction should heighten the transport team's suspicion for tracheobronchial injuries. Treatment is intubation, with placement of the tube distal to the injury site, which most often can involve an intentional right mainstem intubation.

38. **C:** Urinary output is perhaps the most accurate method of evaluating the effectiveness of fluid replacement. Adult burn patients should have an hourly urine output of 30-50 mL/hr, and in the pediatric patient, it should be maintained at 1-2 mL/kg/hr/% BSA below 30 kg. Oliguria is an indication of inadequate fluid volume and should be easily corrected by increasing the rate of fluid administration. An osmotic diuretic, such as mannitol can be administered to avoid acute renal failure when fluid administration has been ineffective.

39. **A:** Hydrofluoric acid (HF) is an extremely corrosive liquid and is a contact poison. Because of the ability of hydrofluoric acid to penetrate tissue, poisoning can occur readily through exposure of skin or eyes, or when inhaled or swallowed. Symptoms of exposure to hydrofluoric acid may not be immediately evident. HF interferes with nerve function, meaning that burns may not initially be painful. Once absorbed into blood through the skin, it reacts with blood calcium and may cause cardiac arrest. Formation

of insoluble calcium fluoride is proposed as the etiology for both precipitous fall in serum calcium and the severe pain associated with tissue toxicity. In some cases, exposures can lead to hypocalcemia. Thus, hydrofluoric acid exposure is often treated with calcium gluconate, a source of Ca^{2+} that sequesters the fluoride ions. HF chemical burns can be treated with a water wash and 2.5% calcium gluconate gel or special rinsing solutions. However, because it is absorbed, medical treatment is necessary; rinsing off is not enough and in some cases, amputation may be necessary.

40. **D:** *Cushing's triad* is the triad of widening pulse pressure (rising systolic, declining diastolic), change in respiratory pattern (irregular respirations), and bradycardia. It is a sign of increased ICP, and it occurs as a result of the Cushing reflex. *Brain herniation,* also known as *cistern obliteration,* is a deadly side effect of very high ICP that occurs when the brain shifts across structures within the skull. Brain herniation frequently presents with abnormal posturing a characteristic positioning of the limbs indicative of severe brain damage. These patients have a lowered level of consciousness, with Glasgow Coma Scores of three to five. One or both pupils may be dilated and fail to constrict in response to light. Vomiting can also occur due to compression of the vomiting center in the medulla oblongata. Routine hyperventilation is not longer recommended in the initial management of the patient with traumatic brain injury. The patient's $EtCO_2$ should be maintained between 35-45 mmHg. Mannitol may be used to treat increasing ICP manifested by deterioration in the patient's neurologic status.

41. **B:** *Neurogenic shock, also known as a type of distributive shock or vasogenic shock,* is an imbalance between parasympathetic and sympathetic nervous stimulation of vascular smooth muscle, resulting in sustained vasodilatation typically, and the heart rate does not increase in the neurogenic shock patient due to loss of sympathetic impulses/stimulation. Vasomotor paralysis below the level of the injury occurs resulting in decreased peripheral vascular resistance. Sympathetic impulses, which would normally stimulate vasoconstriction, are interrupted, leading to widespread vasodilation. Blood collects in the capillary beds, reducing venous

return, cardiac output, and blood pressure. Refer to the table for review of compensatory mechanisms.

Compensatory mechanisms of neurogenic shock	
Body compensates by	Resulting in
Increasing cardiac output	Stimulation of the sympathetic nervous system causes an increase in heart rate, stroke volume, and PVR.
Redistributing the circulating blood volume to vital organs	Vasoconstriction and release of antidiuretic hormone (ADH) and renin to decrease urine production.
Increasing oxygen delivery to cells	Stimulation of the sympathetic nervous system causes bronchodilation, increased respirations, and tidal volume.

42. A: Refer to the table for review of spinal cord injury syndromes

Spinal cord injury syndromes	
Type of syndrome	Clinical manifestations
Anterior cord	Blood supply to the anterior portion of the spinal cord is interrupted, causing a complete motor paralysis below the level of the lesion due to interruption of the corticospinal tract. Loss of pain and temperature sensation at and below the level of the lesion due to interruption of the spinothalamic tract. Retained proprioception and vibratory sensation due to intact dorsal columns. Most often occurs after hyperflexion injury.http://en.wikipedia.org/wiki/Anterior_cord_syndrome—cite_note-0#cite_note-0
Brown-Séquard	Any presentation of spinal injury that is an incomplete lesion can be called a partial Brown-Séquard or incomplete Brown-Séquard syndrome, so long as it has characterized by features of a motor loss and numbness to touch and vibration on the same side of the spinal injury and loss of pain and temperature sensation on the opposite side. Most often occurs from a penetrating injury that has damaged one side of the spinal cord.
Central cord	It is characterized by disproportionately greater motor impairment in upper compared to lower extremities and variable degree of sensory loss below the level of injury. Most often occurs after hyperextension injury.

43. **C:** Circumferential burns to the chest or extremities represent the more easily recognizable complications of burn care. Circumferential burns to the chest wall decrease chest wall compliance, creating respiratory insufficiency and hypoxia, especially in the pediatric patient. The treatment for this problem is an escharotomy, which allows the chest to expand fully for more efficient ventilation. Circumferential burns to the extremities or digits can be equally threatening to the circulatory stability of the affected limb, producing the "five Ps" that represent the signs and symptoms of an arterial injury: pain, pallor, pulselessness, paresthesias, and paralysis. Escharotomies ideally should be performed before transport of the patient and should be performed only under the direction of a medical physician.

44. **C:** Shock is a clinical syndrome which results in a systemic imbalance between oxygen supply and demand. Inadequate blood flow to body organs and tissue causes life-threatening cellular dysfunction. Refer to the table for review of shock stages.

Stages of shock			
Grades/ Class	Stages	Loss of effective blood volume (mL)	Results in
I	Early, reversible, compensatory	<15% (<750)	Mild increase in HR and RR
II	Early, reversible, compensatory	15-30% (750-1,500)	Moderate tachycardia and begins to narrow the pulse pressure, increasing RR and delayed capillary refill time.
III	Intermediate, progressive, decompensated shock	30-40% (1,500-2,000)	Compensatory mechanisms begin to fail and hypotension, tachycardia, and low urine output (< 0.5 mL/kg/hr in adults) are seen. Body switches to anaerobic metabolism and lactic acids are produced.
IV	Irreversible, refractory	>40% (2,000-2,500)	Profound hypotension, DIC, end-organ damage (MODS), and death.

45. **D:** $90 \times 2 = 180$; $180 \times 2 = 360$; 360 divided by $3 = 120$; $120\text{-}25 = 95$

Cerebral prefusion pressure	
Formula	Normal range (mmHg)
MAP = [(DBP × 2) + SBP] divided by 3	80-100
CPP = MAP − ICP	70-90
ICP	0-10

Answer = 95 mmHg

46. **B:** Cardiac tamponade, tension pneumothorax, massive pulmonary embolism, and aortic stenosis are classified as forms of obstructive shock. In these situations, the flow of blood is obstructed, which impedes circulation and can result in circulatory arrest.

47. **B:** $2 \times 100 = 200$; $200 \times 70 = 14,000$; half is administered in the first eight hours = 7,000 mL (is the lower end of the Consensus formula).

Answer = 7,000-14,000 mL

Consensus formula (Parkland and modified Brook formulas combined)
[(2-4 mL × weight in kg) × % TBSA] = Total fluids in twenty-four hours with half of the total fluids calculated administered in the first eight hours and the rest in the subsequent sixteen hours.

48. **A:** *Early signs and symptoms* of a tension pneumothorax can be characterized by increased work of breathing, tachycardia, pulsus paradoxus, narrowing pulse pressure, and breath's sounds diminished on the affected side. *Late signs and symptoms of decompensated obstructive shock* include cyanosis, hypoxemia hypotension, bradycardia, and confusion. The affected side of the chest may be hyper-expanded and show decreased movement, with increased movement on the other side. The breath sounds may be diminished or absent on the affected side, as air in the pleural space dampens sound and percussion of the chest may sound hyperresonant (higher pitched). In very severe cases, the respiratory rate falls sharply,

which may result in further shock and coma. Recent studies have shown that the development of tension features may not always be as rapid as previously thought. Particular clinical signs may also be less useful in the recognition of tension pneumothorax, such as the deviation of the trachea away from the affected side and the presence of increased jugular venous pressure.

49. **B:** *Pulseless electrical activity (PEA)*, also known by the older term *electromechanical dissociation* or *nonperfusing rhythm*, refers to any heart rhythm observed on the ECG that should be producing a pulse, but is not. The most common cause of PEA is hypovolemia. The approach in treatment of PEA is to treat the underlying cause. These possible causes are remembered as the 6 Hs and the 6 Ts or by using the mneumonic PATCH4MD. Refer to the tables for review of causes for PEA.

Causes of PEA	
6 Hs	6 Ts
Hypovolemia	Tablets or Toxins (overdose)
Hypoxia	Tamponade (cardiac)
Hydrogen ions (acidosis)	Tension pneumothorax
Hyper or Hypokalemia	Thrombosis (MI)
Hypoglycemia	Thrombosis (pulmonary embolism)
Hypothermia	Trauma

Causes of PEA—PATCH4MD	
P	Pulmonary embolism
A	Acidosis
T	Tension pneumothorax
C	Cardiac tamponade
H	Hypovolemia
H	Hypoxia
H	Hyper or hypokalemia, hypoglycemia
H	Hypothermia
M	MI
D	Overdose

Where an underlying systemic cause cannot be determined rapidly enough, pulseless electrical activity should be treated as if the patient were in asystole. Treatment is intravenous delivery epinephrine (1:10,000) 1 mg every 3-5 minutes, and, if the underlying rhythm is bradycardia (<60 BPM), Atropine 1 mg IV up to 0.04 mg/kg. Both these drugs should be administered along with appropriate CPR techniques. Defibrillators are not used for this rhythm as the problem lies in the response of the myocardial tissue to electrical impulses.

50. **A:** Cyanide makes the cells of an organism unable to use oxygen, primarily through the inhibition of cytochrome oxidase. Inhalation of high concentrations of cyanide causes coma with seizures, apnea, and cardiac arrest, with death following in a matter of minutes. At lower doses, loss of consciousness may be preceded by general weakness, giddiness, headaches, vertigo, confusion, and perceived difficulty in breathing. A fatal dose for a patient can be as low as 1.5 mg/kg body weight. Blood cyanide concentrations may be measured as a means of confirming the diagnosis in hospitalized patients or to assist in the forensic investigation of a criminal poisoning. *Cyanide toxicity can occur following ingestion of amygdalin (found in almonds and apricot kernels), prolonged administration of nitroprusside, and after exposure to gases produced by the combustion of synthetic materials.* The United States standard cyanide antidote kit first uses a small inhaled dose of amyl nitrite, followed by intravenous sodium nitrite, followed by intravenous sodium thiosulfate. Hydroxocobalamin is newly approved in the US at doses from 2.5 to 10 mg per injection and is available in Cyanokit antidote kits.

Hydroxocobalamin (OHCbl, or B_{12a}) is a natural form of vitamin B_{12}. Pharmaceutically, hydroxycobalamin is usually produced as a sterile injectable solution; it is used for treatment of the vitamin deficiency and also (because of its affinity for cyanide ion) as a treatment for cyanide poisoning. Hydroxocobalamin will bind circulating and cellular cyanide molecules to form cyanocobalamin, which is excreted in the urine.

Bibliography

2005 American Heart Association guidelines for cardiopulmonary resuscitation and emergency cardiovascular care. Part 7.2: Management of Cardiac Arrest. *Circulation.* 2005; 112(24 Suppl): IV 58-66.

Alonso, J, Cardellach, F, López, S, Casademont, J, Miró, O. Carbon monoxide specifically inhibits cytochrome c oxidase of human mitochondrial respiratory chain. *Pharmacol Toxicol.* 2003; 93(3):142-6.

American College of Surgeons. *ATLS, Advanced Trauma Life Support Program for Doctors. Bull Am Coll Surg.* 2008; p. 58.

American College of Surgeons. *Atls, Advanced Trauma Life Support Program for Doctors. Bull Am Coll Surg.* 2008; p. 58.

American College of Surgeons. Chapter 10-Pediatric Trauma. *In: Advanced Trauma Life Support Instructor Course Manual,* Sixth edition, 1997. Chicago, First Impression, pp. 353-375.

Association of Air Medical Services. (2004). *Guidelines for Air Medical Crew Education,* Iowa, Kendall/Hunt Publishing Company.

Ayotte, P, Hébert, M, Marchand, P. Why is hydrofluoric acid a weak acid? *J Chem Phys.* 2005; 123(18):184501.

Baumann, MH, Strange, C, Heffner, JE, et al. Management of spontaneous pneumothorax. American College of Chest Physicians Delphi consensus statement. *Chest* 2001; 119(2):590-602.

Borron, SW, Baud, FJ, Mégarbane, B, Bismuth, C. Hydroxocobalamin for severe acute cyanide poisoning by ingestion or inhalation. *Am J Emerg Med.* 2007; 25(5):551-8.

Bosch, X, Poch E, Grau, JM. Rhabdomyolysis and acute kidney injury. *N Engl J Med.* 2009; 361(1):62-72.

Darovic, G. (1999). *Handbook of Hemodynamic Monitoring,* 2nd edition. Philadelphia, W.B. Saunders.

Dart, RC. Hydroxocobalamin for acute cyanide poisoning. *Clin Toxicol.* 2006; 44(1):1-3.

Dawodu, ST. (2007). Traumatic brain injury: Definition, epidemiology, pathophysiology. emedicine.com.

Greenwood, NN, Earnshaw, A. (1984). *Chemistry of the Elements,* Pergamon, Oxford. p. 921.

Hall, AH, Dart, R, Bogdan, G. Sodium thiosulfate or hydroxocobalamin for the empiric treatment of cyanide poisoning? *Ann Emerg Med.* 2007; 49(6):806-13.

Holleran, R. (1996). *Flight Nursing: Principles and Practice,* 2nd edition. St. Louis, Mosby.

Holleran, R. (2003). *Air and Surface Patient Transport: Principles and Practice,* 3rd edition. St. Louis, Mosby.

Holleran, R. (2009). *ASTNA Patient Transport: Principles and Practice,* 4th edition. St. Louis, Mosby.

Huerta-Alardín, AL, Varon, J, Marik, PE. Bench-to-bedside review: rhabdomyolysis—an overview for clinicians. *Crit Care.* 2005; 9(2):158-69.

Keel, M, Meier, C. Chest injuries—what is new? *Curr Opin Crit Care.* 2007; 13(6):674-9.

Krupa, D. (1997). *Flight Nursing Core Curriculum.* Park Ridge, IL, National Flight Nurses Association.

Lee, C, Revell, M, Porter, K, Steyn, R. The prehospital management of chest injuries: a consensus statement. *J Emerg Med.* 2007; 24(3):220-4.

Leigh-Smith S, Harris T. Tension pneumothorax—time for a re-think? *J Emerg Med.* 2005; 22(1):8-16.

Marik, PE, Corwin, HL. Efficacy of red blood cell transfusion in the critically ill: a systematic review of the literature. *Crit Care Med.* 2008; 36:2667-2674.

Marx, J. (2010). *Rosen's emergency medicine: concepts and clinical practice,* 7th edition. Philadelphia, PA, Mosby/Elsevier. p. 393-396.

Mitochondrion: biogenesis of cytochrome c oxidase, 2005;5(6):363-388.

Pediatric Trauma. In: American College of Emergency Physicians and American Academy of Pediatrics. *Advanced Pediatric Life Support Instructor Manual.* 1998. Dallas, ACEP. pp. 75-87.

Sauret, JM, Marinides, G, Wang, GK. Rhabdomyolysis. *Am Fam Physician.* 2002; 65(5):907-12.

Smith, Jet al. (2006). *Textbook of Surgery.* Wiley-Blackwell. p. 446.

Vanholder, R, Sever, MS, Erek, E, Lameire, N. Rhabdomyolysis. *Clin J Am Soc Nephrol.* 2000; 11(8):1553-61.

Wilkerson, RG, Stone, MB. Sensitivity of bedside ultrasound and supine anteroposterior chest radiographs for the identification of pneumothorax after blunt trauma. *Acad Emerg Med. 2010;*

Yamashita, M, Yamashita, M, Suzuki, M, Hirai, H, Kajigaya, H. Ionophoretic delivery of calcium for experimental hydrofluoric acid burns. *Crit Care Med.* 2001; 29(8):1575-8.

Module 7
Environmental and Toxicology Emergencies

1. You are transporting a thirty-eight-year-old man who is presented to the ER with a history of cocaine-induced tachycardia and is complaining of midsternal chest pain. Vital signs are as follows: temperature 101.2°F, BP 200/100, HR 140, RR 28, SaO$_2$ 97% on 2 liters/min of oxygen via nasal cannula. Which of the following medication is contraindicated for management of this patient?

   A. Nitroglycerin
   B. Morphine Sulfate
   C. Metoprolol
   D. Midazolam

2. You have been requested to transport a fifty-five-year-old mane with a history of CHF who is complaining of blurred vision and visual disturbances. The patient states that he has been seeing green and yellow halos for the last two days. The ECG on the monitor shows the following rhythm. The most likely cause for his visual disturbance is

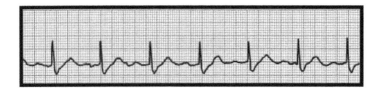

   A. Digitalis toxicity
   B. MI
   C. Pulmonary embolism
   D. Retinal hemorrhage

3. You have been requested to transport a twenty-year-old female with a history of acetylsalicylic acid poisoning two hours prior to your arrival at the sending facility. The patient is complaining of nausea, headache, and tinnitus. When evaluating her ABGs, you would expect which of the following acid-base disturbances to manifest in the early stage of poisoning?

   A. Respiratory alkalosis
   B. Respiratory acidosis
   C. Metabolic alkalosis
   D. Metabolic acidosis

4. All of the following muscle enzymes, if elevated, are a diagnostic hallmark in a heatstroke patient, *except*

   A. SGOT and SGPT
   B. Troponin 1 and 2
   C. LDH
   D. Creatinine phosphokinase

5. Defibrillation is usually not effective until the body core temperature is greater than

   A. 25°C
   B. 28°C
   C. 30°C
   D. 32°C

6. Which of the following rewarming techniques can best avoid the dangers of the afterdrop phenomenon when managing a hypothermic patient?

   A. Passive external
   B. Active internal
   C. Passive internal
   D. Active external

7. You are transporting a patient with history of seizures while on a camping trip in July. Her husband drove her to the closest ER for treatment. She has a history of cardiac heart failure and only takes furosemide daily. Labs reveal CK 27,000, LDH 800, BUN 34, CR 1.1, K 3.1, Hgb 15.3, Hct 44, CO_2 16, and glucose of 62. The foley bag contains urine that appears dark greenish-brown in color with an output of less than 20 mL in the last hour. She is unresponsive with BP 100/40, HR 144, RR 32, and SaO_2 94%. The decrease in urine output and abnormal urine character is most likely the result of which of the following?

   A. CHF secondary to an acute MI
   B. Disseminated intravascular coagulation
   C. Rhabdomyolysis secondary to heatstroke
   D. Acute renal failure secondary to furosemide toxicity

8. Which of the following blood transfusion reaction can occur within minutes of administration?

   A. Hemolytic
   B. Anaphylactic
   C. Febrile
   D. Circulatory overload

9. You are transporting a forty-year-old mane with history of esophageal varices. The sending physician has ordered a unit of PRBC's transfusion to be infused during transport. Transport time to the receiving facility is approximately 20-30 minutes. The patient should be monitored for which of the following during transport?

   A. Volume overload
   B. Citrate toxicity
   C. Vaso-occlusive crisis
   D. Hemolytic reaction

10. What condition would you suspect with the following 12-lead ECG?

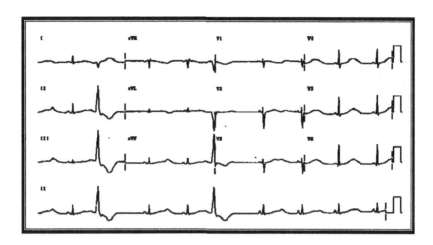

    A. Hypokalemia
    B. Cardiac tamponade
    C. Digitalis toxicity
    D. Tricyclic antidepressant toxicity

11. The treatment for acetaminophen poisoning is

    A. Normal saline
    B. N-acetylcysteine (NAC)
    C. Sodium bicarbonate IV drip
    D. Pyridoxine

12. Antidote for Coumadin overdose is

    A. Protamine sulfate
    B. Glucagon
    C. Vitamin K, FFP
    D. Physostigmine

13. Treatment of Digitalis toxicity would include all of the following, *except*

    A. Digibind
    B. TCP
    C. Magnesium
    D. Beta-blockers

14. When managing a patient with an electrical injury, with the presence of hemochromogen, you should maintain a minimum urine output of

    A. 30-50 mL/hr
    B. 50 mL/hr-100 mL/hr
    C. 1-2 mL/kg/hr
    D. 100 mL/hr

15. The drug of choice for a patient exhibiting signs and symptoms of malignant hyperthermia is

    A. Anectine
    B. Sodium bicarbonate
    C. Dantrolene
    D. Glucagon

16. You are transporting a sixty-five-year-old man who was brought to the emergency department with a history of alcoholism. The staff reports that the patient was found in an alley unresponsive and hypothermic. From the following 12-lead ECG, you would expect the patient's body temperature to be at approximately

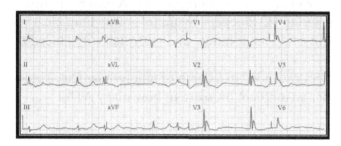

    A. 36°C
    B. 34°C
    C. 30°C
    D. 25°C

17. You have been requested to transport a twenty-year-old female from an ICU with a history of TCA overdose two hours prior to your arrival at the sending facility. Your cardiovascular assessment of the patient would most likely include all of the following with this type of toxicity, *except*

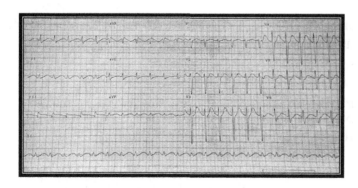

    A. Early sinus bradycardia
    B. Widening QRS
    C. Prolonged QT and PR interval
    D. Early tachycardia

18. The most critical goal and life-saving measure in heat illness is

    A. Cooling the patient to rapidly decrease body temperature
    B. Administering large amounts of fluids and inotropic agents to correct dehydration and hypotension
    C. Immediate endotracheal intubation to prevent aspiration
    D. Administering H2 blockers, mannitol and sodium bicarbonate to prevent acute renal failure and gastrointestinal bleeding

19. A scuba diver descended to a depth of ninety-nine feet. The scuba diver is under an ambient pressure of how many ATA?

    A. 1
    B. 2
    C. 3
    D. 4

20. The most common type of decompression sickness typically seen diving emergencies is

    A. Musculoskeletal
    B. Pulmonary
    C. Arterial gas embolism
    D. Cutaneous

21. Situations that involve a right shift in the oxygen-hemoglobin dissociation curve are all of the following, *except*

    A. Alkalosis
    B. Hypercapnia
    C. Hyperthermia
    D. Increased level of 2,3-DPG

22. Gases in the lungs of a scuba diver expand as ambient pressure decreases during ascent best describes which gas law?

    A. Henry's
    B. Dalton's
    C. Graham's
    D. Boyle's

23. You are transporting a patient who you note has tea-colored urine in small amount in the foley catheter bag. The nurse reports that his output is only 50 mL in the last twenty-four hours. What treatment would you expect to initiate during the two-hour flight?

    A. Rapid fluid resuscitation, sodium bicarbonate drip, and consider Lasix and mannitol
    B. Rapid fluid resuscitation, potassium replacement therapy, and aggressive pain management
    C. Fluid restriction, sodium bicarbonate drip, and consider Lasix and mannitol
    D. Fluid restriction, potassium replacement therapy, and aggressive pain management

24. Your head-injured patient is hypothermic. In what direction does the oxyhemoglobin dissociation curve shift to?

    A. Up
    B. Down
    C. Right
    D. Left

25. Poisoning of the cytochrome oxidase enzyme system may cause

    A. Histotoxic hypoxia
    B. Hypemic hypoxia
    C. Hypoxic hypoxia
    D. Stagnant hypoxia

26. Two types of drug poisoning that cause hallucinations are

    A. Cocaine and PCP
    B. PCP and lysergic acid diethylamide
    C. LSD and benzodiazapines
    D. Methamphetamine and LSD

27. You have been requested to a farming area to transport a forty-year-old man involved in a plane crash. On arrival, the patient is complaining of shortness of breath with increased salivation and blurred vision. Vital signs are BP 100/58, HR 50, RR 36, SaO$_2$ 92%. Management of this patient would include all of the following, *except*

A. Diazepam
B. Atropine
C. Sodium thiosulfate
D. Pralidoxime

28. One of the major organs that must be functional if heat is to be dissipated is the

A. Skin
B. Hypothalamus
C. Kidney
D. Liver

29. ARDS and DIC are a result of what in the hyperthermic patient?

A. Temperature increase
B. Lysosomal enzymes
C. Release of sodium
D. Retention of potassium

30. The antidote for ethanol toxicity is

A. Dextrose
B. Sodium Bicarbonate
C. Fomepizole
D. Naloxone

31. Digitalis toxicity can easily be exacerbated by

A. Acute MI
B. Electrolyte abnormalities
C. Undiagnosed diabetes
D. Beta-blockers

32. All of the following medications are classified as calcium channel blockers, *except*

    A. Diltiazem
    B. Calan, Isoptin
    C. Nicardipine
    D. Metoprolol

33. A patient presenting with a complaint of tinnitus and flulike symptoms will most likely have which of the following diagnosis?

    A. Acetominophen overdose
    B. Beta-blocker overdose
    C. Salicylate overdose
    D. Magnesium toxicity

34. Which of the following lab test is typically ordered four hours postingestion of acetaminophen overdose?

    A. BUN
    B. Liver function
    C. Electrolytes
    D. Coagulation

35. Antidote that can be administered for benzodiazepine overdose is

    A. Naloxone
    B. Romazicon
    C. Deferoxamine
    D. Fomepizole

36. Iron poisoning can be managed with

    A. Naloxone
    B. Romazicon
    C. Deferoxamine
    D. Fomepizole

37. A patient presenting with ethylene glycol ingestion would present with the following signs and symptoms, *except*

    A. Nystagmus
    B. Elevated anion gap
    C. Seizures
    D. Metabolic alkalosis

38. What assessment when managing a patient with iron ingestion would indicate that the treatment is effective?

    A. Urine output appears pink in color
    B. Increased level of consciousness
    C. Appearance of tea-colored urine output
    D. Improvement of metabolic acidosis

39. The administration of Romazicon can cause which of the following adverse reactions?

    A. Respiratory depression
    B. Seizures
    C. Hypotension
    D. Tachycardia

40. Which of the following conditions is commonly associated with ethanol intoxication?

    A. Hyperthermia
    B. Hypoglycemia
    C. Esophageal varices
    D. Increased thiamine production

41. Pralidoxime chloride is administered in the management of

    A. Heparin overdose
    B. Organophosphate exposure
    C. Iron ingestion
    D. Cyanide toxicity

42. Antidote for heparin overdose is

   A. Vitamin K
   B. Fresh frozen platelets
   C. Protamine sulfate
   D. Protopam chloride

43. Normal BUN is

   A. 0-10
   B. 6-23
   C. 15-35
   D. 35-45

44. Elevated BUN can indicate all of the following, *except*

   A. Dehydration
   B. Intra-abdominal hemorrhage
   C. Renal failure
   D. Cerebral vascular accident

45. A patient exposed to organophosphates can present with the following clinical signs/symptoms, *except*

   A. Salivation
   B. Defecation
   C. Mydriasis
   D. Pulmonary edema

46. A patient presenting with tachycardia, pale skin, a change in behavior, and diaphoresis is most likely experiencing which of the following?

   A. Insulin shock
   B. Diabetic ketoacidosis
   C. Alcohol intoxication
   D. Renal failure

47. Organophosphate exposure causes the overproduction of the neurotransmitter acetylcholine by

   A. Deactivation of the acetylcholinesterase enzyme, which is responsible for the breakdown of acetylcholine
   B. Blocking the vagus nerve
   C. Increasing adrenergic stimulation
   D. Activation of the acetycholinesterase enzyme, which is responsible for the production of aceylcholine

48. Management of cyanide toxicity includes all of the following, *except*

   A. Amyl nitrate
   B. Sodium nitrate
   C. Protopam chloride
   D. Sodium thiosulfate

49. Which medication will require the addition of sodium thiosulfate in the infusion bag to prevent thiocyanate toxicity?

   A. Neseritide
   B. Nitroglycerin
   C. Nicardipine
   D. Nitroprusside

50. Your patient ingested an unknown toxin. The electrocardiogram recorded on ER admission shows a minimally irregular wide-QRS tachycardia with a long QT interval. The most likely cause is

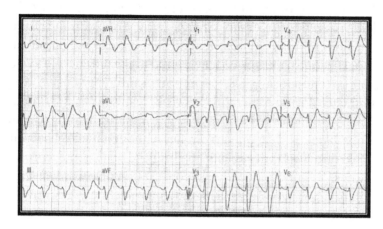

A. TCA overdose
B. Early digitalis overdose
C. Calcium channel blocker overdose
D. Beta-blocker overdose

Answer Key and Rationale

1. **C:** Beta blockers must not be used in the treatment of cocaine, amphetamine, or other alpha adrenergic stimulant overdose. The blockade of only beta receptors increases hypertension and reduces coronary blood flow, left ventricular function, cardiac output, and tissue perfusion by means of leaving the alpha adrenergic system stimulation unopposed. The appropriate antihypertensive drugs to administer during hypertensive crisis, resulting from stimulant abuse are vasodilators like nitroglycerin, diuretics like furosemide and alpha blockers like phentolamine. Although benzodiazepines and NTG are first-line agents in drug-induced acute coronary syndromes, cocaine-induced vasoconstriction also is reversed by phentolamine. Therefore, AHA 2005 Guidelines recommends phentolamine as a second-line agent.

   Cocaine stimulates both the peripheral and central adrenergic nervous system. The drug is metabolized by the liver and excreted by the kidney. With excessive or prolonged use of cocaine, the drug can cause itching, tachycardia, hallucinations, and paranoid delusions. Overdoses cause tachyarrhythmias and a marked elevation of blood pressure. Toxicity results in seizures, followed by respiratory and circulatory depression of medullar origin. This may lead to death from respiratory failure, stroke, cerebral hemorrhage, or heart failure. Cocaine is also highly pyrogenic because the stimulation and increased muscular activity cause greater heat production. Heat loss is inhibited by the intense vasoconstriction. Cocaine-induced hyperthermia may cause muscle cell destruction and myoglobinuria, resulting in renal failure. These can be life-threatening, especially if the user has existing cardiac problems.

2. **A:** The pharmacological actions of digoxin usually results in ECG changes, including ST depression or T wave inversion, which alone may not indicate toxicity. PR interval prolongation, however, may be a sign of digoxin toxicity. Cardiac manifestations are the result of depression through the sinoatrial and atrioventricular nodes and alteration of impulse formation. An often described but rarely seen noncardiac symptom of digoxin toxicity is a disturbance of

color vision (mostly yellow and green color) called xanthopsia. Treatment of digital toxicity includes supportive care, possible correction of electrolyte imbalance, or the administration of Fab fragments if conventional supportive care to life-threatening dysrhythmias and hyperkalemia fails. Fab fragments bind to digoxin, and the Fab-digoxin complex is excreted in the urine.

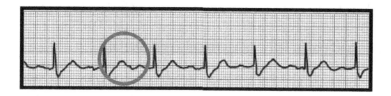

3. **A:** Salicylate toxicity initially manifests in an increased respiratory rate and hyperventilation. Blood gas analysis usually reflects respiratory alkalosis. Clinical manifestations of mild intoxication include headache, vertigo, tinnitus (ringing in the ears), mental confusion, sweating, and thirst. Severe intoxication produces similar symptoms combined with base/electrolyte imbalances. Patients are agitated, restless, and uncommunicative and may have seizures or become comatose. Noncardiac pulmonary edema is observed in severe poisoning, whereas bleeding diatheses are less common. Treatment involves gastric emptying, administration of oral-activated charcoal, and alkaline diuresis. The severely poisoned patient may require hemodialysis. Refer to the table for review of estimated dose ingested and toxic reaction.

Salicylate intoxication assessment based on the estimated dose ingested	
(number of tablets ingested times the milligrams of aspirin per tablet divided by patient weight in kilograms equals the acute ingested dose)	
Ingested amount (mg/kg)	Estimated severity of toxicity
<150	No toxic reaction expected
150-300	Mild to moderate toxic reaction
300-500	Serious toxic reaction
>500	Potentially lethal toxic reaction

. The muscle enzymes, CPK or CK, SGOT, SGPT, and LDH in heatstroke are elevated in the tens of thousands ofdiagnostic hallmark of heatstroke. These enzymes are released by damaged muscle and levels above five times the upper limit of normal indicate rhabdomyolysis. Myoglobin has a short half-life and is, therefore, less useful as a diagnostic test in the later stages. Muscle breakdown occurs from direct thermal injury, clonic muscle activity, or tissue ischemia. CPK or CK levels greater than 20,000 are ominous and are indicative of later DIC, acute renal failure, and potentially dangerous hyperkalemia.

5. **C:** If ventricular fibrillation (VF) is detected, emergency personnel should deliver three shocks to determine fibrillation responsiveness. If VF persists after three shocks, further shocks should be avoided until after rewarming to above 30°C (86°F). CPR, rewarming, and rapid transport should immediately follow the three defibrillation attempts. If core temperature is below 30°C (86°F), successful defibrillation may not be possible until rewarming is accomplished. If the patient fails to respond to initial defibrillation attempts or initial drug therapy, subsequent defibrillations or additional boluses of medication should be avoided until the core temperature rises above 30°C (86°F).

6. **B:** The consensus is that the patient should be rewarmed as quickly as possible because the myocardium is refractory to therapy below 30°C. There are three techniques for rewarming: passive external, active external, and active internal. Only passive external, active external, and limited forms of active internal rewarming measures can be initiated in the prehospital environment. Afterdrop is a dangerous phenomenon that can occur in the initial stages of passive and active external rewarming. Afterdrop is defined as a decline of 1-2°C in the core body temperature when cool blood from the extremities moves to the core. Any action that moves blood rapidly from the extremities to the heart can cause afterdrop and precipitate ventricular fibrillation. Active internal rewarming delivers heat to the body core, thereby avoiding the dangers of

afterdrop. The heart, lungs, and brain are warmed first and in turn rewarm of the rest of the body.

Rewarming techniques	
Type of technique	Definition
Passive external	It is used in mild hypothermia and when the patient can generate heat by shivering and vasoconstriction. The patient is placed in a warm environment, covered with blankets and allowed to rewarm naturally.
Active external	Involves placing heat on the external surface of the body, such as thermal blankets, heat pack to the groin, neck, and axillary areas.
Active internal	Includes heated oxygen, IV fluids, hemodialysis, peritoneal dialysis, gastric, and cardiopulmonary bypass.

7. **C**: Rhabdomyolysis is a common condition which complicates a variety of genetic and acquired diseases. It is characterized by muscle cell necrosis and release of muscle cell components into the circulation, most notably creatinine phosphokinase (CPK), also known as creatinine kinase (CK) and myoglobin. Other muscle enzymes that can be elevated are SGOT, SGPT, and LDH. The primary mechanism through which muscle damage occurs in rhabdomyolysis is sarcoplasmic calcium overload, leading to activation of degradative enzymes. This may occur secondary to a number of processes, including ATP depletion and increased intracellular sodium concentration and direct sarcolemmal injury. The complications of rhabdomyolysis can be potentially life threatening and include cardiac arrest and myoglobinuric acute renal failure. Prompt action must be taken to prevent these complications in a patient with rhabdomyolysis, most importantly aggressive intravenous volume replacement.

Heat-related disorders	
Type of heat-related illness	Clinical manifestations
Heat cramps *(adequate water replacement with inadequate replacement of salts)*	Of heavily exercised muscle occur during and after exercise in a hot environment, which involve painful sustained muscular contractions, most commonly involving the muscles of the lower extremity.
Heat exhaustion *(can result from loss of water, loss of salt or both)*	With sodium and water loss, the patient becomes dehydrated, tachycardic and orthostatic hypotension can occur. The patient retains the ability to sweat, which gives rise to cool, clammy skin. Nausea, vomiting, and diarrhea, with muscle cramps may also be present. Lab values showing classic signs of dehydration include elevated hematocrit, BUN, serum protein, and concentrated urine levels.
Heat stroke *(life-threatening medical emergency in which the body's physiologic heat-dissipating mechanisms fail, and body temperature rises rapidly)*	Central core temperature exceeds 42°C (106°F). Signs and symptoms can include confusion, irrational behavior, coma, seizures, hot, flushed skin, with or without sweating, vomiting, and diarrhea. Respiratory alkalosis, if often present with tetany and hypokalemia. Heatstroke results in high output failure, with cardiac output of 20 L or more.

Hyperthermia is an elevated body temperature due to failed thermoregulation. Hyperthermia occurs when the body produces or absorbs more heat than it can dissipate. When the elevated body temperatures are sufficiently high, hyperthermia is a medical emergency and requires immediate treatment to prevent disability and death. The most common causes are heat stroke and adverse reactions to drugs. Heat stroke is an acute condition of hyperthermia that is caused by prolonged exposure to excessive heat or heat and humidity. The heat-regulating mechanisms of the body eventually become overwhelmed and unable to effectively deal with the heat, causing the body temperature to climb uncontrollably. Hyperthermia is a relatively rare side effect of many drugs, particularly those that affect the central nervous system. Malignant hyperthermia is a rare complication of some types of general anesthesia.

8. **A:** *Acute hemolytic reaction* has the shortest onset and is considered a medical emergency. It results from rapid destruction (hemolysis) of the donor red blood cells by host antibodies, usually related to ABO blood group incompatibility—the most severe of which often involves group A red cells being given to a patient with group O type blood. Properdin then binds to complement, C3, in the donor blood, facilitating the reaction through the alternate pathway cascade. The most common cause is clerical error (i.e., the wrong unit of blood being given to the patient). The symptoms are fever and chills, sometimes with back pain and pink or red urine (hemoglobinuria). The major complication is that hemoglobin released by the destruction of red blood cells can cause acute renal failure. The most important step in treating a presumed transfusion reaction is to stop the transfusion immediately (saving the remaining blood and IV tubing for testing) and to provide supportive care to the patient. More specific treatments depend on the nature and presumed cause of the transfusion reaction.

Types of transfusion reactions	
Form of reaction	**Clinical manifestations**
Acute hemolytic	Onset can occur within minutes of the transfusion. Usually related to ABO blood group incompatibility.
Delayed hemolytic	Onset can occur 5-10 days after transfusion. Features include fever, lower than expected blood hemoglobin concentration, with associated jaundice and urobilinogenuria.
Anaphylactic	Onset can occur 30 minutes after receiving transfusion. These reactions are most common in people with selective IgA deficiency.
Febrile nonhemolytic	Onset can occur 30-90 minutes after receiving transfusion. This is the most common adverse reaction to a blood transfusion. Symptoms include fever and dyspnea. Such reactions are clinically benign, causing no lasting side effects or problems but are unpleasant.
Circulatory overload	Onset can occur anytime after receiving transfusion. Patients with impaired cardiac function (e.g., CHF) can become volume-overloaded as a result of blood transfusion, leading to edema, dyspnea (shortness of breath), and orthopnea (shortness of breath while lying flat).

9. **D:** Acute hemolytic reaction can occur within minutes of the transfusion. The most common immediate adverse reactions to transfusion are fever, chills, and urticaria. The most potentially significant reactions include acute and delayed hemolytic transfusion reactions and bacterial contamination of blood products. During the early stages of a reaction, it may be difficult to ascertain the cause.

Citrate is the anticoagulant used in blood products. It is usually rapidly metabolized by the liver. Rapid administration of large quantities of stored blood may cause citrate toxicity, resulting in hypocalcaemia and hypomagnesemia when citrate binds calcium and magnesium. This can result in myocardial depression or coagulopathy. Patients most at risk are those with liver dysfunction or neonates with immature liver function having rapid large volume transfusion.

10. **D:** TCAs exert a quinidinelike cardiac action that depresses conduction velocity, prolonged QT interval, QRS interval widening, right bundle-branch block, and first-degree heart block are common findings. More than fifty medications, many of them common, can lengthen the Q-T interval in otherwise healthy people and cause a form of acquired long QT syndrome known as drug-induced long QT syndrome. Medications that can lengthen the Q-T interval and upset heart rhythm include certain antibiotics, antidepressants, antihistamines, diuretics, heart medications, cholesterol-lowering drugs, diabetes medications, as well as some antifungal and antipsychotic drugs. An easy way to assess for a prolonged QT interval is to measure the Q-T interval from the beginning of the QRS complex to the end of the T wave. If the length measures greater than 50% the width of an R-R interval, the Q-T interval is prolonged.

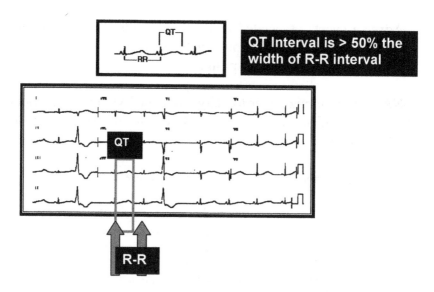

QT Interval is > 50% the width of R-R interval

11. **B:** *N-Acetylcysteine (NAC); trade name Mucomyst, Acetadote* is FDA approved to reduce the extent of liver injury after acetaminophen overdose. The primary toxic effect of acetaminophen is hepatotoxicity caused by the formation of the toxic metabolite N-acetyl-p-benzoquinonimine. Acute ingestion of 200 mg/kg in children or 6.5 grams in adults of acetaminophen may cause hepatotoxicity. Chronic ingestion of acetaminophen often occurs in adults with ongoing pain syndromes or children with febrile illnesses and can also result in hepatoxicity if the recommended daily dose is exceeded. The decision to initiate antidotal therapy following acute ingestion is based on the serum acetaminophen concentration. The Rumack-Matthew nomogram compares the acetaminophen concentration with the time since ingestion to provide guidance on which patients should be considered for antidotal therapy. The nomogram cannot be used to evaluate chronic ingestions. Oral administration is often limited by nausea and vomiting, which results in delayed or ineffective administration of NAC. Intravenous administration of NAC results in 100% bioavailability.

Adverse events associated with IV NAC administration include anaphylactoid type reactions such as flushing, urticaria, rash, hypotension, and bronchospasm.

NAC can minimize liver toxicity associated with acetaminophen and should be administered within 8-10 hours of an acute exposure when possible.

Acetominophen overdose management with Nac	
Route	Recommended dosing for adults and pediatrics
Oral NAC	The FDA approved oral dosing regimen is 140 mg/kg as the loading dose, then 70 mg/kg every 4 hours for 17 doses starting 4 hours after the loading dose. Oral NAC is irritating to the gastrointestinal track and should be diluted to a final concentration of no more than 5% to reduce the risk for vomiting. The oral form of NAC has an unpleasant odor and taste that can also affect compliance with administration.
IV NAC	The recommended adult dosage regimen for the IV formulation is a loading dose of 150 mg/kg in 200 mL of 5% dextrose given over 15 to 30 minutes.

12. **C:** The antidote for an overdose with warfarin (Coumadin) is vitamin K.

In severe cases, blood or plasma transfusions can be given to help reverse a Coumadin overdose. In all cases, the patient should be evaluated for bleeding (including less obvious internal bleeding) and appropriate measures should be taken to control the bleeding. Warfarin is prescribed to people with an increased tendency for thrombosis or as secondary prophylaxis in those individuals that have already formed a blood clot (thrombus). Warfarin treatment can help prevent formation of future blood clots and help reduce the risk of embolism. Heparin is generally used for anticoagulation for the following conditions: acute coronary syndrome (NSTEMI), atrial fibrillation, deep-vein thrombosis, pulmonary embolism, cardiopulmonary bypass for heart surgery, ECMO circuit for extracorporeal life support. Antidote dosage for heparin reversal is Protamine Sulfate 1 mg IV for every 100 IU of active heparin. In patients who are allergic to fish, it can cause significant histamine release, resulting in hypotension and bronchoconstriction, and also causes pulmonary hypertension. Infusion should be slow to minimize these side effects. In large doses, Protamine Sulfate itself has some anticoagulant effect.

Lab value monitoring will include coagulation studies. The *prothrombin time (PT)* and its derived measures of *prothrombin ratio (PR)* and *international normalized ratio (INR)* are measures of the *extrinsic pathway* of coagulation. They are used to determine the clotting tendency of blood, in the measure of warfarin dosage, liver damage, and vitamin K status. The reference range for prothrombin time is usually around 12-15 seconds; the normal range for the INR is 0.8-1.2. PT measures factors I, II, V, VII, and X. It is used in conjunction with the activated partial thromboplastin time (aPTT), which measures the *intrinsic pathway*.

13. **D:** The administration of beta-blockers or calcium channel blockers, which also reduce heart rate, are contraindicated in digitalis toxicity. *Digoxin toxicity* is a poisoning that occurs when excess doses of digoxin (digitalis) are consumed acutely or over an extended period of time. Digoxin toxicity is often divided into acute or chronic. The theraputic level for digoxin is 0.5-2.0 ng/mL. Low potassium levels predispose to digitoxicity and dysrhythmias. The classic dysrhythmia is a paroxysmal atrial tachycardia with block. Symptoms include fatigue, nausea, vomiting, changes in heart rate and rhythm, loss of appetite (anorexia), diarrhea, visual disturbances (yellow or green halos around objects), confusion, dizziness, nightmares, agitation, and/or depression. The primary treatment of digoxin toxicity is digoxin immune Digoxin (Digibind) should not be given if the apical heart rate is below 60 beats per minute. Other treatments that may be tried to treat life-threatening dysrhythmias until digoxin immune fab is acquired are Magnesium, phenytoin, and lidocaine. Atropine is also used in cases of bradydysrhythmias. In severe cases, hemodialysis may be required to reduce the levels of digoxin in the body.

14. **D:** It is essential to maintain higher rates of urinary output because hemoglobinuria and myoglobinuria are common with electrical injuries. The fluid resuscitation must be based on actual urine

flow. A minimum of 50-100 mL/hour of urine output must be maintained; however, in the presence of urinary hemochromagen, the fluid volume must sufficient quantity to maintain a minimum urine output of 100 mL/hr.

15. **C:** The current treatment of choice is the intravenous administration of dantrolene (Dantrium), the only known antidote, discontinuation of triggering agents, and supportive therapy directed at correcting hyperthermia, acidosis, and organ dysfunction. Dantrolene is a muscle relaxant that appears to work directly on the ryanodine receptor to prevent the release of calcium. Treatment must be instituted rapidly on clinical suspicion of the onset of malignant hyperthermia. *Malignant hyperthermia (MH)* is a rare life-threatening condition that is triggered by exposure to certain drugs used for general anesthesia (specifically all volatile anesthetics), nearly all gas anesthetics, and the neuromuscular blocking agent succinylcholine. In susceptible individuals, these drugs can induce a drastic and uncontrolled increase in skeletal muscle oxidative metabolism, which overwhelms the body's capacity to supply oxygen, remove carbon dioxide, and regulate body temperature, eventually leading to circulatory collapse and death if not treated quickly. Malignant hyperthermia develops during or after receiving a general anesthetic, and symptoms are generally identified by operating department staff. Characteristic signs are muscular rigidity, followed by a hypercatabolic state; with increased oxygen consumption, increased carbon dioxide production (hypercapnea, usually measured by capnography), tachycardia (fast heart rate), and an increase in body temperature (hyperthermia) at a rate of up to ~2°C per hour, temperatures up to 42°C (108°F) are not uncommon. Rhabdomyolysis (breakdown of muscle tissue) may develop as evidenced by red-brown discoloration of the urine and cardiological or neurological evidence of electrolyte disturbances.

16. **C:** Hypothermia, defined as core body temperature <95°F (35°C), is associated with ECG changes of diagnostic and prognostic importance. In the initial stages of hypothermia, a sinus tachycardia develops as part of the general stress reaction. As the temperature

drops below 90°F (32°C), a sinus bradycardia supervenes, associated with progressive prolongation of the PR interval, QRS complex, and Q-T interval. With temperature approaching 86°F (30°C), atrial ectopic activity is often noted and can progress to atrial fibrillation. At this level of hypothermia, 80% of patients have Osborn waves, also known as J waves, hypothermic waves, and camel-hump sign that consist of an extra deflection at the end of the QRS complex.

Osborn waves are positive deflections occurring at the junction between the QRS complex and the ST segment, where the S point, also known as the J point, has a MI-like elevation. The Osborne waves are best seen in the inferior and lateral precordial leads on the 12-lead ECG. They become more prominent as the body temperature drops, and they regress gradually with rewarming. Prolongation of the Q-T interval and the presence of Osborn waves are directly related to the severity of the hypothermia. With temperature <86°F (30°C), a progressive widening of the QRS complex and prolonged Q-T interval increases the risk of ventricular fibrillation. When the temperature drops to 60°F (15°C), asystole supervenes.

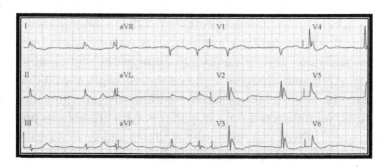

How to convert temperature	
Fahrenheit to celsius	Subtract 32 from the Fahrenheit temperature then divide by 1.8
Celsius to fahrenheit	Multiply the celsius temperature by 1.8 then add 32

17. **A:** Sinus tachycardia is the most common cardiac disturbance seen following TCA overdose. TCAs remain widely prescribed for depression and an increasing number of other indications, including anxiety disorders. TCA overdose is a significant cause of fatal drug poisoning. The severe morbidity and mortality associated with these drugs is well documented due to their cardiovascular and neurological toxicity. Additionally, it is a serious problem in the pediatric population due to their inherent toxicity and the availability of these in the home when prescribed for bed wetting and depression. An overdose on TCA is, especially, fatal as they are rapidly absorbed from GI tract in the alkaline conditions of the small intestines. As a result, toxicity often becomes apparent in the first hour after an overdose. However, symptoms may take several hours to appear if a mixed overdose has caused delayed gastric emptying.

Many of the initial signs are those associated to the anticholinergic effects of TCAs such as dry mouth, blurred vision, urinary retention, constipation, dizziness, emesis, tachycardia, mydriasis (pupil dilation), fever, and flushing (skin redness). Treatment depends on severity of symptoms and can include the administration of IV fluids, and pressor agents (alpha-adrenergic agents are preferred). GI decontamination may be helpful within the first several hours postingestion because TCAs can slow gastric emptying through the anticholinergic activity. Activated charcoal reduces the absorption of TCAs. It may also be beneficial in cases of multi-substance ingestion. It should be administered only in patients who are able to protect the airway. If there is a metabolic acidosis and/or ECG changes present (prolonged QT interval, QRS widening), infusion of sodium bicarbonate is recommended. Physostigmine is *not* an antidote to cyclic antidepressant poisoning and should not be used on these patients. Commonly known TCAs, among others, are *amitriptyline* (Elavil, Tryptizol, Laroxyl); *doxepin* (Adapin, Sinequan); *imipramine* (Tofranil, Janimine, Praminil); *nortriptyline* (Pamelor, Aventyl).

TCA overdose	
System	Clinical manifestations
Cardiac	Hypertension (early and transient, should not be treated), tachycardia, and hypotension, dysrhythmias (including ventricular tachycardia and ventricular fibrillation, most serious consequence), ECG changes include prolonged Q-T and P-R intervals, QRS widening, and RBBB because TCAs exert a quinidinelike cardiac action depresses conduction velocity. Acidosis can occur because of cardiac and respiratory depression.
CNS	Syncope, confusion, anxiety, seizure, coma, myoclonus, hyperreflexia.
Respiratory	Hypoventilation resulting from CNS depression.
GI	Decreased or absent bowel sounds.

The toxic effects of tricyclics are results of the following four main pharmacologic properties:

1. Inhibition of norepinephrine and serotonin reuptake at nerve terminals
2. Anticholinergic action
3. Direct alpha-adrenergic blockade
4. Membrane-stabilizing effect on the myocardium by blocking the cardiac myocyte fast sodium channels

18. **A:** Cooling can be accomplished by first removing the patient from the hot environment. The transport team should remove the patient's clothing and wet down the patient. Covering the patient with cool fluid and increasing the movement of air over the patient enhance heat loss by increasing the evaporative gradient. The transport team should open the windows of the ambulance or make use of the air circulation of helicopter rotors during transport to further increase air movement over the patient. Controversy surrounds the question of which method is ideal for cooling the patient with heatstroke. Several methods are considered to be of therapeutic benefit. Packing the patient in ice and immersing the body in cold water are historic methods of cooling. Other therapies involve the use of room-temperature water evaporated from the patient's skin surface by circulating air from a fan. The field treatment measure of ice packs placed

in areas of maximum heat transfer (neck, axillae, and inguinal areas) may also be continued with caution. Cooling measures are ceased when body core temperature reaches 39°C (102°F). Refractory hyperthermia will require move-invasive methods. Iced-water gastric lavage, iced peritoneal lavage, hemodialysis, and cardiopulmonary bypass have been used as end attempts in severely refractory hyperthermia.

19. **D:** *Atmospheric pressure* is the force per unit area exerted against a surface by the weight of air above that surface in the earth's atmosphere. A column of air one square inch in cross-section, measured from sea level to the top of the atmosphere, would weigh approximately 14.7 lbs per square inch (psi) or 760 mmHg (torr), which is defined as 1 atmosphere of pressure (ATM). Because the density of water is uniform throughout, the proportional relationship of pressure and depth remains constant; pressure increases 1 ATM for every thirty-three-foot column of seawater. At the given depth underwater, the total pressure will be the sum of the barometric pressure exerted by the column of air above plus the hydrostatic pressure exerted by the column of water. This is the concept of absolute pressure or atmospheres absolute (ATA). Therefore, a scuba diver at a depth of thirty-three feet will experience an ambient pressure of 2 ATM absolute pressure, or 2 ATA (air column plus water column).

20. **B:** *Decompression illness (DCI)* describes a collection of symptoms arising from decompression of the body. DCI is caused by two different mechanisms, which result in overlapping sets of symptoms. The two mechanisms are the following:

Decompression Sickness (DCS), which results from gas dissolved in body tissue under pressure, precipitating out of solution and forming bubbles on decompression. It typically afflicts scuba divers on poorly managed ascent from depth or aviators flying in inadequately pressurized aircraft. *Arterial gas embolism (AGE),* which is gas bubbles in the bloodstream. In the context of DCI these may form either as a result of precipitation of dissolved gas into the blood on depressurization, as for DCS above, or by gas entering the blood mechanically as a result of pulmonary barotrauma. Pulmonary barotrauma is a rupturing of the lungs by internal overpressurization caused by the expansion of air held in the lungs on depressurization such as a scuba diver ascending while holding the breath or the explosive decompression of an aircraft cabin or other working environment.

Diving and altitude emergencies	
Condition	Clinical manifestation
Decompression sickness (DCS)	Musculoskeletal decompression illness (Type I DCS), better known as the "bends," is the most common type of DCS, which may comprise limb or joint pain (shoulder and elbow pain most common), skin rash, pruritus, and joint swelling ("skin bends"). Type II DCS comprises more serious manifestations such as headache, fatigue, visual disturbances, motor/sensory neurologic impairment/deficits, confusion, seizures, coma, and death.
Pulmonary decompression illness	Otherwise known as the "chokes" or type IV DCS, is a result of large volumes of emboli occluding end arteries in the pulmonary circulation, altering the gas exchange and resulting in symptoms of dyspnea, chest pain, and nonproductive cough.
Arterial gas embolism (AGE)	Signs and symptoms of AGE are consistent with strokelike presentation. The most common symptom of AGE is asymmetric multiplegia or paralysis involving the lower extremities. Always suspect AGE whenever a scuba diver presents with an altered level of consciousness, respiratory distress, or signs of cerebral decompression illness.

Differentiating between DCS and AGE	
Decompression sickness (DCS)	Arterial gas embolism (AGE)
The dive must be of sufficient duration to saturate tissues	Any type of dive can cause AGE
Onset is latent (0-36 hours)	Onset is immediate (<10-120 minutes)
Neurologic deficits manifest in spinal cord and brain.	Neurologic deficits manifest in only the brain

Immediate treatment of DCS and AGE are to establish basic and advanced life-support measures, place the patient in left lateral decubitus position (Durante position) has been recommended to minimize further passage of air emboli to the brain and transport to the closest hyperbaric treatment facility for recompression. Patients should be transported in an aircraft with cabin pressurized to 1 ATA. If the aircraft cannot be pressurized to 1 ATA, such as a helicopter, it should be flown at the lowest and safest altitude possible, preferably below 1,000 feet above sea level.

21. **A:** The oxygen-hemoglobin dissociation curve illustrates the relationship between hemoglobin saturation and PaO_2. This curve depicts the ability of hemoglobin to bind and release oxygen into the tissues. Various physiologic states change the relationship between hemoglobin saturation and PaO_2.

Oxyhemoglobin diassociation curve	
Right shift	Left shift
Causes a decrease in the affinity of hemoglobin to oxygen. This makes it harder for the hemoglobin to bind to oxygen, but it makes it easier for the hemoglobin to release bound oxygen.	Causes an increase in the affinity, making the oxygen easier for the hemoglobin to pick up but harder to release.
R stands for raised/releases oxygen	L stands for low/holds onto oxygen
High temperature (hyperthermia)	Low temperature (hypothermia)
High 2,3-DPG levelsProduction increases with hypoxemia, chronic lung disease, anemia, and CHF	Low 2,3-DPG levels Production decreases with septic shock and hypophosphatemia
High pCO_2	Low pCO_2
There is *no* "L" in ACIDOSIS	There is an "L" in ALKALOSIS

22. **D:** As a diver descends from or ascends to the water's surface the effect of increasing ambient pressure on the scuba diver involve an understanding of the behavior of gases under conditions of varying pressure and volume. The following table is a brief description of the primary gas laws of diving.

Gas laws of diving	
Name	Definition
Boyle's law	States that at a constant temperature and mass the volume of a gas is inversely proportional to the total pressure. In simple terms, volume decreases as pressure increases; conversely, the volume increases as pressure decreases.
Henry's law	States that solubility is proportional to the partial pressure of a gas. As the pressure increases or decreases, the gas goes into or comes of solution. This is known as the "soda bottle" phenomenon. When you release the pressure from the bottle by removing the cap, the dissolved gas comes out of the solution.
Dalton's law	States that the total pressure of a mixture of gases equals the sum of partial pressures exerted by the constituent gases. Air comprises approximately 78% nitrogen, 21% oxygen, and 1% other gases. By increasing the total pressure of the mixture, the pressure of each constituent gas is increased proportionately. When a scuba diver is at a depth of 66 feet, the scuba diver is under an ambient pressure of 3 ATA and is breathing compressed air with partial pressures of nitrogen and oxygen 3 times their value at the surface.

23. **A:** The main goal of treatment is to treat shock and preserve kidney function. Initially this is done through the administration of generous amounts of intravenous fluids, usually saline. This will ensure sufficient circulating volume to deal with the muscle cell swelling (which typically commences when blood supply is restored) and to prevent the deposition of myoglobin in the kidneys. Amounts of six to twele liters over twenty-four hours are recommended. While many sources recommend mannitol, which acts by osmosis to ensure urine production and may prevent heme deposition in the kidney, there are no studies directly demonstrating its benefit. Similarly, the addition of bicarbonate to the fluids is intended to improve acidosis and thereby prevent cast formation in the kidneys, but there is limited evidence that it has benefits above saline alone. Furosemide, a loop diuretic, is often used to ensure sufficient urine production.

http://en.wikipedia.org/wiki/Rhabdomyolysis—cite_note-Vanholder2000-2#cite_note-Vanholder2000-2

24. **D:** Hypothermia causes the oxygen-hemoglobin dissociation curve to shift to the left. Remember everything that is low is left. Refer to the table in question no. 21.

25. **A:** *Histotoxic hypoxia* interferes with the utilization phase of respiration because of metabolic poisoning or dysfunction. Cyanide, sulfide, azide, and carbon monoxide all bind to cytochrome oxidase, thus competitively inhibiting the protein from functioning, which results in chemical asphyxiation of cells. Methanol [methylated spirits] is converted into formic acid, which also inhibits the same oxidase system.

Types of hypoxia	
Name	Definition
Hypoxic	Is a deficiency in alveolar oxygen exchange. Specific causes include breathing air at reduced barometric pressure, strangulation, respiratory arrest, laryngospasm, severe asthma, hypoventilation, breathing gas mixtures with insufficient oxygen, and malfunctioning oxygen equipment at altitude. Causes of reduction in the gas exchange area include pneumonia, drowning, atelectasis, chronic obstructive pulmonary disease, pneumothorax, pulmonary embolism, congenital heart defects, and physiologic shunting.
Hypemic	Is a reduction in the oxygen-carrying capacity of blood. Specific causes include anemia, hemorrhage, hemoglobin abnormalities, use of drugs (sulfa, nitrates), and intake of chemicals (cyanide, carbon monoxide).
Stagnant	Occurs when conditions exist that result in reduced total cardiac output, pooling of the blood within certain regions of the body, a decreased blood flow to the tissues, or restriction of blood flow. Specific causes include heart failure, shock, continuous positive-pressure breathing, acceleration (G forces), and pulmonary embolism.
Histotoxic	Considered to be tissue poisoning, occurs when metabolic disorders or poisoning of the cytochrome oxidase enzyme system results in a cell's inability to use molecular oxygen. Specific causes include respiratory enzyme, poisoning or degradation, and the intake of carbon monoxide, cyanide, or alcohol.

26. **B:** *Lysergic acid diethylamide (LSD)* is the most potent hallucinogen known. *Phencyclidine (PCP),* also known as *angel*

dust and other street names, is a recreational, dissociative drug formerly used as an anesthetic agent, exhibiting hallucinogenic and neurotoxic effects. Patients may become hostile, beligerent, and destructive. A common neurologic sign of PCP intoxication is nystagmus. Extreme caution should be taken during transport; use of ear protection, sedation, and restraints may be necessary prior to transport. In extreme situations, sedation and neuromuscular blocking agents, with airway control, may be necessary to safely transport these patients.

27. **C:** Many organophosphates are potent nerve agents, functioning by inhibiting the enzyme action of acetylcholinesterase (AChE) in nerve cells. They are one of the most common causes of poisoning worldwide and are frequently intentionally used in suicides in agricultural areas. The effects of organophosphate poisoning are recalled using the mnemonic SLUDGE (salivation, lacrimation, urination, defecation, gastrointestinal motility, emesis). These side effects occur because of the excess acetylcholine (AcH) that results from blocking acetylcholinesterase (enzyme responsible for the breakdown of AcH). In addition, bronchospasm, blurred vision, and bradycardia may result. Treatment includes the administration of Atropine (drying effect) and the antidote is pralidoxime (2-pam). Pralidoxime reversibly binds to the enzyme acetylcholinesterase, competing with organophosphate binding. Since barbiturates are potentiated by the anticholinesterases, they should be used cautiously in the treatment of seizures; diazepam is the recommended drug of choice.

28. **A:** One of the major organs that must be functional if heat is to be dissipated is the skin. The primary mechanism for heat dissipation is the evaporation of sweat. Vasodilation maximizes the cooling surface and greatly decreases peripheral vascular resistance.

29. **B:** Muscle damage is evidenced by rhabdomyolysis. Elevated creatine phophokinase (CPK) values are a diagnostic hallmark of heatstroke because of the rhabdomyolytic process. The release of destructive *lysosomal enzymes* occurs as a result of extensive muscle damage, which can lead to ARDS, DIC, and ATN.

30. **C:** *Ethylene glycol* is an organic compound widely used as an automotive antifreeze. In its pure form, it is an odorless, colorless, syrupy, sweet-tasting liquid. The major danger is due to its sweet taste. Because of that, children and animals are more inclined to consume large quantities of it than they are other poisons. The primary source of ethylene glycol in the environment is from run-off at airports where it is used in de-icing agents for runways and airplanes. Upon ingestion, ethylene glycol is oxidized to glycolic acid which is, in turn, oxidized to oxalic acid, which is toxic. This and its toxic byproducts first affect the central nervous system, then the heart, and finally the kidneys. Ingestion of sufficient amounts can be fatal if untreated. Serum blood levels guide treatment for ethylene glycol ingestion. Ethanol IV administration blocks the conversion of ethylene glycol to its toxic form. Fomepizol (Antizol) is an antidote for ethanol toxicity, which prevents the formation of toxic metabolites.

31. **D:** A group of medicines extracted from foxglove plants are called "digitalin." The use of *digitalis purpurea* extract containing cardiac glycosides for the treatment of heart conditions is used to increase cardiac contractility (positive inotrope) and as an antiarrhythmic agent to control the heart rate, particularly in atrial fibrillation. Digitalis is often prescribed for patients in atrial fibrillation, especially if they have been diagnosed with CHF. Digitalis works by inhibiting sodium-potassium ATPase. This results in an increased intracellular concentration of sodium, which in turn increases intracellular calcium by passively decreasing the action of the sodium-calcium exchanger in the sarcoplasmic reticulum. The increased intracellular calcium gives a positive inotropic effect. Digitalis poisoning can cause heart block and either bradycardia or tachycardia, depending on the dose and the condition of the patients heart. The classic drug of choice for VF (ventricular fibrillation) in the emergency setting, amiodarone, can worsen the dysrhythmia caused by digitalis; therefore, the second-choice drug lidocaine is more commonly used.

32. **D:** *Metoprolol* is classified as a beta-blocker, which blocks the action of endogenous catecholamines (epinephrine and

norepinephrine) in particular, on β-adrenergic receptors, part of the sympathetic nervous system, which mediates the "fight or flight" response. There are three known types of beta receptors, designated β_1 *(one heart)*, β_2 *(two lungs)* and β_3 receptors. β_1-adrenergic receptors are located mainly in the heart and in the kidneys. β_2-adrenergic receptors are located mainly in the lungs, gastrointestinal tract, liver, uterus, vascular smooth muscle, and skeletal muscle. β_3-adrenergic receptors are located in fat cells. Some beta-blockers such as, labetalol and carvedilol, exhibit mixed antagonism of both β—and α_1-adrenergic receptors, which provides additional arteriolar vasodilating action. *Calcium channel blockers* are a class of drugs and natural substances that disrupt the calcium (Ca^{2+}) conduction of calcium channels.

33. **C:** The main undesirable side effects of aspirin are gastrointestinal ulcers, stomach bleeding, and tinnitus, especially in higher doses. In children and adolescents, aspirin is no longer used to control flulike symptoms or the symptoms of chickenpox or other viral illnesses because of the risk of Reye's syndrome. Aspirin overdose can be acute or chronic. In acute poisoning, a single large dose is taken; in chronic poisoning, higher than normal doses are taken over a period of time. Toxicity is managed with a number of potential treatments, including activated charcoal, intravenous dextrose, normal saline, sodium bicarbonate, and dialysis.

34. **B:** The most effective way to diagnose aceteminophen poisoning is by obtaining a blood acetominophen level. A drug nomogram developed in 1975, called the Rumack-Matthew nomogram, estimates the risk of toxicity based on the serum concentration of acetominophen at a given number of hours after ingestion. Use of a timed serum paracetamol level plotted on the nomogram appears to be the best marker, indicating the potential for liver injury. Acetominophen level drawn in the first four hours after ingestion may underestimate the amount in the system because acetominophen may still be in the process of being absorbed from the gastrointestinal tract. Therefore, a serum level taken before four hours is not recommended. The toxic dose of acetominophen is highly variable. In adults, single doses above 10 grams or 200 mg/kg of bodyweight, whichever is lower, have a reasonable

likelihood of causing toxicity. In children acute doses above 200 mg/kg could potentially cause toxicity.

Damage to the liver, or hepatotoxicity results not from Tylenol itself but from one of its metobolites, N-acetyl-p-benzoquinonemine (NAPQI). NAPQI depletes the liver's natural antioxidant glutathione and directly damages cells in the liver, leading to liver failure. Treatment is aimed at removing the acetominophen from the body and replacing glutathione. Activated charcoal can be used to decrease absorption of acetominophen if the patient presents for treatment soon after the overdose; the antidote *N-acetylcysteine (NAC)* acts as a precursor for glutathione, helping the body regenerate enough to prevent damage to the liver. A liver transplant is often required if damage to the liver becomes severe.

Acetominiphen toxicity phases	
Phase	Clinical manifestations
I	The first phase begins within hours of overdose and consists of nausea, vomiting, pallor, and sweating. Patients often have no specific symptoms or only mild symptoms in the first 24 hours of poisoning.
II	The second phase occurs between 24 and 72 hours following overdose and consists of signs of increasing liver damage. In general, damage occurs in hepatocytes as they metabolize the acetominophen. Signs and symptoms can include right upper quadrant pain, acute renal failure; laboratory studies may show evidence of hepatic necrosis with elevated AST, ALT, bilirubin, and prolonged coagulation times, particularly an elevated prothrombin time (PT).
III	The third phase follows at 3 to 5 days, and is marked by complications of massive hepatic necrosis, leading to fulminant hepatic failure with complications of coagulation defects, hypoglycemia, kidney failure, hepatic encephalopathy, cerebral edema, sepsis, multiple organ failure, and death.

35. **B:** *Flumazenil* (also known as trade names *Anexate, Lanexat, Mazicon, Romazicon)* is a competitive benzodiazepine receptor antagonist that can be used as an antidote for benzodiazepine overdose. It reverses the effects of benzodiazepines by competitive inhibition at the benzodiazepine binding site on

the GABA receptor. Flumazenil is very effective at reversing the CNS depression associated with benzodiazepines but is less effective at reversing respiratory depression. There are many complications that must be taken into consideration when used in the acute care setting. Its use, however, is controversial as it has numerous contraindications. It is contraindicated in patients who are on long-term benzodiazepines, those who have ingested a substance that lowers the seizure threshold, or in patients who have tachycardia, widened QRS complex, anticholinergic signs, or a history of seizures. Due to these contraindications and the possibility of it causing severe adverse effects, including seizures, adverse cardiac effects, and death, in the majority of cases, there is no indication for the use of flumazenil in the management of benzodiazepine overdose as the risks generally outweigh any potential benefit of administration. It also has no role in the management of unknown overdoses. Additionally, if full airway protection has been achieved, a good outcome is expected and therefore, flumazenil administration is unlikely to be required.

36. **C:** The specific antidote for moderate to severe cases of iron poisoning is deferoxamine, a chelator that binds the ferric ion and forms a ferrioxamine complex, a water-soluble compound that is excreted in the urine (thereby reducing the iron load). Serious iron poisoning usually causes symptoms within six hours of the overdose. The symptoms of iron poisoning typically occur in five stages. In stage 1 (within 6 hours after the overdose), symptoms include vomiting, vomiting blood, diarrhea, abdominal pain, irritability, drowsiness, unconsciousness, and seizures. Deferoxamine mesylate, for injection, is an iron-chelating agent, available in vials for intramuscular, subcutaneous, and intravenous administration. Deferoxamine mesylate is contraindicated in patients with severe renal disease or anuria, since the drug and the iron chelate are excreted primarily by the kidney. Excretion of the resulting ferrioxamine complex results in *pink-red urine* that is classically called "vin-rosé urine."

37. **D:** Symptoms of ethylene glycol poisoning usually follow a three-step progression, although poisoned individuals will not

always develop each stage. Other laboratory abnormalities may suggest poisoning, especially the presence of a metabolic acidosis, particularly if it is characterized by a large anion gap. Large anion gap acidosis is usually present during the initial stage of poisoning.

Ethylene glycol toxicity stages	
Stages	Clinical manifestations
I	Stage 1 (0.5 to 12 hours) consists of neurological and gastrointestinal symptoms; patients may appear to be intoxicated, exhibiting symptoms such as dizziness, incoordination of muscle movements, nystagmus, headaches, slurred speech, and confusion. Irritation to the stomach may cause nausea and vomiting.
II	Stage 2 (12 to 36 hours) is a result of accumulation of organic acids formed by the metabolism of ethylene glycol and consists of increased heart rate, high blood pressure, hyperventilation, and metabolic acidosis. Additionally low calcium levels in the blood, overactive muscle reflexes, muscle spasms, prolonged Q-T interval, and congestive hear failure may occur. If untreated, death most commonly occurs during this period.
III	Stage 3 (24 to 72 hours) of ethylene glycol poisoning is the result of kidney injury. Symptoms include acute tubular necrosis, red blood cells in the urine, excess proteins in the urine, lower back pain, decreased production of urine, anuria, hyperkalemia, and acute kidney failure. If kidney failure occurs, it is typically reversible, although weeks or months of supportive care, including hemodialysis may be required before kidney function returns.

38. **A:** Excretion of the resulting ferrioxamine complex results in *pink-red urine* that is classically called "vin-rosé urine."

39. **B:** Romazicon has the possibility of causing severe adverse effects including seizures, adverse cardiac effects, and death. In the majority of cases, there is no indication for the use of flumazenil in the management of benzodiazepine overdose as the risks generally outweigh any potential benefit of administration. Additionally, if full airway protection has been achieved, a good outcome is expected and therefore, flumazenil administration is unlikely to be required.

40. **B:** Alcohol and *hypoglycemia* are the two things that really do not go together. Sometimes people with hypoglycemia or "low blood sugar" are mistaken for drunks. This is because their reaction to sugar and alcohol can be very similar. The high sugar content of some alcoholic drinks alone can cause blood sugar to drop so fast that they appear intoxicated. This is because over consumption of sugar causes the pancreas to release insulin into the blood stream. Because insulin has a much longer half-life (the time of a substance to reduce itself by half) than sugar, the insulin will remain longer in the blood than the sugar.

Wernicke-Korsakoff syndrome is a neurological condition, caused by an acute deficiency of the vitamin thiamine, often related to acute and chronic alcohol use. Symptoms include confusion, profound short-term memory loss, incoordination, and abnormalities of eye movement (gaze palsies). Excessive prolonged use of alcohol can damage the stomach lining (gastritis), esophagus (esophageal varices), liver (liver failure, cirrhosis), pancreas (pancreatitis), and heart (cardiomyopathy). Ethanol enhances cutaneous blood flow, which causes heat loss through vasodilation.

41. **B:** The mainstays of medical therapy in organophosphate (OP) poisoning include Atropine, *pralidoxime (2-PAM, Protopam),* and benzodiazepines. Pralidoxime is a nucleophilic agent that reactivates the phosphorylated AChE by binding to the OP molecule. Used as an antidote to reverse muscle paralysis, resulting from OP AChE pesticide poisoning but is not effective once the OP compound has bound AChE irreversibly (aged). Current recommendation is administration within forty-eight hours of OP poisoning. Because it does not significantly relieve depression of respiratory center or decrease muscarinic effects of AChE poisoning, administer Atropine concomitantly to block these effects of OP poisoning. Signs of atropinization might occur earlier with addition of 2-PAM to treatment regimen. 2-PAM administration is not indicated for carbamate exposure since no aging occurs.

42. **C:** *Protamine sulfate* is a drug that reverses the anticoagulant effects of heparin by binding to it.

List of antidotes	
Antidote	**Toxicity/Overdose/Exposure Indication/s**
Activate charcoal	Many oral toxins
Atropine	Organophosphate, carbamate insecticides, some mushrooms
Beta-blockers	Theophylline
Calcium chloride	Black widow spider bites
Calcium gluconate	Hydrofluoric acid
Chelators	Heavy metal poisoning
Cyanide Kit (amyl nitrite, sodium nitrite, or thiosulfate)	Cyanide poisoning
Deferoxamine mesylate	Iron poisoning
Digoxin immune fab antibody (digibind and digifab)	Digoxin poisoning
Diphenhydramine	Extrapyramidal reactions (dystonic) associated with antipsychotic or phenothiazine medications
Ethanol or Fomepizole	Ethylene glycol poisoning and methanol poisoning
Flumazenil	Benzodiazepine poisoning
Glucagon	Beta-blocker and calcium channel blocker poisoning
Hyperbaric Oxygen Therapy	Carbon monoxide and cyanide poisoning
Insulin	Beta-blocker and calcium channel blocker poisoning
Methylene Blue	Methemoglobinemia
Naloxone	Opioid poisoning
N-acetylcysteine	Acetaminophen poisoning
Octreotide	Oral hypoglycemic agents, gastrointestinal bleeding secondary to esophageal varices
Pralidoxime chloride (2-PAM)	Organophosphate insecticide poisoning
Protamine Sulfate	Heparin poisoning
Prussian blue	Thallium poisoning
Physostigmine sulfate	Anticholinergic poisoning
Pyridoxine	Isoniazide (INH) poisoning, ethylene glycol
Phytomenadione (vitamin K) and fresh frozen plasma	Warfarin poisoning
Sodium bicarbonate	Aspirin, tricyclic antidepressants with wide QRS

43. **D:** BUN:creatinine ratio is usually >20:1 in prerenal and postrenal azotemia, and <12:1 in acute tubular necrosis.

Laboratory values		
Lab test	Normal range	Clinical manifestations
Sodium	135-145	<120 or >160 can cause seizures.
Potassium	3.5-4.5	>7 can cause ventricular dysrhythmias; ECG findings peaked/tented T wave >5 mm in height.
Calcium	8.8-10.4	Trouseau's and Chvostek's signs can indicate hypocalcemia.
CO_2	24-30	<20 can indicate acidosis; look for cause; calculate anion gap.
BUN	6-23	Elevated BUN can indicate dehydration, blood in the gut or renal failure.
Creatinine	0.6-1.4	Elevated indicates renal failure; BUN will be elevated.
Glucose	70-110	Assess for changes in behavior
Serum Os	285-295	Maintain <320 in the head-injured patient.
Magnesium	1.5-2.5	Levels of 4-8 are therapeutic levels in the preeclampsia obstetrical patient to prevent seizures. Levels >10 can be toxic and may require the administration of calcium.
Ammonia	Adult: 15-45 Pediatric: 40-80	Increased levels with Reye's syndrome and hepatic encepholapathy. Evacuate the bowel of any blood (blood contains protein which increases ammonia levels).
BNP	<100	Measurable peptide used to diagnosis CHF but can be nonspecific. Levels >500 CHF diagnosis.
Hemoglobin	12-18	Low indicates anemia; high many causes
Hematacrit	36-52%	Low indicates anemia; high can indicate dehydration and other conditions
Platelets	150-400	Low platelets (thrombocytopenia), high platelets (thrombosis).
WBC	4.5-10.5	Are more elevated in the pediatric patient, but is considered normal range.
CK/CPK	60-400	>20,000 are ominous and is indicative of later DIC, acute renal failure and potentially dangerous hyperkalemia in heatstroke.

44. **D:** Increased BUN levels suggest impaired kidney function. This may be due to acute or chronic kidney disease, damage, or failure. It may also be due to a condition that results in decreased blood flow to the kidneys, such as CHF, shock, stress, recent MI, or severe burns, conditions that cause obstruction of urine flow or dehydration. BUN concentrations may be elevated when there is excessive protein breakdown (catabolism), significantly increased protein in the diet, or gastrointestinal bleeding (because of the proteins present in the blood).

45. **C:** Many organophosphates are potent nerve agents, functioning by inhibiting the action of acetylcholinesterase (AChE) in nerve cells. They are one of the most common causes of poisoning worldwide, and are frequently intentionally used in suicides in agricultural areas. The effects of organophosphate poisoning are recalled using the mnemonic *SLUDGE* (salivation, lacrimation, urination, defecation, gastrointestinal motility, emesis). These side effects occur because of the excess acetylcholine that results from blocking acetylcholinesterase. In addition, bronchospasm, blurred vision, and bradycardia may result. Another mnemonic is *DUMBBELSS,* which stands for diarrhea, urination, *miosis,* bradycardia, bronchoconstriction, excitation (as of muscle in the form of fasciculations and CNS), lacrimation, salivation, and sweating.

46. **A:** Hypoglycemic *(insulin shock)* symptoms and manifestations can be divided into those produced by the counter-regulatory hormones (epinephrine and glucagon) triggered by the falling glucose, and the neuroglycopenic effects produced by the reduced brain sugar.

Hypoglycemia clinical manifestations		
Adrenergic	Glucagon	Neuroglycopenic
Shakiness, anxiety, nervousness, palpitations, tachycardia, diaphoresis, feeling of warmth, pallor, coldness, dilated pupils (mydriasis), feeling of numbness "pins and needles" (parasthesia).	Hunger, nausea, vomiting, abdominal discomfort, and headache.	Abnormal mentation, impaired judgment, nonspecific dysphoria, anxiety, personality changes, belligerence, combativeness, fatigue, weakness, apathy, lethargy, ataxia, incoordination, sometimes mistaken for "drunkenness," and seizures.

47. **A:** The primary mechanism of action of organophosphate pesticides is inhibition of carboxyl ester hydrolases, particularly acetylcholinesterase (AChE). AChE is an enzyme that degrades the neurotransmitter acetylcholine (ACh) into choline and acetic acid. ACh is found in the central and peripheral nervous system, neuromuscular junctions, and red blood cells (RBCs). Organophosphates inactivate AChE by phosphorylating the serine hydroxyl group located at the active site of AChE. The phosphorylation occurs by loss of an organophosphate leaving group and establishment of a covalent bond with AChE. Once AChE has been inactivated, ACh accumulates throughout the nervous system, resulting in overstimulation of muscarinic and nicotinic receptors. Clinical effects are manifested via activation of the autonomic and central nervous systems and at nicotinic receptors on skeletal muscle. Organophosphates can be absorbed cutaneously, ingested, inhaled, or injected. Although most patients rapidly become symptomatic, the onset and severity of symptoms depend on the specific compound, amount, route of exposure, and rate of metabolic degradation.

48. **C:** *Pralidoxime chloride* (2-PAM, protopam) is a nucleophilic agent that reactivates the phosphorylated AChE by binding to the OP molecule.

49. **D:** *Sodium nitroprusside* is an antihypertensive agent used frequently in the critical care setting. Recently, the Food and Drug Administration (FDA) published a report that led to a labeling change, emphasizing the pharmacokinetics of nitroprusside with metabolism to highly toxic cyanide. Although evidence validates that cyanogenesis occurs with nitroprusside administration, prevention and treatment of cyanide poisoning is rarely instituted in clinical practice. Simultaneous infusion of thiosulfate with nitroprusside provides the sulfur donor necessary to prevent cyanide accumulation. Cyanide combines with thiosulfate to form the less toxic sodium thiocyanate, which is then excreted. A 10:1 ratio of nitroprusside to thiosulfate in the infusion eliminates the possibility of cyanide intoxication without altering the efficacy of nitroprusside.

50. **A:** *Tricyclic antidepressants,* (commonly called TCAs) have been prescribed since the 1950s for depression. Examples of TCAs are imipramine (Tofranil), amitriptyline (Elavil) and nortriptyline (Pamelor). Sinus tachycardia, the result of anticholinergic effects, often occurs with therapeutic doses of tricyclic antidepressants and has been a poor marker for serious toxicity. In a small study of patients with an acute overdose of tricyclic antidepressants, QRS prolongation, probably a manifestation of the quinidinelike effects of the drugs, was a better predictor of seizures and ventricular arrhythmias than was a serum drug level. Sodium loading may be the most important factor in the reversal of the symptoms of cyclic antidepressant toxicity. Prolonged QRS is most often the indication for serum alkalinization in TCA toxicity.

Although beta-blockers were once contraindicated in CHF, as they have the potential to worsen the condition, studies in the late 1990s showed their positive effects on morbidity and mortality in CHF. Bisoprolol, carvedilol, and sustained-release metoprolol are specifically indicated as adjuncts to standard ACE inhibitor and diuretic therapy in CHF.

Beta-blockers are primarily known for their reductive effect on heart rate, although this is not the only mechanism of action of importance in CHF. Beta-blockers, in addition to their sympatholytic B1 activity in the heart, influence the renin/angiotensin system at the kidneys. Beta-blockers cause a decrease in renin secretion, which, in turn, reduce the heart oxygen demand by lowering extracellular volume and increasing the oxygen-carrying capacity of blood. Beta-blockers' sympatholytic activity reduce heart rate, thereby increasing the ejection fraction of the heart despite an initial reduction in ejection fraction.

Glucagon has been used in the treatment of overdose. Glucagon has a positive inotropic action on the heart and decreases renal vascular resistance. It is, therefore, useful in patients with beta-blocker cardiotoxicity. Cardiac pacing should be reserved for patients unresponsive to pharmacological therapy.

The most widespread clinical usage of calcium channel blockers is to decrease blood pressure in patients with hypertension, with particular efficacy in treating elderly patients. With a relatively low blood pressure, the afterload on the heart decreases; this decreases the amount of oxygen required by the heart. Calcium channel blockers, frequently, are used to control heart rate, prevent cerebral vasospasm, and reduce chest pain due to angina pectoris. Most calcium channel blockers decrease the force of contraction of the myocardium. Calcium channel blockers work by blocking voltage-gated calcium channels in cardiac muscle and blood vessels. This decreases intracellular calcium, leading to a reduction in muscle contraction. In the heart, a decrease in calcium available for each beat results in a decrease in cardiac contractility. It is because of the negative inotropic effects of most calcium channel blockers that they are avoided (or used with caution) in individuals with cardiomyopathy. Many calcium channel blockers also slow down the conduction of electrical activity within the heart by blocking the calcium channel during the plateau phase of the action potential of the heart. This results in a negative chronotropic effect, resulting in a lowering of the heart rate and the potential for heart block. The negative chronotropic effects of calcium channel blockers make them a commonly used class of agents in individuals with atrial fibrillation or flutter in whom control of the heart rate is an issue. Treatment of calcium channel blocker toxicity involves intravenous calcium, atropine, fluids, insulin, and inotropes. Insulin is required because, at high doses, calcium channel blockers block the effect of insulin.

Bibliogaphy

2005 American Heart Association guidelines for cardiopulmonary resuscitation and emergency cardiovascular care. Part 7.2: Management of Cardiac Arrest. *Circulation.* 2005; 112 (24 Suppl): IV 58-66.

Acetadote® package insert. Issued March 2004. Cumberland Pharmaceuticals, Nashville, TN.

Alonso, J, Cardellach, F, López S, Casademont J, Miró O. Carbon monoxide specifically inhibits cytochrome c oxidase of human mitochondrial respiratory chain. *Pharmacol Toxicol.* 2003; 93(3):142-6.

Arthur, DC, Margulies, RA. A short course in diving medicine. *Ann Emerg Med.* 1987; 16:689-701.

Association of Air Medical Services. (2004). *Guidelines for Air Medical Crew Education,* Iowa, Kendall/Hunt Publishing Company.

Aydin, M, Gursurer, M, Bayraktaroglu, T, Kulah, E, Onuk, T. Prominent J wave (Osborn wave) with coincidental hypothermia in a 64-year-old woman. *Tex Heart Inst J.* 2005; 32(1):105.

Ayotte, P, Hébert, M, Marchand, P. Why is hydrofluoric acid a weak acid? *J Chem Phys.* 2005; 123(18):184501.

Barceloux, DG, Krenzelok, EP, Olson, K, Watson, W. American academy of clinical toxicology practice guidelines on the treatment of ethylene glycol poisoning. Ad hoc committee. *Clin toxicol.* 1999; 37(5):537-60.

Bartlett, D. Acetaminophen toxicity. *Journal of emergency nursing: JEN: official publication of the Emergency Department Nurses Association* 30 (3): 281-3.

Bizovi, KE, Smilkstein, MJ. (2002). Analgesics and nonprescription medications. In: Goldfrank, LR, Flomenbaum, NE, Lewin, NA, Howland, MA, Hoffman, RS, Nelson, LS, (Eds). *Goldfrank's Toxicologic Emergencies.* 7th edition. New York, NY: McGraw-Hill. pp. 480-501.

Borron, SW, Baud, FJ, Mégarbane, B, Bismuth, C. Hydroxocobalamin for severe acute cyanide poisoning by ingestion or inhalation. *Am J Emerg Med.* 2007; 25(5):551-8.

Bosch, X, Poch, E, Grau, JM. Rhabdomyolysis and acute kidney injury. *N Engl J Med.* 2009; 361(1):62-72.

Brent, J. Current management of ethylene glycol poisoning. *Drugs.* 2001; 61(7):979-88.

Bronstein, AC, Spyker, DA, Cantilena, LR Jr, Green JL, Rumack BH, Heard, SE. 2007 Annual Report of the American Association of Poison Control Centers' National Poison Data System (NPDS): 25th Annual Report. *Clin Toxicol (Phila).* Dec 2008; 46(10):927-1057.

Bronstein, AC, Spyker, DA, Cantilena, LR Jr, Green, JL, Rumack, BH, Heard, SE. 2007 Annual Report of the American Association of Poison Control Centers' National Poison Data System (NPDS): 25th Annual Report. *Clin Toxicol (Phila).* Dec 2008; (10):927-1057.

Buckley, NA, Dawson, AH, Whyte, IM, O'Connell, DL. Relativ Wiley CC, Wiley JF (1998). Pediatric benzodiazepine ingestion resulting in hospitalization. *J Toxicol Clin Toxicol.* 36(3):227-31. etoxicity of benzodiazepines in overdose. *BMJ* 310(6974):219-21.

Burr, W, Sandham, P, Judd, A (June 1989). Death after flumazepil. *BMJ.* 298(6689):1713.

Caravati, EM, Erdman, AR, Christianson, G, et al. Ethylene glycol exposure: an evidence-based consensus guideline for out-of-hospital management. *Clin toxicol, (Philadelphia, Pa.).* 2005; 43(5):327-45.

Chuang, FR, Jang, SW, Lin, JL, Chern, MS, Chen, JB, Hsu, KT. QTc prolongation indicates a poor prognosis in patients with organophosphate poisoning. *Am J Emerg Med.* 1996; 14(5):451-3.

Clark, RF. Insecticides: Organic Phosphorus compounds and Carbamates. In: Goldfrank LR, Flomenbaum NE, Lewin NA, Nelson LS, Howland MA, Hoffman RS, (Eds.). *Goldfrank's Toxicologic Emergencies. Stamford, Ct: Appleton & Lange.* 8th edition. 2006. pp.1497-1512.

Clay, KL, Murphy, RC. On the metabolic acidosis of ethylene glycol intoxication. *Toxicol Appl pharmacol.* 1977; 39(1):39-49.

Cohen, MJ, Hanbury, R, Stimmel, B. Abuse of amitriptyline. *JAMA.* 1978; 240(13):1372-3.

Dargan, PI, Wallace, CI, Jones, AL. An evidenced based flowchart to guide the management of acute salicylate (aspirin) overdose. *Emerg Med J.* 2002; 19(3):206-9.

Darovic, G. (1999). *Handbook of Hemodynamic Monitoring,* 2nd edition. Philadelphia, W.B. Saunders.

Dart, RC. Hydroxocobalamin for acute cyanide poisoning. *Clin Toxicol.* 2006; *44(1):1-3.*

Ferguson, RK, Boutros, AR. Death following self-poisoning with aspirin. *J Am Med Assoc.* 1970; 213(7):1186-8.

Flowers, D, Clark, JF, Westney, LS. Cocaine intoxication associated with abruptio placentae. *J Natl Med Assoc.* 1991; 83(3):230-2.

Gabow, PA, Clay, K, Sullivan, JB, Lepoff, R. Organic acids in ethylene glycol intoxication. *Ann Intern Med.* 1986; 105(1):16-20.

Goldfrank LR, ed. *Goldfrank's Toxicologic Emergencies.* 8th ed. New York, NY: McGraw Hill; 2006.

Goldfrank, LR. (2002). *Goldfrank's toxicologic emergencies.* New York, McGraw-Hill Medical Publ. Division.

Green, RD, Leitch, DR. Twenty years of treating decompression sickness. *Aviat Space Environ Med.* 1987; 58:362-6.

Greenwood, NN, Earnshaw, A. (1984). *Chemistry of the Elements.* Pergamon, Oxford. p. 921.

Hall, AH, Dart, R, Bogdan, G. Sodium thiosulfate or hydroxocobalamin for the empiric treatment of cyanide poisoning. *Ann Emerg Med.* 2007; 49(6):806-13.

Halsall, PJ, Hopkins, PM. Malignant hyperthermia. *Continuing Education in Anaesthesia, Critical Care and Pain.* 2003; 3(1):5-9.

Harrigan, RA, Brady, WJ. ECG abnormalities in tricyclic antidepressant ingestion. *Am J Emerg Med.* 1999; 17(4):387-93.

Heard, K, Cain, BS, Dart, RC, Cairns, CB. Tricyclic antidepressants directly depress human myocardial mechanical function independent of effects on the conduction system. *Acad Emerg Med.* 2001; 8(12):1122-7.

Heard, KJ. Acetylcysteine for acetaminophen poisoning. *N Engl J Med.* 2008; 359(3):285-92.

Höjer, J, Baehrendtz, S, Gustafsson, L. Benzodiazepine poisoning: experience of 702 admissions to an intensive care unit during a 14-year period. *J Intern Med.* 1989; 226(2):117-22.

Holleran, R. (1996). *Flight Nursing: Principles and Practice,* 2nd edition. St. Louis, Mosby.

Holleran, R. (2003). *Air and Surface Patient Transport: Principles and Practice,* 3rd edition. St. Louis, Mosby.

Holleran, R. (2009) *ASTNA Patient Transport: Principles and Practice,* 4th edition. St. Louis, Mosby.

Huerta-Alardín, AL, Varon, J, Marik, PE. Bench-to-bedside review: rhabdomyolysis—an overview for clinicians. *Crit Care.* 2005; 9(2):158-69.

Hugh A McAllister Jr, Imad AA, Mohammed K, Edward JB Jr, 2000 American Heart Association, Inc. Obsorn Waves of Hypothermia. *Circulation.* 2000; 101:e233.

Isbister, GW, I, Dawson, A. Pediatric acetaminophen overdose. *Journal of toxicology. Clin toxicol.* 2001; 39(2):169-72.

Johnston, RP, Broome, JR, Hunt, PD, et al. Patent foramen ovale and decompression illness in divers (letter). *Lancet.* 1996; 348:1515.

Jones, A. Over-the-counter analgesics: a toxicology perspective. *Am J Ther.* 2002; 9(3):245-57.

King, JO, Denborough, MA, Zapf, PW. Inheritance of malignant hyperpyrexia. *Lancet.* 1972; 1(7746):365-70.

Knauth, M, Ries, S, Pohimann, S, et al. Cohort study of multiple brain lesions in sport divers: role of a patent foramen ovale. *BMJ.* 1997; 314:701-703.

Kolb, ME, Horne, ML, Martz, R. Dantrolene in human malignant hyperthermia. *Anesthesiology* 1982; 56(4):254-62.

Kot, J, Sicko, Z, Michalkiewicz, M, Lizak, E, Góralczyk, P. Recompression treatment for decompression illness: 5-year report (2003-2007) from National Centre for Hyperbaric Medicine in Poland. *Int Marit Health.* 2008; 59(1-4):69-80.

Krause, T, Gerbershagen, MU, Fiege, M, Weisshorn, R, Wappler, F. Dantrolene—a review of its pharmacology, therapeutic use and new developments. *Anaesthesia.* 2004; 59 (4):364-73.

Krupa, D. (1997), *Flight Nursing Core Curriculum.* Park Ridge, IL, National Flight Nurses Association.

Lawrence, DT. Toxicity, Iron. *eMedicine Journal* [serial online]. Last updated October 30, 2006.

Liebelt, EL, Francis, PD, Woolf, AD. ECG lead aV_R versus QRS interval in predicting seizures and arrhythmias in acute tricyclic antidepressant toxicity. *Ann Emerg Med.* 1995; 26(2):195-201.

Litman, R, Rosenberg, H. Malignant hyperthermia: update on susceptibility testing. *JAMA.* 2005; 293(23):2918-24.

Lynn, BB. *Toxicity, Cocaine: Treatment and Medication.* Emergency Medicine, Last updated March 19, 2010

Melanson, SE, Lewandrowski, EL, Griggs, DA, Flood, JG. Interpreting tricyclic antidepressant measurements in urine in an emergency department setting: comparison of two qualitative point-of-care urine tricyclic antidepressant drug immunoassays with quantitative serum chromatographic analysis. *J Anal Toxicol.* 2007; 31(5):270-5.

Mitchell, JR, Jollow, DJ, Potter, WZ, Gillette, JR, Brodie, BB. Acetaminophen-induced hepatic necrosis. IV. Protective role of glutathione. *J Pharmacol Exp Ther.* 1973; 187(1):211-7.

Mitchell, SJ, Doolette, DJ. Selective vulnerability of the inner ear to decompression sickness in divers with right-to-left shunt: the role of tissue gas supersaturation. *J Appl Physiol.* 2009; 106(1):298-301.

Monteban-Kooistra, WE, van den Berg, MP, Tulleken, JE. Brugada electrocardiographic pattern elicited by cyclic antidepressants overdose. *Intensive Care Med.* 2006; 32(2):281-5.

Newton, HB, Burkart J, Pearl, D, Padilla, W. Neurological decompression illness and hematocrit: analysis of a consecutive series of 200 recreational scuba divers. *Undersea Hyperb Med.* 2008; 35(2):99-106.

Ngo, AS, Anthony, CR, Samuel, M, Wong, E, Ponampalam, R. Should a benzodiazepine antagonist be used in unconscious patients presenting to the emergency department? *Resuscitation.* 2007; 74(1):27-37.

Prescott, LF, Balali-Mood, M, Critchley, JA, Johnstone, AF, Proudfoot, AT. Diuresis or urinary alkalinization for salicylate poisoning? *Br Med J (Clin Res Ed).* 1982; 285 (6352):1383-6.

Rang, HP, Dale, MM, Ritter, JM, Moore, PK. (2003). *Pharmacology,* 5th edition. Edinburgh, Churchill Livingstone.

Rosenbaum, T, Kou, M. Are one or two dangerous? Tricyclic antidepressant exposure in toddlers. *J Emerg Med.* 2005; 28(2):169-74.

Sauret, JM, Marinides, G, Wang, GK. Rhabdomyolysis. *Am Fam Physician.* 2002; 65(5):907-12.

Schmidt, LE, Dalhoff, K, Poulsen, HE. Acute versus chronic alcohol consumption in acetaminophen-induced hepatotoxicity. *Hepatology.* 2002; 35(4):876-82.

Spanierman, C. Toxicity, Iron. *eMedicine Journal* [serial online]. Last updated January 8, 2007.

Spiller, HA, Sawyer, TS. Impact of activated charcoal after acute acetaminophen overdoses treated with N-acetylcysteine. *J Emerg Med* 2007; 33(2):141-4.

Teicher, M, Glod, C, Cole, J. Antidepressant drugs and the emergence of suicidal tendencies. *Drug Saf.* 1993; 8(3):186-212.

Thanacoody, HK, Thomas, SH. Tricyclic antidepressant poisoning: cardiovascular toxicity. *Toxicol Rev.* 2005; 24(3):205-14.

Hall, VA, Guest, JM. Sodium nitroprusside-induced cyanide intoxication and prevention with sodium thiosulfate prophylaxis; *Am J Crit Care.* 1992; 1(2):19-25.

Vanholder, R, Sever, MS, Erek, E, Lameire, N. Rhabdomyolysis. *J Am Soc Nephrol.* 2000; 11(8):1553-61.

Wang, J, Corson, K, Minky, K, Mader, J. Diver with acute abdominal pain, right leg paresthesias and weakness: a case report. *Undersea Hyperb Med.* 2002; 29(4):242-6.

Weinstein, RS, Cole, S, Knaster, HB, Dahlbert, T. Beta blocker overdose with propranolol and with atenolol. *Ann Emerg Med.* 1985; 14(2):161-3.

Williams, ST, Prior, FG, Bryson, P. Hematocrit change in tropical scuba divers. *Wilderness Environ Med.* 2007; 18(1):48-53.

Yamashita, M, Yamashita, M, Suzuki, M, Hirai, H, Kajigaya, H. Ionophoretic delivery of calcium for experimental hydrofluoric acid burns. *Crit Care Med.* 2001; 29(8):1575-8.

Yang, T, Riehl, J, Esteve, E, et al. Pharmacologic and functional characterization of malignant hyperthermia in the R163C RyR1 knock-in mouse." *Anesthesiology.* 2006; 105(6):1164-75.

Yurumez, Y, Durukan, P, Yavuz, Y, et al. Acute organophosphate poisoning in university hospital emergency room patients. *Intern Med.* 2007; 46(13):965-9.

Module 8
High-Risk Obstetrical Emergencies

1. You arrive on the scene of twenty-one-year-old woman involved a single roll-over accident, who is approximately twenty-eight weeks pregnant. Your assessment reveals palpation of fetal parts over the abdomen. What is your diagnosis of the patient?

   A. Liver laceration
   B. Uterine rupture
   C. Placenta previa
   D. Abruptio placenta

2. The patient is in a breech presentation and delivery appears to be halted upon delivery of the head. The appropriate action would be to

   A. Initiate rapid transport, placing mother in a knee-chest position
   B. Administer tocolytic agents
   C. Perform Trousseau's maneuver
   D. Perform Mauriceau's maneuver

3. Your patient is experiencing hypertonic uterine contractions. Appropriate therapy would be to

   A. Turn the patient on their side
   B. Discontinue all tocolytic medications
   C. Discontinue any oxytocin administration
   D. Administer Celestone

4. The patient fetus is exhibiting variable decelerations. This is most likely due to

   A. Uterine insufficiency
   B. Cord problems (prolapse, nuchal, short, compression)
   C. Placenta abruption
   D. Normal neurological waveform

5. Late decelerations may indicate

 A. Cord compression
 B. Acidosis
 C. Anemia
 D. Uterine placental insufficiency

6. The second stage of labor ends with

 A. Crowning
 B. Onset of contractions
 C. Dilation of the cervix
 D. Delivery of the infant

7. The fetus of a pre-eclamptic mother during labor will commonly experience

 A. Tachycardia
 B. Late decelerations
 C. Sinusoidal waveform
 D. None of the above

8. Normal magnesium level value is

 A. 0.6-1.4
 B. 3.5-4.5
 C. 1.5-2.5
 D. 6-23

9. Preeclampsia is characterized by of the following, *except*

 A. Hypertension
 B. Edema
 C. Proteinuria
 D. Seizures

10. The fetus's variability is

    A. The best indicator of fetal viability
    B. Normally 10-15 beats per minute
    C. Expected to increase during active labor
    D. All of the above

11. Sinusoidal patterns are commonly associated with all of the following, *except*

    A. Fetal hypovolemia or anemia
    B. Accidental tap of the umbilical cord during amniocentesis
    C. Pregnancy-induced hypertension
    D. Placental abruption

12. You are transporting a twenty-five year-old G1, PO female who is twenty-eight weeks gestation with a history of presenting to the ER department with headache, hyperreflexia, nausea, vomiting, epigastric pain, and dyspnea. Assessment revealed moist rales on auscultation, wheezing with tachycardia seen on the cardiac monitor. When evaluating her lab results, consumptive thrombocytopenia unaccompanied by any other coagulation factor abnormalities is characteristic of HELLP syndrome, which is defined as a platelet count of less than

    A. $200,000/mm^3$
    B. $140,000/mm^3$
    C. $100,000/mm^3$
    D. $50,000/mm^3$

13. After administering fluid resuscitation, performing vigorous fundal massage and giving oxytocin, your patient continues with postpartum hemorrhage. Which drug would be indicated to decrease blood loss?

    A. Apresoline
    B. Methergine
    C. Terbutaline
    D. Magnesium sulfate

14. When administering magnesium sulfate, the following adverse reactions can occur, *except*

    A. Transient drop in blood pressure
    B. Flushing
    C. Increase in FHR variability
    D. Nausea and vomiting

15. Hemolytic disease of the newborn can be prevented by the administration of which of the following to a Rhesus negative mother who had a pregnancy with a Rhesus positive infant?

    A. Albumin
    B. Rho(D) immune globulin
    C. Steroids
    D. Indomethacin

16. Frequency of a contraction is defined as

    A. End of a contraction to the beginning of the next contraction
    B. End of contraction to the end of the next contraction
    C. Beginning of contraction to the end of the contraction
    D. Beginning of the contraction to the beginning of the next contraction

17. Duration of a contraction is defined as

    A. End of a contraction to the beginning of the next contraction
    B. End of contraction to the end of the next contraction
    C. Beginning of contraction to the end of the contraction
    D. Beginning of the contraction to the beginning of the next contraction

18. Gravida means

    A. Total number of live births
    B. Total number of pregnancies
    C. Term gestation thirty-seven weeks and greater
    D. Total number of miscarriages

19. You are transporting a twenty-three-year-old female from a small rural hospital with a diagnosis of preterm labor. Her fundal height is measured just slightly above the umbilicus. Your patient is approximately in how many weeks' gestation?

    A. 16-20 weeks
    B. 20-24 weeks
    C. 24-28 weeks
    D. 28-32 weeks

20. The most common site for an ectopic pregnancy to occur is the

    A. Os
    B. Uterus
    C. Fallopian tube
    D. Cervix

21. When managing preterm labor, all of the following medications can decrease or stop uterine activity, *except*

    A. Apresoline
    B. Magnesium sulfate
    C. Terbutaline
    D. NSAIDs

22. The administration of which of the following medications can help decrease the chance that the fetus will have respiratory distress syndrome when born?

    A. Magnesium sulfate
    B. Ritodrine
    C. Betamethasone
    D. Indomethacin

23. When evaluating the following FHR strip, you would interpret the strip as having

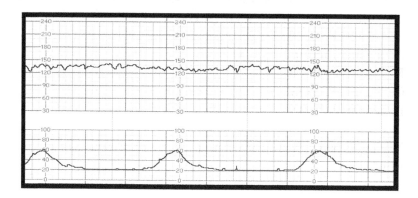

   A. Moderate baseline variability
   B. Late decelerations
   C. Fetal bradycardia
   D. Variable decelerations

24. Which of the following terms best describes an intermittent, painless contraction that may occur every ten to twenty minutes after the first trimester of pregnancy?

   A. Abruptio placenta
   B. Placenta previa
   C. True labor
   D. Braxton Hicks

25. Regular and rhythmic contractions that produce progressive cervical changes after the twentieth week of gestation and before the thirty-seventh week is known as

   A. Braxton Hicks contractions
   B. False labor
   C. Preterm labor
   D. True labor

26. A small amount of fluid is spread on a slide and allowed to dry completely. A frond crystallization pattern of dried amnionitc fluid (with high concentration of sodium chloride) will be seen under microscopic examination. The test finding is called

A. Positive ferning
B. Positive pooling
C. Positive SROM
D. Positive PROM

27. Nitrazine paper will turn what color in the presence of amniotic fluid?

A. Yellow
B. Red
C. Green
D. Blue

28. Labetalol—

A. Acts at the neuromuscular junction to slow transmission of impulses.
B. Is a selective mixed alpha-beta adrenergic antagonist agent that decreases systemic vascular resistance without changing cardiac output.
C. Acts by relaxing arterioles and decreasing vasospasm, which results in reducing blood pressure and stimulating cardiac output.
D. Is a vasodilator used to relax a hypertonic uterus during delivery.

29. A patient exhibiting signs and symptoms of magnesium sulfate toxicity can present with all of the following, *except*

A. Deteriorating loss of consciousness
B. Respiratory depression
C. Depressed deep tendon reflexes
D. Increased deep tendon reflexes

30. You are transporting a twenty-four-year-old female, twenty-eight-week gestation, G2, P1, who presents to the ER department complaining of lower abdominal contractions every 5-10 minutes. She has a history of myasthenia gravis and gestational diabetes. Which of the following medications would *not* be administered to control uterine activity?

    A. Magnesium sulfate
    B. Terbutaline
    C. Nifidipine
    D. Nicardipine

31. A patient presenting with shoulder pain and lower abdominal pain with a history of having her last menses approximately 6-8 weeks, is most likely exhibiting which of the following?

    A. Missed abortion
    B. Ectopic pregnancy
    C. Pelvic inflammatory disease
    D. Spleen injury

32. Which of the following can be a serious complication if, Terbutaline is administered to an insulin-dependent pregnant diabetic patient?

    A. Hypoglycemia
    B. Hypocalcemia
    C. Hemolysis, elevated liver enzymes and low platelets
    D. Transient hyperglycemic response

33. Macrosomia refers to

    A. Intrauterine growth restriction
    B. A fetus that is large for gestational age, with increased fat deposition, and an enlarged spleen and liver
    C. Fetal distress
    D. Hydramnios

34. Inversion of the uterus may occur with any of the following, *except*

    A. Hypertonic uterus
    B. Excessive cord traction
    C. Fundal pressure
    D. Uterine atony

35. Which of the following has been recognized as a primary cause of preterm labor?

    A. Hypertonic uterus
    B. Trauma
    C. Infection
    D. No prenatal care

36. Signs and symptoms of preeclampsia include all of the following, *except*

    A. Headache
    B. Epigastric pain
    C. Visual disturbances
    D. Seizures

37. The baseline variability for the following fetal tracing is

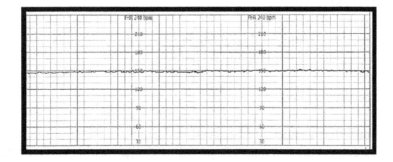

    A. Absent
    B. Mild
    C. Moderate
    D. Marked

38. Interpret the following fetal tracing

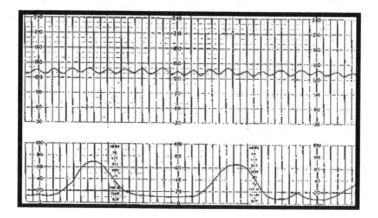

   A. Variable decelerations
   B. Late decelerations
   C. Sinusoidal pattern
   D. Hypertonic contractions

39. Preeclampsia most commonly occurs during

   A. First trimester
   B. End of second trimester, beginning of third trimester
   C. Third trimester
   D. End of third trimester

40. Placental abruption can be defined as

   A. An overt cord prolapse that slips down into the vagina or appears externally after the amniotic membranes have ruptured.
   B. A spontaneous or traumatic disruption of the uterine wall.
   C. A blood loss in excess of 500 mL after delivery.
   D. The premature detachment of a normally implanted placenta from the uterine wall.

41. You are preparing to transport a twenty-year-old female, twenty-four weeks gestation, G3, P1, AB 1. The mother is being placed in lateral recumbent position to prevent which of the following?

    A. Decrease uterine contractions
    B. Supine hypotensive syndrome
    C. Hypertension
    D. Relieve bladder distention

42. The diastolic blood pressure goal when managing pregnancy-induced hypertension is

    A. <80 mmHg
    B. 80-90 mmHg
    C. 90-100 mmHg
    D. 110-120 mmHg

43. You are transporting a nineteen-year-old female, thirty weeks gestation, G2, P1, who is presented in a small rural ER department with abdominal pain after receiving a blow to the abdomen two hours prior. The sending staff is concerned that the patient may be exhibiting signs and symptoms of a placental abruption. Which of the following would assist the transport team in recognizing that the presence of concealed bleeding may be increasing?

    A. Administering tocolytics
    B. Assessing vital signs every fifteen minutes or more if needed
    C. Marking and determining the fundal height frequently
    D. Assessing for contractions and external vaginal hemorrhage every fifteen minutes or more if needed

44. Interpret the following fetal tracing

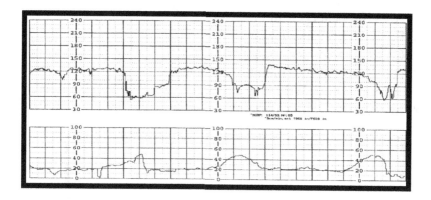

    A. Late decelerations
    B. Variable decelerations
    C. Early decelerations
    D. Sinusoidal FHR pattern

45. Interpret the following fetal tracing

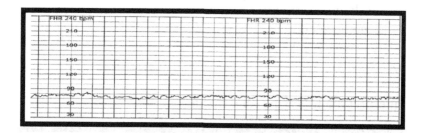

    A. Normal
    B. Fetal bradycardia
    C. Fetal tachycardia
    D. Sinusoidal FHR pattern

46. The most common cause of postpartum hemorrhage (PPH) is

    A. Placenta previa
    B. Abruption placenta
    C. Uterine inversion
    D. Uterine atony

47. Acute fetal tachycardia is defined as

    A. >100 beats per minute
    B. >120 beats per minute
    C. >160 beats per minute
    D. >180 beats per minute

48. Interpret the following fetal tracing

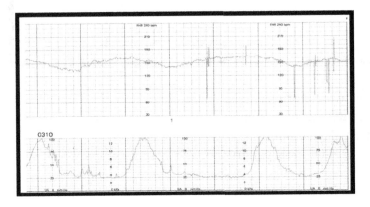

    A. Early decelerations
    B. Late decelerations
    C. Variable decelerations
    D. Normal

49. Interpret the following fetal tracing

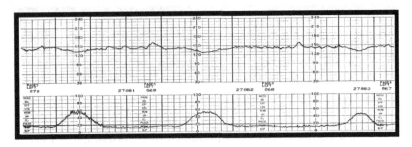

    A. Early decelerations
    B. Sinusoidal pattern
    C. Variable decelerations
    D. Late decelerations

50. Leopold's maneuver can be used to

    A. Assess cervical dilation
    B. Assess fetal position
    C. Assess strength of contractions
    D. Assess gestational age

Answer Key and Rationale

1. **B:** Signs and symptoms of uterine rupture include severe, sudden, continual abdominal pain and signs of hypovolemic shock. Contractions may cease or may increase in intensity and frequency. Shoulder (referred pain known as Kehr's sign) or chest pain as a result of the collection of blood under the diaphragm, generalized tenderness with rebound, *an abdominal mass with fetal parts easily felt,* or vaginal bleeding is likely when the rupture occurs in the lower uterine segment. Most bleeding is intra-abdominal and the abdomen may be distended.

2. **D:** *Mauriceau's maneuver* is a method of delivering the head in an assisted vaginal breech delivery in which the infant's body is supported by the right forearm while traction is made upon the shoulders by the left hand. The fetal head is maintained in a flexed position by using the Mauriceau's maneuver, which is performed by placing the index and middle fingers over the maxillary prominence on either side of the nose. The fetal body is supported in a neutral position, with care to not overextend the neck. In the breech presentation, the baby enters the birth canal with the buttocks or feet first as opposed to the normal head first presentation. Certain factors can encourage a breech presentation. Prematurity is likely the chief cause. There are either three or four main categories of breech births, depending upon the source.

Breech presentations	
Type of Breech	Definition
Frank	Buttocks comes first, and legs are flexed at the hip and extended at the knees (with feet near the ears). 65-70% of breech babies are in the frank breech position.
Complete	Hips and knees are flexed so that the baby is sitting cross-legged (yoga position), with feet beside the buttocks.
Footling	One or both feet come first, with the buttocks at a higher position. This is rare at term but relatively common with premature births.
Kneeling	Kneeling position, with one or both legs extended at the hips and flexed at the knees. This is extremely rare and is excluded from many classifications.

Total breech extraction is where the fetal feet are grasped, and the entire fetus is extracted. Total breech extraction should be used only for a noncephalic second twin; it should not be used for a singleton fetus because the cervix may not be adequately dilated to allow passage of the fetal head.

3. **C:** A hyperstimulated uterus may have fewer than five contractions in ten minutes, but the interval between contractions is less than one minute. Another term used to describe long, strong contractions is "titanic." An overdose of oxytocin may cause this type of uterine activity.

4. **B:** Variable decelerations can occur at any time during a contraction. The shape may also vary and is frequently V-shaped or W-shaped. Cord compression is responsible for these decelerations, which have a very characteristic appearance; frequently a short acceleration is observed, followed by a rapid deceleration for some seconds, then a rapid rise and a short acceleration before there is a return to the fetal heart rate (FHR) baseline. There are two keys in to interpreting FHR tracings: one is to focus on assessment of variability and second is to accurately identify the type of deceleration.

Decelerations	
Type of deceleration	Definition
Early deceleration	A transient decrease in heart rate that coincides with the onset of a uterine contraction *"mirror-image of the contraction."*
Late deceleration	A transient decrease in heart rate occurring at or after the peak of a uterine contraction, which may indicate fetal hypoxia.
Variable deceleration	A transient series of decelerations that vary in intensity, duration, and relation to uterine contraction, resulting from vagus nerve, firing in response to a stimulus such as umbilical cord compression in the first stage of labor.

Periodic Changes: These are accelerations or decelerations in the fetal heart rate that occur in direct association with uterine contractions.

Episodic Changes: These are accelerations or decelerations in the fetal heart rate that occur independent of uterine contractions. Example: A deceleration or acceleration in response to a vaginal exam, maternal vomiting, or fetal movement.

Early Deceleration

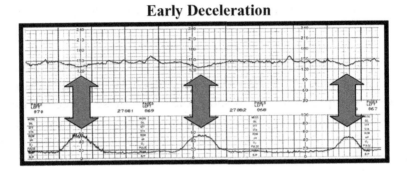

Based on visual assessment, an early deceleration is defined as an apparent gradual decrease in fetal heart rate and return to baseline associated with uterine contractions. *Early deceleration is caused by vagal simulation from head compression and is a reassuring pattern that may be prevented by avoiding early rupture of membranes.*

- Early decelerations are not considered ominous
- In association with a uterine contraction, a visually apparent, gradual (onset to nadir 30 seconds or more) decrease in FHR with return to baseline.
- Nadir of the deceleration occurs at the same time as the peak of the contraction.

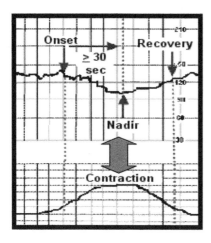

Late Deceleration

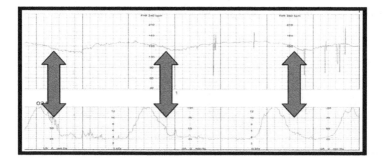

Based on visual assessment, a late deceleration is defined as an apparent gradual decrease in fetal heart rate and return to baseline associated with uterine contractions. *Late deceleration is associated with uteroplacental insufficiency and is a result of hypoxia and metabolic abnormalities.*

- Late decelerations are one of the most ominous fetal heart rate patterns.
- In association with a uterine contraction, a visually apparent, gradual (onset to nadir 30 seconds or more) decrease in FHR with return to baseline. The nadir of the deceleration occurs after the peak of the contraction.
- Onset, nadir, and recovery of the deceleration occur after the beginning, peak and end of the contraction.

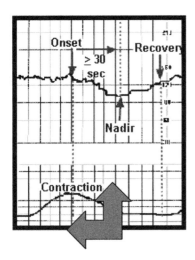

Variable Deceleration

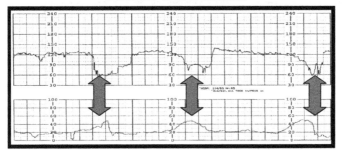

Based on visual assessment, a variable deceleration is defined as an apparent abrupt decrease in fetal heart rate below the baseline which may or may not be associated with uterine contractions. When variable decelerations occur in conjunction with uterine contractions, the onset, depth and duration vary with each succeeding uterine contraction. *Variables are transitory decreases in the fetal heart rate caused by umbilical cord compression.*

- They coincide with contractions and may appear V-shaped, U-shaped or W-shaped. The significance of the variables depends upon how often they occur, how deep they go, and how long they last. What is also crucial is how the fetus responds in their presence.
- An abrupt decrease in FHR of >15 BPM, measured from the most recently determined baseline rate. The onset of decelerations to nadir is less than thirty seconds; lasts >15

seconds but <2 minutes in duration from onset to return to baseline.

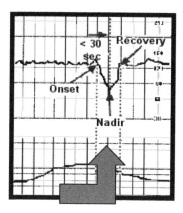

Prolonged Deceleration

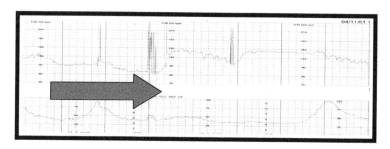

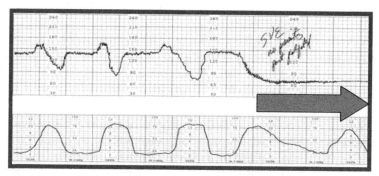

Based on visual assessment, a prolonged deceleration is defined as an apparent decrease in fetal heart rate below the baseline.

- A decrease in FHR of >15 beats per minute measured from the most recently determined baseline rate.

- The deceleration lasts >2 minutes but less than ten minutes from onset to return to baseline.
- A prolonged deceleration that is sustained for ten minutes or more is a baseline change.

5. **D:** A late deceleration is one that begins close to the apex of the contraction, gradually decelerates, and gradually returns to the FHR baseline after the contraction is over. Late decelerations always indicate *uteroplacental insufficiency;* there is inadequate oxygen exchange in the placenta during a contraction. When a contraction is stronger, the insufficiency is greater and the deceleration is proportional. Late decelerations are one of the most ominous fetal heart rate patterns.

New National Institute of Child Health and Human Development (NICHD) guidelines divide all FHR patterns into three categories. Refer to the table to review guidelines.

NICHD fetal heart rate pattern guidelines	
Categories	Definition
Category I—Normal	*Category I has the following 4 characteristics:* ✓ Baseline rate: 110-160 BPM ✓ Moderate variability: 6-25 BPM ✓ Absence of late or variable decelerations ✓ Absence or presence of early decelerations or accelerations
Category II—Intermediate	Category II comprises of all FHR patterns not in category I or III. Category II tracings are not predictive of abnormal fetal acid—base status. When a category II tracing is identified, a fetal scalp stimulation test may help identify fetuses in which acid-base status is normal.
Category III—Abnormal	The new NICHD guidelines label four FHR patterns as abnormal. One of the abnormal patterns is a sinusoidal heart rate, defined as a pattern of regular variability, resembling a sine wave, with fixed periodicity of 3-5 cycles/minute and amplitude of 5-40 BPM. A sinusoidal pattern may indicate fetal anemia caused by feto-maternal hemorrhage or alloimmunization.

Accelerations

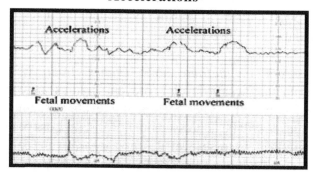

Based on visual assessment, an acceleration is defined as an apparent abrupt increase in fetal heart rate above the baseline.

- Onset to peak is <30 seconds of fetal heart rate above baseline. Peak is >15 BPM. Duration is >15 seconds and is <2 minutes from onset to return to baseline.
- In pregnancies less than thirty-two weeks gestation, accelerations are defined as an increase of ten beats per minute or more above baseline which lasts ten seconds or more. (peak of 10 BPM and duration of 10 seconds)
- An acceleration is classified as prolonged if the duration is two minutes or more but less than ten minutes in duration. Accelerations that are ten minutes or more are considered a baseline change.

6. **D:** The four stages of the childbirth process are based on changes in the uterus and cervix as labor progresses. The first stage of labor begins at the onset of labor and ends when the cervix is 100% effaced and completely dilated to 10 centimeters. This is the longest stage of labor and can last 12-17 hours. *The second stage begins when the cervix is completely effaced and dilated and ends with the birth of the baby, lasting about 1-2 hours.* The third stage begins with the birth of the baby and ends with the delivery of the placenta. This is the shortest stage of labor, lasting 15-20 minutes. The fourth stage begins with delivery of the placenta and ends 1-2 hours after delivery.

7. **B:** Uteroplacental insufficiency may result from pregnancy-induced hypertension (PIH), diabetes mellitus (DM), cardiovascular or kidney disease, chorioamnionitis, smoking, and a fetus that is past

maturity. It may also result from decreased placental perfusion in placental abruption or previa, uterine hypertonus as a result of oxytocin stimulation and hypotension.

8. **C:** *Normal serum magnesium level ranges from 1.5-2.5.* Therapeutic serum magnesium levels to prevent seizures range from approximately 4-8 mEq/L. When therapeutic levels are achieved, deep tendon reflexes will be depressed but not absent. Loss of deep tendon reflexes indicates a toxic level. Respiratory arrest and cardiac arrest are seen with high toxic levels >15 mEq/L. While a patient is receiving intravenous magnesium sulfate, frequent assessment of deep tendon reflexes is essential. Respirations should also be closely monitored and the infusion stopped if less than twelve breaths per minute. Pulse oximetry should be used during transport. The antidote for magnesium sulfate toxicity is calcium gluconate. Calcium stimulates the release of acetylcholine, stimulating nerve transmission to the muscle. The recommended dosage of calcium gluconate is 1 gram of a 10% solution administered intravenously over at least three minutes. If administered too rapidly, bradycardia and dysrhythmias may occur.

9. **D:** Pregnancy-induced hypertension (PIH) refers to a group of hypertensive disorders that have their onset during pregnancy and resolve after pregnancy. Gestational hypertension develops after twenty weeks gestation without evidence of hypertension. Preeclampsia is characterized by hypertension, proteinuria, and edema. Eclampsia refers to the development of clonic and tonic seizures.

"The Big Three" in assessing PIH	
Problem	Definition
Hypertension	A rise in systolic blood pressure of 30 mmHg or a rise in diastolic blood pressure of 15 mmHg on the basis of previously known pressure or a blood pressure of 140/90 or higher. The diastolic blood pressure is a more reliable predictor of the disease process.
Edema	Nondependent edema of the eyelids, face, and hands is characteristic of PIH. Pitting edema of the lower extremities is common.
Proteinuria	Usually develops after hypertension, and edema is evident when proteinuria is present.

10. **D:** Normal variability is indicative of an adequately oxygenated autonomic nervous system. Variability is the single most important factor in predicting fetal well-being. *Variability* is defined as fluctuations in the fetal heart rate baseline that are two cycles per minute or more and that are irregular in amplitude. The visual quantification of the amplitude from peak to trough in beats per minute is as follows:

Fetal heart rate patterns variability		
Amplitude Range	Classification	Variability FHR Tracings
Undetectable	Absent	
Undetectable to <5 BPM	Minimal	
6 to 25 BPM	Moderate	
More than 25 BPM *(may be an early sign of hypoxia)*	Marked	

11. **C:** A uniform sine wave pattern indicates fetal hypovolemia or anemia and may occur in cases of erythroblastosis fetalis, accidental

tap of the umbilical cord during amniocentesis, fetomaternal transfusion, placental abruption, or another type of accident. Variability will be absent or minimal and accelerations are not seen. When this pattern is recognized, rapid delivery is usually recommended. A pseudosinusoidal or undulating pattern may be identified and can be associated to maternal drug administration of narcotics.

Sinusoidal or Sine Wave FHR Pattern

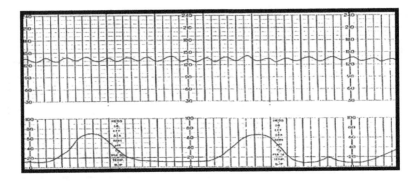

Sinusoidal FHR patterns, which are excluded from the definition of variability are described as a smooth, sine wave-like pattern of regular frequency and amplitude.

Pseudosinusoidal or Undulating FHR Pattern

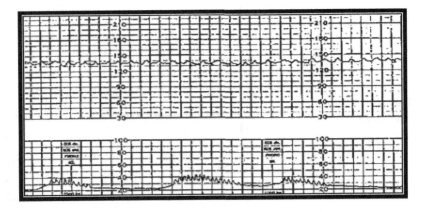

The *pseudo-sinusoidal* FHR pattern appears very similar to the sinusoidal pattern; however, this pattern shows less regularity in the shape and amplitude of the variability waves. This type of pattern is benign and transient and can occur in the presence of narcotics.

Saltatory FHR Pattern

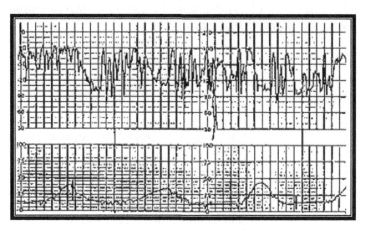

A *saltatory* FHR pattern is rapidly occurring couples of acceleration and deceleration causing relatively large oscillations of the baseline fetal heart rate. This pattern is usually caused by acute hypoxia or mechanical compression of the umbilical cord. It is considered a nonreassuring pattern, but it is not usually an indication for immediate delivery.

A *reassuring FHR pattern* is the presence of fetal heart rate accelerations. This usually indicates there is no academia and is generally indicative of fetal well-being. In most cases, moderate variability is also reassuring but few studies exist to support this contention.

When the fetal heart has absent or minimal variability without spontaneous accelerations and the fetal heart rate status does not change despite intervention, these findings are nonreassuring. A *nonreassuring FHR pattern* is the standard terminology to be used to describe threats to fetal well-being or indicators of fetal compromise. This term replaces such terms as fetal distress or fetal stress.

12. **C:** HELLP syndrome *(hemolysis, elevated liver enzymes, and low platelets)* is considered a complication of severe preeclampsia. HELLP syndrome is a life-threatening obstetric complication usually considered to be a variant of preeclampsia. Both conditions usually occur during the later stages of pregnancy or sometimes after childbirth. *A platelet count lower than 100,000/mm^{-3} is characteristic of HELLP syndrome.*

HELLP syndrome	
Problem	Definition
H = hemolysis	Is confirmed by evidence of red cell fragments and irregularly shaped red cells on peripheral blood smears.
EL = elevated liver enzymes	Hyperbilirubinemia is frequently seen and jaundice may be present. The serum transaminase levels may be elevated to as high as 4,000 U/L, but milder elevations are typical.
LP = low platelet count	Thrombocytopenia; platelet count lower than 100,000 mm^{-3}.

Complications of PIH include eclampsia, placental abruption, pulmonary edema, DIC, hemolytic anemia, thrombocytopenia, preterm delivery, prematurity, IUGR, and HELLP. The only effective treatment is prompt delivery of the baby. Several medications have been investigated for the treatment of HELLP syndrome, but evidence is conflicting as to whether magnesium sulfate decreases the risk of seizures and progress to eclampsia. The DIC is treated with fresh, frozen plasma to replenish the coagulation proteins, and the anemia may require blood transfusion. In mild cases, corticosteroids and antihypertensives (labetalol, hydralazine, nifedipine) may be sufficient. Intravenous fluids are generally required.

13. **B:** *Methylergonovine* (Methergine), 0.2 mg administered intramuscularly or intravenously, is recommended. Methylergonovine should be used cautiously in patients with PIH because of the pressor effects that may result in further elevated blood pressure. Methylergonovine is a blood vessel constrictor and smooth muscle agonist most commonly used to prevent or control

excessive bleeding following childbirth and spontaneous or elective abortion. It also causes uterine contractions to aid in expulsion of retained products of conception after a missed abortion and to help deliver the placenta after childbirth. Side effects can include nausea, vomiting, diarrhea, cramping, dizziness, pulmonary hypertension, coronary artery vasoconstriction, and severe systemic hypertension (especially in patients with preeclampsia).

14. **C:** *Magnesium sulfate* is not an antihypertensive agent. However, a transient drop in blood pressure after initiation of treatment is frequently seen and can be attributed to smooth muscle relaxation. Adverse reactions include flushing, diaphoresis, nausea, vomiting, and drowsiness. *A decrease in FHR variability may be observed.* The drug is primarily excreted in the urine; toxicity may develop rather rapidly in the patient with significantly impaired kidney function.

15. **B:** The commonly used terms *Rh factor, Rh positive,* and *Rh negative* refer to the *D antigen* only. *Rho(D) immune globulin* is a medicine solution of IgG anti-D (anti-RhD) antibodies used to prevent the immunological condition known as Rhesus disease (or hemolytic disease of newborn). The disease ranges from mild to severe. When the disease is mild, the fetus may have mild anemia with reticulocytosis. When the disease is moderate or severe, the fetus can have a more marked anemia and erythroblastosis (erythroblastosis fetalis). When the disease is very severe, it can cause morbus hemolyticus neonatorum, hydrops fetalis, or stillbirth.

During any pregnancy, a small amount of the baby's blood can enter the mother's circulation. If the *mother is Rh negative* and the baby is Rh positive, the mother produces antibodies (including IgG) against the Rhesus D antigen on her baby's red blood cells. During this and subsequent pregnancies, the IgG is able to pass through the placenta into the fetus and if the level of it is sufficient, it will cause destruction of Rhesus D positive fetal red blood cells, leading to the development of Rh disease. The medication has an FDA Pregnancy Category C. It is given by intramuscular injection as part of modern routine antenatal care at about twenty-eight weeks of pregnancy, and within seventy-two hours after childbirth.

It is also given after antenatal pathological events that are likely to cause a fetomaternal hemorrhage.

16. **D:** *Frequency* shows how far apart your contractions are.

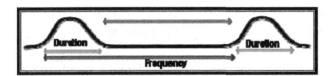

17. **C:** *Duration* shows how long your contractions last.

18. **B:** *Gravida* indicates the total number of pregnancies a woman has had, regardless of whether they were carried to term. Para indicates the number of viable (>20 weeks) births. Note: pregnancies consisting of multiples, such as twins or triplets, count as *one* birth.

19. **B:** The fundal height is measured from the top of the pubic bone to the top of the uterus and is generally measured in centimeters. It's a measurement, as you might suspect, that should increase as the pregnancy continues toward the estimated date of confinement (EDC). The fundal height can be out of sync with what's expected for the gestational age due to abnormal conditions such as, oligohydramnios (too little fluid, taking away from the entire mass effect, leading to a smaller fundal height), hydramnios, polyhydramnios (too much fluid, indicating possibly genetic problems or anatomical problems with the baby), and abnormal position of the baby close to term.

Fundal Height of Uterus by Weeks

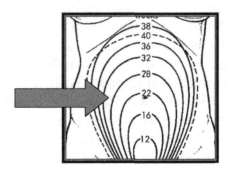

20. **C:** *Most ectopic pregnancies occur in the fallopian tube (so-called tubal pregnancies),* but implantation can also occur in the cervix, ovaries, and abdomen. An ectopic pregnancy is a potential medical emergency, and, if not treated properly, can lead to death. Clinical presentation of ectopic pregnancy occurs at a mean of 7.2 weeks after the last normal menstrual period, with a range of five to eight weeks. *Shoulder pain (Kehr's sign)* is caused by free blood tracking up the abdominal cavity and irritating the diaphragm and is an ominous sign.

21. **A:** *Hydralazine (Apresoline)* acts by relaxing arterioles and decreasing vasospasm, and as a result, it reduces blood pressure and stimulates cardiac output. Hydralazine is recommended when the diastolic blood pressure is 100 mmHg or greater. Two milligrams administered intravenously every five minutes until the diastolic blood pressure ranges between 90-100 mmHg.

22. **C:** *Betamethasone (Celestone)* is a steroid used to stimulate fetal lung maturation (prevention of ARDS) and to decrease the incidence and mortality from intracranial hemorrhage in premature infants. It is given to the pregnant mother as an injection into muscle tissue. The use of betamethasone can decrease the chance that the fetus will have respiratory distress syndrome when born. It is usually used if preterm delivery is a concern. Dexamethasone (Decadron) can also been used, which is very similar. Side effects may include sleeplessness and higher blood sugar levels for the mother and decreased fetal movement for the baby.

23. **A:** The presence of *moderate variability* is strongly predictive of normal fetal acid-base status.

24. **D:** A Braxton Hicks contraction might get closer together but not consistently, or they may feel stronger but go away with activity and/or rest. These contractions were first described in 1872 by British gynecologist John Braxton Hicks. Sometimes these contractions are also called prelabor contractions or Hicks sign. Not everyone will notice or experience these contractions, and some pregnant mothers will have them frequently.

25. **C:** *Preterm* is defined at before the thirty-seventh week. Preterm labor does not always result in preterm delivery. Generally true labor contractions will get longer in length, closer in frequency, and stronger in intensity.

Contractions False labor versus true labor	
Braxton Hick	**True labor**
Contractions don't get closer together.	Contractions do get closer together.
Contractions don't get stronger.	Contractions do get stronger.
Contractions tend to be felt only in the front.	Contractions tend to be felt all over.
Contractions don't last longer.	Contractions do last longer.
Walking has no effect on the contractions.	Walking makes the contractions stronger.
Cervix doesn't change with contractions.	Cervix opens and thins with contractions.

26. **A:** This test is based on the ability of amniotic fluid to form a fern pattern when air-dried on a glass slide; this phenomenon in part due to the fluid's protein and sodium chloride content. A vaginal liquid pool specimen is obtained, allowed to dry completely in room air, and examined microscopically. A positive screen is depicted by the presence of fernlike patterns characteristic of amniotic fluid crystals.

27. **D:** Nitrazine paper is impregnated with an indicator dye Phenaphthazine. The color changes as pH changes, giving a broad range of colors from yellow through blue. It is used to test vaginal pH during late pregnancy to determine the breakage of the amniotic sac. While vaginal pH is normally acidic, a pH above 7.0 can indicate that the amniotic sac has ruptured *(nitrazine paper will turn blue)*. More sensitive than litmus paper, nitrazine indicates pH in the range of 4.5 to 7.5. An elevated vaginal pH can also be associated with bacterial vaginosis.

28. **B:** *Labetalol (Normodyne, Trandate)* is a mixed alpha/beta adrenergic antagonist, which is used to treat high blood pressure. It has a particular indication in the treatment of pregnancy-induced hypertension which is commonly associated with preeclampsia. It is also used to treat chronic hypertension of pheochromocytoma and hypertensive crisis. It works by blocking these adrenergic receptors, which decreases peripheral vascular resistance without significantly altering heart rate or cardiac output. The standard dosage when managing pregnancy-induced hypertension is 20 mg administered by intravenous push over two minutes and may be repeated as needed every ten minutes with 40-80 mg until the maximum dose of 300 mg has been administered.

29. **D:** Excess magnesium sulfate results in magnesium sulfate toxicity, which results in both respiratory depression and a *loss of deep tendon reflexes (hyporeflexia)*. The kidneys are efficient at excreting excess magnesium and it is unlikely that the mineral will accumulate to toxic levels. A high intake of magnesium might impair absorption and use of calcium. Frequently monitor patients' vital signs, oxygen saturation, deep tendon reflexes, and level of consciousness (also fetal heart rates and maternal uterine activity if the drug is used for preterm labor). Assess patients for signs of toxicity (e.g., visual changes, somnolence, flushing, muscle paralysis, respiratory depression, loss of patellar reflexes) or pulmonary edema. Calcium *gluconate* is the antidote for magnesium sulfate toxicity. Rapid intravenous injections of calcium gluconate may cause vasodilation, cardiac arrhythmias, decreased blood pressure, and bradycardia. Intramuscular injections may lead to local necrosis and abscess formation. Extravasation of calcium gluconate can lead to cellulitis.

30. **A:** Myasthenia gravis and renal failure are contraindications for the use of *magnesium sulfate*. The recommended dose is 4-6 grams intravenous bolus given slowly over 15-30 minutes, followed by a maintenance infusion drip of 1-5 grams/hour on an infusion pump (average infusion is 2 grams/hour).

Tocolytics	
Drug name	Classification
Terbutaline (Brethine)	*Beta-Sympathomimetic:* Relaxes smooth muscle in the uterus to inhibit uterine contractions.
Nifedipine (Procardia, Adalat) Nicardipine (Cardene)	*Calcium Channel Blockers:* Antagonizes the action of calcium within the myometrial cells to reduce its contractility. The primary calcium channel blocker used as a tocolytic is nifedipine, but nicardipine has also been used.
Magnesium Sulfate	*Electrolyte:* Intracellular calcium is displaced by magnesium ions, leading to inhibition of uterine contractions. *Myasthenia Gravis and renal failure* are contraindications.
Indomethacin (Indocin) Ketorolac (Toradol) Sulindac (	*NSAIDS:* Limiting the use of any NSAID to 48 hours will usually eliminate the potential for fetal toxicity. NSAIDs should not be used in women with significant renal or hepatic disease, active peptic ulcer disease, coagulation disorders, thrombocytopenia, NSAID-sensitive asthma, or other sensitivity to NSAIDs.
Nitroglycerin (Tridil)	*Vasodilator:* Has been used to relax a hypertonic uterus during delivery, thereby allowing safe delivery of the fetus.

31. **B:** An *ectopic pregnancy* is a complication of pregnancy in which the pregnancy implants outside the uterine cavity. With rare exceptions, ectopic pregnancies are not viable. Furthermore, they are dangerous for the mother, internal bleeding being a common complication. Clinical presentation of ectopic pregnancy occurs at a mean of 7.2 weeks after the last normal menstrual period, with a range of five to eight weeks. *Shoulder pain (Kehr's sign)* is caused by free blood tracking up the abdominal cavity, irritating the diaphragm and is an ominous sign.

32. **D:** Tocolytics are medicines that attempt to stop labor. The typical dosage of Terbutaline (brethine) is 0.25 mg subcutaneously every twenty minutes to three hours. The drug is discontinued if the maternal heart rate exceeds 120 beats/minute. Terbutaline is contraindicated if the mother has cardiac dysrhythmia. The principal maternal adverse effects are *hyperglycemia,* cardiac dysrhythmias,

myocardial ischemia, pulmonary edema, hypotension, and tachycardia. The infrequent fetal and newborn adverse effects are fetal tachycardia, hyperinsulinemia, hyperglycemia, myocardial and septal hypertrophy, and myocardial ischemia. Because of the risk of hyperinsulinemia, newborns may develop hypoglycemia.

33. **B:** The term *macrosomia* is used to describe a newborn with an excessive birth weight. It is seen more commonly when the mother has gestational diabetes mellitus (GDM) or diabetes mellitus (DM) without vasculopathy. Macrosomia, as defined by birth weight greater than 4,000-4,500 g (8 lb 13 oz to 9 lb 15 oz), occurs with higher frequency in prolonged pregnancies that continue beyond the expected delivery date. It has also been defined as greater than 90% for gestational age after correcting for neonatal sex and ethnicity. Based on these definitions, macrosomia affects 1-10% of all pregnancies. *Cephalo-pelvic disproportion* exists when the capacity of the pelvis is inadequate to allow the fetus to negotiate the birth canal. This may be due to a small pelvis, a nongynecoid pelvic formation, a large fetus, or a combination of these factors.

34. **A:** *Uterine inversion is a rare medical emergency in which the corpus turns inside out and protrudes into the vagina.* The uterus is *most commonly inverted when too much traction is applied to the umbilical cord in an attempt to deliver the placenta.* Excessive pressure on the fundus during delivery of the placenta, a flaccid uterus, or placenta accreta (abnormally adherent placenta) can contribute.

Treatment is immediate manual reduction by pushing up on the fundus until the uterus is returned to its normal position. If the uterus has contracted, a tocolytic agent can relax the uterus to allow replacement. If the placenta is still attached, the uterus should be replaced before the placenta is removed. Removing the placenta before attempting to replace the uterus may increase hemorrhage. Because of discomfort, IV analgesics and sedatives or a general anesthetic are sometimes needed. Once the uterus is replaced and the placenta has been delivered, *oxytocin (Pitocin)* infusion should be started. Refer to the table for review of delivery complications.

Delivery complications	
Type of complication	
Breech presentation	The second most common abnormal presentation is breech. There are several types of breech presentations: Frank, complete, footling. *Refer to the table in question no.2.*
Uterine rupture	Factors that predispose to uterine rupture include previous surgery involving the myometrium, previous C-section with a higher incidence of a "classic" vertical scar being involved, use of labor stimulant medications, trauma, previous rupture, overdistension of the uterus as a result of multiple gestation or hydramnios.
Fetal dystocia	Fetal dystocia is abnormal fetal size or position, resulting in difficult delivery. The most common abnormal presentation is occiput posterior. The fetal neck is usually somewhat deflexed; thus, a larger diameter of the head must pass through the pelvis. Many occiput posterior presentations require operative vaginal delivery or cesarean delivery.
Shoulder dystocia	Presentation is vertex, but the anterior fetal shoulder is lodged behind the symphysis pubis, preventing vaginal delivery. Shoulder dystocia is recognized when the fetal head is delivered onto the perineum but appears to be pulled back tightly against the perineum *(turtle sign).*
Precipitate	Abnormally rapid labor with strong contractions, rapid cervical dilation, rapid descent of the presenting part and delivery usually occurs in 2 hours from the start of the contractions.
Retained placenta	Normally separates from the uterus spontaneously in 5-20 minutes after delivery. Signs of separation include lengthening of the exposed cord and a gush of blood; the uterus appears to "ball up." Retained placental parts can result in hemorrhage.
Umbilical cord prolapse	Actions to take in the event of cord prolapse include elevating the presenting part off the cord with a hand in the vagina to prevent further cord compression *(must be maintained during transport)* and positioning the patient in a Trendelenburg's or knee-chest position to further reduce pressure on the cord. Tocolytics should be given to slow contractions and reduce the pressure on the cord during contractions.

35. **C:** *Infection* has been recognized as a primary cause of preterm labor. Sources of infection may include urinary tract infection, pyelonephritis, vaginitis, chorioamnionitis, and viral infection.

36. **D:** *Eclampsia* can occur befor labor, during labor, or early into the postpartum period. Headache, visual disturbances, epigastric pain, apprehension, anxiety, and hyperreflexia with clonus in a patient with severe preeclampsia are signs of impending eclampsia. Seizures are characterized by clonic and tonic activity and usually begin around the mouth in the form of facial twitching.

37. **A:** *Absent and minimal variability* may be precipitated by fetal hypoxia, administration of drugs to mother, smoking, extreme prematurity, and fetal sleep. The fetus will have frequent sleep periods ranging from 20-40 minutes. Marked variability of more than twenty-five beats per minute may be one of the earliest signs of hypoxia. The presence of moderate variability is strongly predictive of normal fetal acid-base status. Absent variability is an ominous finding, especially when it occurs in conjunction with late or variable declerations. Assessment of variability is an important part of interpreting a fetal heart rate (FHR) pattern. Baseline FHR is defined as fluctuations in the baseline of irregular amplitude and frequency. These fluctuations are quantified in terms of the amplitude of the peak-to-trough in beats per minute (BPM). Baseline FHR variability is determined on a ten-minute segment of the FHR strip. FHR variability is assigned to one of four possible categories:

Baseline FHR variability	
Category	Definition
Absent	No peak-to-trough changes in FHR detected
Minimal	Amplitude is >0 and ≤5 BPM
Moderate	Amplitude is 6-25 BPM
Marked	Amplitude is >25 BPM

38. **C:** *Sinusoidal FHR pattern,* which are excluded from the definition of variability are described as a smooth, sine wave-like pattern of regular frequency and amplitude.

39. **B:** Preeclampsia is a disease characterized by high blood pressure, swelling of the face and hands, and protein in the urine *after the twentieth week of pregnancy.*

The most common symptom and hallmark of preeclampsia is high blood pressure. This may be the first or only symptom. Blood pressure may be only minimally elevated initially or can be dangerously high; symptoms may or may not be present. The blood pressure is considered to be elevated if the systolic pressure has increased by 30 mmHg or more, or if the diastolic pressure has increased by 15 mmHg or more, above the blood pressure obtained during the first trimester. Generally, a blood pressure of 140/90 mmHg or more is considered above the normal range.

40. **D:** *Placental Abruption,* also known as abruptio placenta, is a separation of the placenta from the uterine wall that can occur over a small area with little evidence or can separate totally with devastating results. The primary cause of placental abruption is largely unknown. Hypertension, whether chronic or PIH, and previous abruption are two factors that are known to greatly increase the risk of placental abruption. No vaginal bleeding will be observed if the hemorrhage is completely concealed behind the placenta. When vaginal bleeding is observed, the blood is usually dark because of the rapid clotting. As the hemorrhage continues and a retroplacental clot forms, enough pressure may be exerted to force blood through the membranes, giving the amniotic fluid a port wine color or into the myometrium, causing a condition called Couvelaire uterus. The uterine tone is increased and irritability will be noted.

Hemorrhagic complications	
Placental abruption	Placenta previa
Sudden severe abdominal pain "tearing pain" may be indicative of retroplacental hemorrhage into the myometrium.	Occurs when the placenta becomes implanted in the lower uterine segment and as a result covers or partially covers the internal cervical os (opening).
Boardlike uterus that fails to relax in between contractions (sustained tone) will aid in the assessment.	The onset usually occurs during or after the hemorrhage because of increased uterine irritability. Bright red vaginal bleeding will be observed; it is usually painless and is not initially associated with contractions.
Hypertonic and tetanic contractions can occur because of increased uterine tone.	Contractions may or may not be present.
Treat for shock	Treat for shock

41. **B:** Aortocaval compression syndrome is compression of the abdominal aorta and inferior vena cava by the gravid uterus when a pregnant woman lies in the supine position. It is a frequent cause of low maternal blood pressure (hypotension). Aortocaval compression is thought to be the cause of *supine hypotensive syndrome*. Supine hypotensive syndrome is characterized by pallor, bradycardia, sweating, nausea, hypotension, and dizziness and occurs when a pregnant woman lies on her back and resolves when she is turned on her side or by displacement of uterus.

42. **C:** The diastolic blood pressure is a more reliable predictor of the disease process. The blood pressure should be taken with the pregnant patient in the left lateral recumbent position. Hypertension associated with PIH is labile and may change in the time it takes to retake the blood pressure. The patient should be monitored closely to rapidly identify preeclampsia and its life-threatening complications (HELLP syndrome and eclampsia). Drug treatment options are limited as many antihypertensives may negatively affect the fetus; methyldopa, hydralazine, and labetalol are most commonly used for severe pregnancy hypertension. *The end goal treatment is to achieve a diastolic blood pressure of 90-100 mmHg.*

The fetus is at increased risk for a variety of life-threatening conditions, including pulmonary hypoplasia.

There exist several hypertensive states of pregnancy:

- Gestational hypertension = usually defined as a BP over 140/90
- Preeclampsia = gestational hypertension (BP > 140/90), and proteinuria (>300 mg of protein in a 24-hour urine sample). Severe preeclampsia involves a BP over 160/110 (with additional signs)
- Eclampsia = seizures in a preeclamptic patient
- HELLP syndrome = Hemolytic anemia, elevated liver enzymes and low platelet count
- Acute fatty liver of pregnancy is sometimes included in the preeclamptic spectrum.

43. **C:** Determination of fundal height and marking the fundus can assist the transport team in recognition of concealed bleeding will be confirmed by noting an increase in the fundal height. Because of normal physiologic changes of pregnancy, early symptoms of hypovolemia may be masked.

44. **B:** *Variable decelerations* can occur at any time during a contraction. The shape may also vary and is frequently V-shaped or W-shaped. Cord compression is responsible for these decelerations, which have a very characteristic appearance; frequently a short acceleration is observed, followed by a rapid deceleration for some seconds. Then there is a rapid rise and a short acceleration before there is a return to the FHR baseline. Signs that the fetus is losing the ability to tolerate the stress of repeated cord compression or that the cord compression is becoming more severe include a deeper deceleration that last longer, a slow return to baseline, an "overshoot" increase in FHR baseline immediately after the deceleration, loss of shoulders, and decreased variability.

45. **B:** The mean fetal heart rate is rounded to increments of five beats per minute during a ten-minute segment, excluding periodic/episodic changes, periods of marked variability or baseline segment that differ by more than twenty-five beats per minute. In any given ten-minute window, the minimum baseline duration must be at least two minutes. Otherwise, it is considered indeterminate. In these instances, review of the previous ten-minute segment should be the basis on which to determine the baseline. In determining the baseline rate, a minimum of a ten-minute period of monitoring is necessary for confirmation of the rate.

The fetal baseline rate is classified as follows:

Classification of baseline fetal heart rate (FHR)	
FHR	Definition
Normal	110-160 beats per minute
Bradycardia	Less than 100 beats per minute
Tachycardia	Over 160 beats per minute

Fetal bradycardia is a response of increased parasympathetic tone and is reflected by a decrease in fetal cardiac output in the presence of hypoxia. The fetus can tolerate sustained bradycardia for only a short length of time before becoming acidotic. Bradycardia can be a result of severe cord compression and can occur minutes before delivery, when the cord is drawn into the pelvis in the second stage of labor or with a cord prolapse. Bradycardia can also occur with hypertonic or titanic contractions and maternal hypotension. Whatever the mechanism of insult to the fetus, the plan of action when presented with possible fetal distress is intrauterine resuscitation. The "key" formula LOCK is as follows:

Intrauterine resuscitation "LOCK"	
Key	**Definition**
L	Place the patient in the *Le*ft lateral recumbent position if possible; manual displacement of the uterus can also be done.
O	Provide 100% supplemental *O*xygen by nonrebreather mask or mechanical ventilation.
C	*C*orrect or improve contributing factors, such as fluid resuscitation for hypotension, discontinue oxytocin infusion if hypertonic, or tetanic contractions are observed; consider tocolytics to decrease uterine contractions; assess for cord prolapse, placental abruption, etc.
K	*K*eep reassessing the FHR and intervene when indicated.

46. **D:** *Uterine atony* is the major cause of postpartum hemorrhage. Uterine atony is a loss of tone in the uterine musculature. Normally, contraction of the uterine muscle compresses the vessels and reduces flow. This increases the likelihood of coagulation and prevents bleeds. Thus, lack of uterine muscle contraction can cause an acute hemorrhage. Clinically, 75-80% of postpartum hemorrhages are due to uterine atony. Blood loss in excess of 500 mL after delivery is defined as postpartum hemorrhage (PPH). The blood loss frequently occurs in the first few hours after delivery but can occur more than twenty-four hours later.

47. **C:** A FHR of more than 160 beats per minute for a period of ten minutes or longer is defined as *fetal tachycardia*. Fetal tachycardia is a response of increased sympathetic tone and is reflected by a compensatory mechanism to increase cardiac output in the presence of transient hypoxia. A decreased variability is generally associated with tachycardia. Factors that contribute to tachycardia include maternal fever, smoking, use of beta-sympathomimetic agents, fetal anemia, fetal hypovolemia, chorioamnionitis, and maternal hyperthyroidism. Whatever the mechanism of insult to the fetus, the plan of action when presented with possible fetal

distress is intrauterine resuscitation. Refer to table in question no. 45 to review the "key" formula LOCK.

48. **B:** *Late decelerations* always indicate uteroplacental insufficiency; there is inadequate oxygen exchange in the placenta during a contraction. Uteroplacental insufficiency may result from *pregnancy-induced hypertension (PIH),* diabetes mellitus (DM), cardiovascular or kidney disease, chorioamnionitis, smoking, and a fetus that is past maturity. It may also result from decreased placental perfusion in *placental abruption or previa,* uterine hypertonus as a result of oxytocin stimulation, and hypotension. Signs of fetal decompensation include back-to-back decelerations, loss of variability, lack of spontaneous accelerations, tachycardia, and subtle decelerations. Standard interventions that may help to resolve the abnormal pattern (and that may also be warranted for some category II tracings) include supplemental oxygen to the mother, a change in maternal position, discontinuation of oxytocin, and resolution of maternal hypotension. In most situations, expeditious delivery is likely warranted if an abnormal pattern persists.

49. **A:** *Early decelerations* are innocuous decelerations that begin very close to the beginning of the contraction, appear almost as a "mirror image" of the contraction, and end close to the end of the contraction. *Head compression* with vagus stimulation causes the deceleration.

50. **B:** *Leopold's Maneuvers* are a common and systematic way to determine the *position of a fetus* inside the woman's uterus. The maneuvers consist of four distinct actions, each helping to determine the position of the fetus. Refer to the table.

Leopold's manuevers			
Assessment steps	Purpose	Procedure	Findings
First Manuever: Fundal grip	To determine fetal part lying in the fundus and presentation.	Using both hands, feel for the fetal part lying in the fundus.	*Head* is more firm, hard, and round and moves independently of the body. *Breech* is less well defined that moves only in conjunction with the body.
Second Manuever: Umbilical grip	To identify location of fetal back and position.	One hand is used to steady the uterus on one side of the abdomen while the other hand moves slightly on a circular motion from top to the lower segment of the uterus to feel for the fetal back and small fetal parts. Use gentle but deep pressure.	*Fetal back* is smooth, hard, and resistant surface. *Knees and elbows* of fetus feel with a number of angular nodulation.
Third Manuever: Pawlik's grip	To determine engagement of presenting part.	Using thumb and finger, grasp the lower portion of the abdomen above symphysis pubis; press in slightly and make gentle movements from side to side.	The presenting part is engaged if it is not movable. It is not yet engaged if it is still movable.
Fourth Manuever: Pelvic grip	To determine the degree of flexion of fetal head. To determine attitude or habitus.	Facing foot part of the patient, palpate fetal head, pressing downward about 2 inches above the inguinal ligament. Use both hands.	*Good attitude*—if brow correspond to the side (2nd maneuver) that contained the elbows and knees. *Poor attitude*—if examining fingers will meet an obstruction on the same side as fetal back (hyperextended head). Also palpates infant's anteroposterior position. If brow is very easily palpated, fetus is at posterior position (occiput pointing toward patient's back).

Bibliography

Alarab, M, Regan, C, O'Connell, MP, Keane, DP, O'Herlihy, C, Foley, ME. Singleton vaginal breech delivery at term: still a safe option. *Obstet Gynecol.* 2004; 103(3):407-12.

American College of Obstetricians and Gynecologists. ACOG committee opinion. Mode of term singleton breech delivery. Number 265, December 2001. *Int J Gynaecol Obstet.* 2002; 77(1):65-6.

American College of Obstetricians and Gynecologists. ACOG Practice Bulletin. Clinical Management Guidelines for Obstetrician-Gynecologists, Number 70, December 2005 (Replaces Practice Bulletin Number 62, May 2005). Intrapartum fetal heart rate monitoring. Obstet Gynecol. 2005; 106:1453-1460.

Apothecon, Princeton, NJ, Nitrazine Paper, p0083-00, p0084-00 52520. Communication from Bristol-Myers Squibb Company, March 28, 1997.

Association of Air Medical Services. (2004). *Guidelines for Air Medical Crew Education,* Iowa, Kendall/Hunt Publishing Company.

Bucher, H, Guyatt, G, Cook, RJ, Hatala, R, Cook, DJ, Lang, JD, et al. Effect of calcium supplementation on pregnancy-induced hypertension and preeclampsia: a meta-analysis of randomized controlled trials. *JAMA.* 1996; 275:1113-7.

Drug Therapy During Labor and Delivery: Premature Labor. *Am J Health Sys Pharm.* 2006; 63(12):1131-1139.

Eller, DP, VanDorsten, JP. Route of delivery for the breech presentation: a conundrum. *Am J Obstet Gynecol.* 1995; 173(2):393-6; discussion 396-8.

Hacker, Neville, Moore, JG, Joseph, G. (2004). Essentials of Obstetrics and Gynecology. 4th edition. Vol. 1. Philadelphia, Elsevier Inc. p. 151.

Hellman, LM, et al. (1971). *Williams Obstetrics,* 14th edition. New York, Appleton-Century-Crofts. pp. 405-406.

Hickok, DE, Gordon, DC, Milberg, JA, Williams, MA, Daling, JR. The frequency of breech presentation by gestational age at birth: a large population-based study. *Am J Obstet Gynecol.* 1992; 166(3):851-2.

Hofmeyr, GJ. Interventions to help external cephalic version for breech presentation at term. *Cochrane Database Syst Rev*. 2004; (1):CD000184.

Holleran, R. (1996). *Flight Nursing: Principles and Practice,* 2nd edition. St. Louis, Mosby.

Holleran, R. (2003). *Air and Surface Patient Transport: Principles and Practice,* 3rd edition. St. Louis, Mosby.

Holleran, R. (2009). *ASTNA Patient Transport: Principles and Practice,* 4th edition. St. Louis, Mosby.

Krupa, D. (1997). *Flight Nursing Core Curriculum.* Park Ridge, IL, National Flight Nurses Association.

Macones, GA, Hankins, GDV, Spong, CY, Hauth, J, Moore, T. The 2008 National Institute of Child Health and Human Development workshop report on electronic fetal monitoring: update on definitions, interpretation, and research guidelines. *Obstet Gynecol*. 2008; 112:661-666.

Magann, EF, Chauhan, SP, Naef, RW, Blake, PG, Morrison, JC, Martin, JN Jr. Standard parameters of preeclampsia: can the clinician depend upon them to reliably identify the patient with the HELLP syndrome? *Aust N Z J Obstet Gynaecol*. 1993; 33:122-6.

Martin, JN, Blake, PG, Lowry, SL, Perry, KG, Files, JC, Morrison JC. Pregnancy complicated by preeclampsia-eclampsia with the syndrome of hemolysis, elevated liver enzymes, and low platelet count: how rapid is postpartum recovery? *Obstet gynecol*. 1990; 76(5 Pt 1):737-41.

Mulik, V, Usha Kiran, TS, Bethal, J, Bhal, PS. The outcome of macrosomic fetuses in a low risk primigravid population. *Int J Gynaecol Obstet*. 2003; 80(1):15-22.

Okun, N, Verma, A, Mitchell, BF, Flowerdew, G. Relative importance of maternal constitutional factors and glucose intolerance of pregnancy in the development of newborn macrosomia. *J Matern Fetal Med*. 1997; 6(5):285-90.

Omu, AE, Al-Harmi, J, Vedi, HL, Mlechkova, L, Sayed, AF, Al-Ragum, NS. Magnesium sulphate therapy in women with pre-eclampsia and eclampsia in Kuwait. *Med Princ Pract*. 2008; 17(3):227-32.

Page, EW, Villee, CA, Villee, DB. (1976). *Human Reproduction,* 2nd Edition. Philadelphia, W. B. Saunders. p. 211.

Portis, R, Jacobs, MA, Skerman, JH, Skerman, EB. HELLP syndrome (hemolysis, elevated liver enzymes, and low platelets) pathophysiology and anesthetic considerations. *AANA J.* 1997; 65:37-47.

Richards, DA, Tuckman, J, Prichard, BN. Assessment of alpha—and beta-adrenoceptor blocking actions of labetalol. *Br J Clin Pharmacol.* 1976; 3(5):849-855.

Riva, E, Mennini, T, Latini, R. The alpha—and beta-adrenoceptor blocking activities of labetalol and its RR-SR (50:50) stereoisomers. *Br J Pharmacol.* 1991; 104(4):823-8.

Sibai, BM, Frangieh, AY. Management of severe preeclampsia. *Curr Opin Obstet Gynecol.* 1996; 8:110-3.

Sibai, BM. Acute renal failure in pregnancies complicated by HELLP. *Am J Obstet Gynecol.* 1993; 168:1682.

Spellacy, WN, Miller, S, Winegar, A, Peterson, PQ. Macrosomia—maternal characteristics and infant complications. *Obstet Gynecol.* 1985; 66(2):158-61.

Speroff, L, Glass, RH, Kase, NG. (1999). *Clinical Gynecological Endocrinology and Infertility,* 6th edition. Lippincott Williams & Wilkins. p. 1149.

Tay, JI, Moore, J, Walker, JJ. Ectopic pregnancy. *West J Med.* 2000; 173(2):131-4.

Tomsen, TR. HELLP syndrome (hemolysis, elevated liver enzymes, and low platelets) presenting as generalized malaise. *Am J Obstet Gynecol.* 1995; 172:1876-90.

Vendittelli, F, Rivière, O, Crenn-Hébert C, Rozan, MA, Maria B, Jacquetin, B. Is a breech presentation at term more frequent in women with a history of cesarean delivery? *Am J Obstet Gynecol.* 2008; 198(5):521. e1-6.

Weinstein, L. Syndrome of hemolysis, elevated liver enzymes, and low platelet count: a severe consequence of hypertension in pregnancy. *Am J Obstet Gynecol.* 1982; 142 (2): 159-67.

Yui-Ming Lam, Hung-Fat Tse, Chu-Pak Lau. Continuous calcium chloride infusion for massive nifedipine overdose. *Chest.* 119(4):1280-1282.

Module 9
Neonatal and Pediatric Emergencies

1. Pediatric dose for Epinephrine is

   A. 0.1 mg/kg IV
   B. 0.01 mg/kg ETT
   C. 1 mg IV
   D. 0.01 mg/kg IV

2. The pediatric patient may be pretreated with which medication prior to administering Anectine for the purpose of preventing bradycardia?

   A. Etomidate
   B. Atropine
   C. Oxygen
   D. Vecuronium

3. You are transporting a thirty-two-week premature neonate with respiratory distress. Which drug may be administered in preparation for transport?

   A. Antibiotics
   B. Surfactant
   C. D10
   D. Prostaglandin

4. A neonate who is experiencing repetitive motions of a bicycling type action with lip smacking is presenting with what type of seizure?

   A. Subtle
   B. Tonic
   C. Clonic
   D. Myoclonic

5. Your patient is PDA dependent. This would indicate likely require the administration of which of the following drugs?

   A. Indomethacin
   B. Progesterone
   C. Prostaglandin
   D. Synthetic surfactant

6. Which of the following would calculate an appropriate ETT size for a pediatric patient?

   A. (age + 12)/4
   B. Age + (16/4)
   C. (Age + 16)/4
   D. Age/4+4

7. Some pediatric endotracheal tubes are cuffless, which prevents

   A. Gastric insufflation
   B. Right mainstem intubation
   C. Aspiration
   D. Subglottic stenosis and ulcerations

8. Persistent Pulmonary Hypertension (PPHN) is a syndrome characterized by persistent elevated pulmonary vascular resistance resulting in

   A. Right-to-left shunt
   B. Left-to-right shunt
   C. Apnea
   D. Systemic hypotension

9. The most common side effect, complicating transport of a newborn with the use of Prostaglandin E1 is

   A. Hypoglycemia
   B. Apnea, hypoventilation
   C. Hypotension
   D. Diarrhea

10. A medication utilized in the neonate that accelerates closure of the PDA is

   A. Ibuprofen, Indomethacin
   B. Dobutamine
   C. PGE1
   D. Oxytocin

11. A pediatric patient presents to the ED in acute respiratory distress, with increased work of breathing and reduced oxygen saturation. The patient is treated with multiple rounds of nebulized albuterol, ipratropium, oxygen supplementation, and parental steroids, with none to minimal improvement in clinical and objective evidence of respiratory distress. Which of the following medications is recommended for sedation prior to intubation because of the bronchodilatory effect it possesses?

   A. Etomidate
   B. Ketamine
   C. Versed
   D. Fentanyl

12. You are transporting a nine-year-old man weighing 40 kg with diagnosis of status asthmaticus on a ventilator. $EtCO_2$ is 60. Ventilator settings are at Vt 250, FIO_2 1.0, Rate 16, I:E 1:3, PEEP 5, PIP 48. How will you manage this patient?

   A. Increase tidal volume
   B. Increase I:E ratio
   C. Increase PEEP
   D. Increase respiratory rate

13. Recommended urinary output when caring for a pediatric patient should be

   A. 100 mL/hr
   B. 30-50 mL/hr
   C. 1-2 cc/kg/hr
   D. >200 mL/hr

14. You are transporting a three-year-old boy who was struck by a vehicle two hours prior to your arrival in the ER department. Your assessment reveals BP 60/38, HR 54, RR 36, SaO_2 92%, skin condition is cool, with a delayed capillary refill. He is awake but is restless and irritable. Which of the following should always be recognized as ominous signs and should be treated aggressively in the pediatric patient?

    A. Tachypnea and bradycardia
    B. Delayed capillary refill and cool skin
    C. Decreased level of consciousness and hypotension
    D. Hypotension and bradycardia

15. You are transporting a 20-kg patient presenting with second- and third-degree burns to his entire face, anterior torso, and complete left arm. How much fluid should the patient receive in the first eight hours using the Parkland formula?

    A. 2,880 mL
    B. 1,960 mL
    C. 1,440 mL
    D. 3,650 mL

16. You are transporting a newborn who was delivered vaginally in a small ER about six hours prior to your arrival with a history of bilious vomiting, abdominal distention, feeding intolerance, and lack of stools for the last twenty-four hours. Initial management would include

    A. Endotracheal intubation and ventilation
    B. Needle decompression to correct underlying pulmonary leak
    C. Decompression of the bowel with intermittent large-bore gastric suction
    D. Request contrast studies for further evaluation prior to transport

17. You are managing a four-year-old boy presenting lethargic with nystagmus. You note he has depressed DTRs and has a profound anion-gap. The patient should be managed with which of the following?

    A. IV ethanol drip
    B. Calcium
    C. Potassium supplement
    D. Sodium bicarbonate

18. The fetus was delivered with obvious meconium staining. His one-minute APGAR is 8. Endotracheal suctioning

    A. Should be performed via nose, then mouth
    B. Should be performed via mouth, then nose
    C. Should be performed endotracheally, then mouth, then nose
    D. Should not be performed

19. Which of the following lab test is used to diagnose Reye's syndrome?

    A. Liver function tests
    B. Ammonia
    C. BUN
    D. Potassium

20. During transport, management of a thirty-seven week newborn diagnosed with persistent pulmonary hypertension (PPHN) may include which of the following to prevent right-to-left shunting?

    A. Maintaining a $pCO_2 > 45$ mmHg
    B. Continuous monitoring of the blood pressure; support blood pressure with fluid volume replacement, and a vasopressor as needed
    C. Continuous monitoring of the serum glucose
    D. Administration of surfactant

21. Pediatric airway anatomy differs from adult anatomy in the following ways, *except*

   A. Airway diameter in children is smaller than adults
   B. The larynx is located more anterior in infants and children
   C. The epiglottis is long and narrow and angled away from the trachea
   D. In children, younger than six years of age, the narrowest portion of the trachea is at the cricoid process.

22. Primary cause of bradycardia in the neonate and pediatric patient is

   A. Hypoglycemia
   B. Hypoxia
   C. Hypovolemia
   D. Hemorrhage

23. Drug of choice for profound hypotension in septic shock is

   A. Isotonic crystalloid solution
   B. Levophed
   C. Nipride
   D. Dobutamine

24. You are managing a four-year-old boy who is requiring intubation. The appropriate size ET tube for this patient would be

   A. 3.5
   B. 4.0
   C. 4.5
   D. 5.0

25. What finding would you expect to see on a chest x-ray for a patient presenting with laryngotracheobronchitis?

   A. Macdonald's sign
   B. Angel wing sign
   C. Steeple sign
   D. Thumb print sign

26. Vt is calculated at

    A. 3-5 mL/kg
    B. 5-8 mL/kg
    C. 6-10 mL/kg
    D. 10-15 mL/kg

27. A scaphoid abdomen, unequeal breath sounds, dyspnea, and a shift in the PMI are a classic presentation of which of the following in the neonate patient?

    A. Tension pneumothorax
    B. Diaphragmatic hernia
    C. Aspiration pneumonia
    D. RDS, formerly known as hyaline membrane disease

28. Hypoglycemia in the neonate can be treated with

    A. D 25% 2-4 mL/kg
    B. D 10% 2-4 mL/kg
    C. D 10% 5-10 mL/kg
    D. D 5% 2-4 mg/kg

29. You are transporting a ten-year-old boy with a history of being struck by a vehicle while riding his bicycle. Your assessment reveals a deteriorating neurologic status, hypotension, and bradycardia. Your management of the this patient would include all of the following, *except*

    A. Elevation of the backboard to 30 degrees
    B. Fluid resuscitation
    C. Serum glucose determination
    D. Nasal intubation

30. A full-term newborn weighing 2,800 grams should be intubated with what size endotracheal tube?

    A. 2.5
    B. 3.0
    C. 3.5
    D. 4.0

31. An eight-year-old child was hit by a car. Your assessment reveals radiation of pain to the left shoulder, ecchymosis, and abrasions to the retroperitoneal area bilaterally and abdominal distention. What injury do you suspect?

    A. Liver
    B. Spleen
    C. Pneumothorax
    D. Kidney

32. What finding would you expect to see on the lateral neck x-ray to confirm suspicion of epiglottitis?

    A. McDonald's sign
    B. Steeple sign
    C. Angel wing sign
    D. Thumb print sign

33. Fluid resuscitation in a neonate patient should be administered at

    A. 5 mL/kg
    B. 10 mL/kg
    C. 15 mL/kg
    D. 20 mL/kg

34. You are transporting a four-year-old boy trauma patient. You are preparing to administer a weight per kg based medication. How many kilograms does patient weigh approximately?

    A. 10 kg
    B. 12 kg
    C. 15 kg
    D. 20 kg

35. Expected endotracheal tube centimeter depth for a neonate can best be determined by using which of the following formulas?

    A. 6 + weight in kg
    B. 16 + age in years divided by 4
    C. 10 + weight in kg
    D. 3 + weight in kg

36. When identifying vessels on the umbilical stump, the umbilical vein, as compared to the umbilical arteries, is usually located at what position?

    A. 10 o'clock
    B. 4 o'clock
    C. 12 o'clock
    D. 8 o'clock

37. The circulating blood volume in a child is

    A. 10-20 mL/kg
    B. 20-40 mL/kg
    C. 50-60 mL/kg
    D. 70-80 mL/kg

38. A surgical airway can be placed through the cricothyroid membrane on children over the age of

    A. 8 years
    B. 10 years
    C. 11 years
    D. 12 years

39. In an emergency situation, an umbilical vein catheter when placed correctly should only be inserted as far as necessary to obtain blood and should not go beyond which of the following?

    A. Level of the right atrium
    B. Liver
    C. Kidneys
    D. Ductus venonus

40. Noninitiation or discontinuation of newborn resuscitation as recommended by the International Guidelines for Neonatal Resuscitation include all of the following, *except*?

    A. Birthweight < 500 grams
    B. Confirmed trisomy 13 or 18
    C. Gestational age < 28 weeks
    D. Severe fetal growth restriction or congenital hydrocephalus

41. One of the most common causes of new-onset wheezing in children is

    A. Croup
    B. Bronchiolitis
    C. Epiglottitis
    D. Pneumonia

42. Which of the following is not indicated for the treatment of bronchiolitis?

    A. Adequate hydration
    B. Supplemental oxygen
    C. Corticosteroids
    D. Nebulized albuterol aerosols

43. You are transporting a five-year-old boy with a diagnosis of sepsis secondary, a localized necrotic skin area of unknown etiology. The "bull's-eye" appearing necrotic area is noted to the left upper thigh area. Which of the following may be the most likely cause?

   A. Black widow spider bite
   B. Brown recluse spider bite
   C. Snake bite
   D. Scorpion sting

44. A ten-year-old boy presents to the emergency department with a history of feeling a "sharp" pinprick, dull numbing pain to the right foot, muscle cramping, with intense abdominal pain that started about thirty minutes prior. Which of the following may be the most likely cause

   A. Black widow spider bite
   B. Brown recluse spider bite
   C. Snake bite
   D. Scorpion sting

45. You have been called to the scene for a six-year-old girl with a history of snake bite to the left lower extremity while on a camping trip. Management of this patient would include all of the following, *except*

   A. Immobilization of the affected extremity in neutral position
   B. Measuring the leg girth every fifteen minutes and marking the line of demarcation
   C. Administration of pain analgesia, antihistamines, and anti-inflammatory medications
   D. Application of ice to the affected area

46. A newborn who is hypoxic in room air but demonstrates a partial pressure of oxygen greater than 150 in 100% oxygen is more likely to have which of the following?

    A. Heart disease
    B. Pulmonary disease
    C. Esophageal atresia
    D. Necrotizing enterocolitis

47. Gastroschisis in a newborn is best described as

    A. Ischemia of the bowel
    B. An arrest of the development of the abdominal wall, with the abdominal contents remaining externalized, which is covered by a membrane
    C. Persistent elevated pulmonary vascular resistance resulting in a right-to-left shunt at the ductus arteriosus or the foramen ovale, leading to hypoxemia
    D. A defect in the abdominal wall that has otherwise completed its development and allows protrusion of abdominal contents which is not covered by a membrane

48. When transporting a neonate suspected of having esophageal atresia, you should immediately

    A. Obtain vascular access and administer fluids
    B. Elevate the head of the bed to prevent gastric reflux
    C. Provide positive-pressure ventilation
    D. Obtain a chest x-ray

49. Which of the following scenarios would be most suspicious for possible child abuse?

   A. three year old who present with tibial fracture after reportedly falling down a few steps
   B. two year old who presents with a forehead hematoma after reportedly falling out of stroller
   C. Four month old who presents with a nondisplaced femur fracture after reportedly rolling off of the changing table
   D. Four year old who presents with a spiral fracture of the tibia after reportedly getting his leg twisted while falling off a tricycle

50. You have been requested to transport a five-year-old who was involved in a single rollover accident two hours prior to your arrival at the referring facility. Your exam reveals the following vital signs: Temp. 37.0, P160, RR ventilated via the tracheal tube at 20, BP 100/80, oxygen saturation 97%. He is still unresponsive and being ventilated via the tracheal tube. His pupils are briskly reactive to light. There is excellent chest wall rise and fall via ventilation through the tracheal tube. There are numerous abrasions over his face, chest, abdomen, and lower extremities. The abdomen is distended with decreased bowel sounds. His pelvis is stable, but his right thigh is obviously swollen and tense. Distal perfusion to all four extremities seems adequate. The remainder of his physical examination is unremarkable. The child is clinically presenting with which of the following?

   A. Decompenstated shock
   B. Early decompensated shock
   C. Irreversible shock
   D. Compensated progressive shock

Answer Key and Rationale

1. **D:** *Epinephrine (adrenaline)* is a hormone and neurotransmitter. It increases heart rate (beta 1 and inotropic effect), contracts blood vessels (alpha property), dilates air passages (beta-2 property), and participates in the fight-or-flight response of the sympathetic nervous system. A pediatric dosage of 0.01 mg/kg (intravenous or intraosseous route) is recommended every 3-5 minutes as needed. Endotracheal tube route dosage is 0.1 mg/kg body weight (0.1 mL of a 1:1,000 solution). Adrenaline is used as a drug to treat cardiac arrest and other cardiac dysrhythmias resulting in diminished or absent cardiac output. Its primary action initially is to increase peripheral resistance via alpha receptor-dependent vasoconstriction and secondly is to increase cardiac output via its binding to beta-receptors.

2. **B:** Bradydysrhythmia is a complication that frequently is associated with succinylcholine (Anectine) use, especially in the pediatric patient, but may also occur in adults. *Pretreatment with atropine (0.02 mg/kg)* is advised in children to prevent bradycardia, and pretreatment with lidocaine (1.5 mg/kg) in patients with suspected or known head injury has been shown to attenuate the rise in ICP associated with endotracheal initubation. *Atropine* is a tropane alkaloid extracted from deadly nightshade (*Atropa belladonna*), jimsonweed (*Datura stramonium*), mandrake (*Mandragora officinarum*), and other plants of the family Solanaceae. Atropine increases firing of the sinoatrial (SA) node and conduction through the atrioventricular (AV) node of the heart, opposes the actions of the vagus nerve, blocks acetylcholine receptor sites, and decreases bronchial secretions. It is classified as a parasympatholytic *(lytic—blocks)*. It is usually not effective in second-degree heart block (Mobitz type 2) and in third-degree heart block with a low Purkinje or ventricular escape rhythm. Atropine is contraindicated in ischemia-induced conduction block (widened QRS), because the drug increases oxygen demand of the AV nodal tissue, thereby aggravating ischemia and the resulting heart block.

3. **B:** The most common cause of respiratory distress in *the preterm infant (born before 28-32 weeks of gestation)* is respiratory distress syndrome (RDS), formerly known as hyaline membrane

disease (HMD). This condition is primarily caused by a *deficiency of surfactant*. Surfactant decreases the surface tension in the alveolus during expiration, allowing the alveolus to maintain a functional residual capacity. The absence of surfactant results in poor lung compliance and atelectasis. Goal treatment for the use of exogenous surfactant is to increase pulmonary compliance, to prevent atelectasis at the end of expiration, and to facilitate recruitment of collapsed airways. The cornerstone of treatment of RDS is supplemental oxygen to maintain a PaO_2 of 60-70 mmHg and an arterial saturation of 92-95%.

4. **A:** *Subtle seizures* are a type of seizure that is frequently overlooked by health-care providers. It may consist of repetitive mouth or tongue movement, bicycling movements, eye deviations, repetitive blinking, staring, or apnea. To treat neonatal seizures, it is important to attempt to identify the cause. The glucose level should be checked immediately, and if hypoglycemia is present (serum glucose < 40 mg/dL), it should be corrected immediately with 10% of dextrose (2 mL/kg) administering followed with a maintenance infusion drip of 10% of dextrose (80 mL/kg/24 hours). The serum glucose should be checked within 20-30 minutes. Seizures can be managed with different medications to include phenobarbital (luminal), phenytoin (dilantin), and lorazepam (ativan).

Seizures	
Category of seizure	Clinical manifestation
Subtle	It may consist of repetitive mouth or tongue movement, bicycling movements, eye deviations, repetitive blinking, staring, or apnea.
Clonic	Characterized by repetitive jerky movement of the limbs, which may move from limb-to-limb in a disorganized fashion.
Tonic	May resemble posturing seen in older infants and children. It can be accompanied by disturbed respiratory patterns; it may include tonic extension of limb or limbs, or tonic flexion of upper limbs and extension of the lower limbs.
Myoclonic	Characterized by multiple jerking motions of the upper (common) or lower (rare) extremities.

5. **C:** *Prostaglandins* are normally used during transport when the patient's condition is deteriorating, as indicated by the presence of metabolic acidosis, or when deterioration is anticipated before the completion of the transport. Prostaglandin E_1 (PGE 1) is indicated for those heart defects that may be dependent on ductal patency for pulmonary blood flow. These heart defects include transposition without ventricular septal defect (VSD), pulmonary or tricuspid atresia, and critical pulmonary stenosis, including tetralogy of Fallot (TOF). Coarctation of the aorta and hypoplastic left heart syndrome may also require the use of PGE 1 for stabilization for transport. Keeping the patent ductus arteriosus (PDA) open using this medication allows stabilization of the newborn until more definitive treatment, usually surgical, can be carried out.

6. **C:** The proper endotracheal tube (ETT) size can be determined in several ways. It can be approximated by the size of the child's little finger or nares. Refer to table to review more precise methods to ensure proper ETT size and ensure proper tube depth placement.

Methods of calculating proper ET tube size		
Age	ETT size (mm)	ETT depth (cm)
Preterm	3.0 (Preterm infants less than 28 weeks may require a smaller ET tube, 2.5)	6 + weight per kg
Full-term	3.5	6 + weight per kg
One year and above	(Age in years) + 16 divided by 4	ETT size × 3 in the orally intubated patient or 10 + age in years at the gums

7. **D:** *Pediatric tubes that are cuffless prevent subglottic stenosis and ulceration,* and they range in size from 2.5-6.5 mm. Cuffless tubes are recommended in *children younger than eight years of age* because the *cricoid cartilage is the narrowest portion of the trachea,* and if the tube used is of proper size, it serves as a physiologic cuff. A tube that is too large will not pass through the cricoid cartilage. A tube that is too small will not provide total airway protection.

8. **A:** Persistent pulmonary hypertension of the newborn (PPHN) results in a *right-to-left shunt* at the ductus arteriosus or the foramen ovale, leading to hypoxemia in the presence of a structurally normal heart. Demonstration of right-to-left shunting at the ductus using preductal and postductal simultaneous arterial blood gas (ABG) levels is helpful in the diagnosis.

9. **B:** *Apnea and hypoventilation* are the most common side effects complicating transport with the use of PGE 1. The length of transport and the difficulty of placing an ETT during transport must be considered in the decision of whether to place an ETT before transport when prostaglandins are begun. Other side effects can include fever, vasodilation with flushing, and diarrhea. Uncommonly, the vasodilation may result in systemic hypotension requiring intervention.

10. **A:** In newborns, a medication such as *indomethacin or ibuprofen* can be given to accelerate closure of the PDA. These medications are given in the stomach and can constrict the muscle in the wall of the PDA and promote closure. These drugs do have side effects, however, such as kidney injury or bleeding, so not all infants can receive them. Because of the potential side effects, the infant must have lab values checked before medications can be given. If the lab values are not normal or if the medications do not work, surgery can be performed and the PDA tied off (ligated).

In some heart defects, such as pulmonary atresia (an underdeveloped or blocked pulmonary valve), the PDA supplies the only adequate source of blood flow to the lungs so that oxygen can be delivered to the blood. In these patients, the ductus arteriosus supplies blood to the lungs from the aorta. In other anomalies, such as underdeveloped or severely narrowed aorta (such as seen in hypoplastic left heart syndrome), the PDA is crucial to allow adequate blood flow to the body. In these patients, the ductus arteriosus supplies blood to the body from the pulmonary artery.

The presence of the characteristic murmur, along with symptoms of heart failure, in a premature infant most frequently leads to the diagnosis of PDA. The chest radiograph will exhibit an enlarged heart and evidence of an excessive amount of blood flow to the lungs. An echocardiogram is taken to confirm the diagnosis. This will demonstrate the size of the ductus arteriosus and will demonstrate if the heart chambers have become enlarged due to the extra blood flow. In older children, the chest radiograph typically normal.

TOF is the most common cyanotic heart defect, and the most common cause of blue baby syndrome. There is anatomic variation between the hearts of individuals with TOF. Primarily, the degree of right ventricular outflow tract obstruction varies between patients and generally determines clinical symptoms and disease progression. TOF results in low oxygenation of blood due to the mixing of oxygenated and deoxygenated blood in the left ventricle via the VSD and preferential flow of the mixed blood from both ventricles through the aorta because of the obstruction to flow through the pulmonary valve. This is known as a right-to-left shunt. The primary symptom is low blood oxygen saturation with or without cyanosis from birth or developing in the first year of life. If the baby is not cyanotic, then it is sometimes referred to as a "pink tet." Other symptoms include a heart murmur, which may range from almost imperceptible to very loud, difficulty in feeding, failure to gain weight, retarded growth and physical development, dyspnea on exertion, clubbing of the fingers and toes, and polycythemia.

Tetralogy of Fallot (PROV)	
Type of anomaly	Definition
Pulmonary stenosis	A narrowing of the right ventricular outflow tract and can occur at the pulmonary valve (valvular stenosis) or just below the pulmonary valve (infundibular stenosis).
Right ventricular hypertrophy	The right ventricle is more muscular than normal, causing a characteristic boot-shaped appearance as seen by chest x-ray. Due to the misarrangement of the external ventricular septum, the right ventricular wall increases in size to deal with the increased obstruction to the right outflow tract.
Overriding aorta	An aortic valve with biventricular connection, that is, it is situated above the VSD and connected to both the right and the left ventricle.
Ventricular septal defect (VSD)	A hole between the two bottom chambers (ventricles) of the heart.

Children with TOF may develop "tet spells." The precise mechanism of these episodes is in doubt, but presumably results from a transient increase in resistance to blood flow to the lungs with increased preferential flow of desaturated blood to the body. Tet spells are characterized by a sudden, marked increase in cyanosis followed by syncope, and may result in hypoxic brain injury and death. Older children will often squat during a tet spell, which increases systemic vascular resistance and allows for a temporary reversal of the shunt.

11. **B:** Children experiencing severe asthma exacerbations may deteriorate to respiratory failure requiring endotracheal intubation and mechanical ventilation. Mechanical ventilation is often life saving in this setting, but also exposes the asthmatic child to substantial iatrogenic risk. *Ketamine* does have proven bronchodilation effects and is the anesthesia of choice for patients in respiratory distress. Ketamine does appear to have a beneficial role in reducing the length of intubation or hospital admission and level of respiratory distress in pediatric asthma patients already intubated or admitted to the ICU using multiple standard and nonstandard treatment modalities.

12. **B:** The primary goal of asthma management is reversal of hypoxemia as well as control of contributing inflammatory responses. Too much oxygen or mechanical force may result in lung injury. Insufficient oxygen or mechanical force will result in hypoxia and hypoventilation. The starting respiratory rate (RR) is in part age determined, commonly 30-50 in neonates, 25-30 in infants, 20 in children, and 10-15 in teenagers. The rate is also dependent on the disease process. For example, patients who have air trapping or hyperinflation disorders (such as asthma) need a longer expiratory phase and therefore, a slower rate. The inspiratory time (IT or I-time) is also age and rate dependent and will also need to be altered depending on the child's disease. A guideline is 0.4-0.7 seconds for infants and 0.5-1 seconds for children and adults. Longer I-times increase mean airway pressure (MAP) (by prolonging the inspiratory cycle) and therefore usually improve oxygenation. In choosing a tidal volume (TV) or PIP, the most important tenant to remember is, in general, to use a volume

or pressure that causes good visible chest rise and air entry on auscultation. For TV ventilation, the starting range is usually about 5-8 mL/kg.

Adjusting the FIO_2 will only affect the pO_2 and oxygen saturation. Increasing the ventilator rate will increase the minute ventilation, so this decreases the pCO_2 (and hence increases the pH). These are the two most basic changes that occur in ventilator management. One could also increase the minute ventilation (which would decrease the pCO_2) by increasing the TV (on a volume ventilator) or the PIP (on a pressure ventilator). Also realize that any parameter change which increases the MAP will also increase the pO_2. One could increase the MAP by increasing the positive end-expiratory pressure (PEEP), the IT, or the PIP. Increasing the TV on a volume ventilator, in essence, increases the PIP, so this also increases the MAP.

In nonventilated patients, the glottis opens and closes during spontaneous respirations. Partial closure of the glottis provides a physiologic "PEEP" of 3-4 mmHg by preventing complete emptying of the airway. In patients with good oxygenation and little pulmonary disease, a PEEP of 3-5 mmHg is adequate. Higher PEEPs are necessary for the patient with pulmonary edema, pneumonia, or atelectasis. High PEEP may also be useful for the postoperative heart patient with surgical bleeding. Be aware that increasing PEEP increases MAP. Patients with high MAPs may require volume infusions to maintain venous return and cardiac output. Inotropic support may also be needed in patients requiring very high PEEP of > 10 mmHg.

13. **C:** End-organ perfusion will decrease with fluid or blood loss and will be reflected by oliguria or anuria. *Maintenance of 1-2 mL/kg of urine output* is the goal of circulatory support in the pediatric patient. Urinary output varies with age.

Urine output parameters		
Newborns to one year	Toddlers	Older children
2 mL/kg/hr	1.5 mL/kg/hr	1 mL/kg/hr

After fluid resuscitation, maintenance fluids must be provided on a kilogram body weight basis. Prevention of hypothermia as a result of fluid resuscitation is imperative.

Intravenous maintenance fluid formula		
First 10 kg of body weight	Second 10 kg of body weight	Any weight > 20 kg
100 mL/kg/24 hr	50 mL/kg/24 hr	20 mL/kg/24 hr

Example: Following this formula, a 30 kg pediatric patient would require 1,700 mL over 24 hours (1,000 mL for the first 10 kg, 500 mL for the second 10 kg, and 200 mL for the remaining 10 kg), hourly rate set at 70 mL/hr on the infusion pump.

14. **D:** The initial compensatory mechanism that the transport team should look for during the early stages of hemorrhagic shock is tachycardia. The other compensatory mechanism that occurs to maintain normal perfusion and blood pressure is an increase in the systemic vascular resistance, which is manifested clinically by mottled or cool extremities, weak or thready distal pulses, delayed capillary refill time, and a narrowed pulse pressure.

Hypotension and bradycardia should always be recognized as ominous signs and aggressively treated in the pediatric patient. After ventilation and oxygenation has been addressed, fluid resuscitation should quickly follow. Resuscitation begins with a 20 mL/kg bolus of warmed Ringer's lactate or normal saline. Because only approximately one-third of crystalloid infusions remain in the intravascular space, this bolus may need to repeated twice or thrice. If more than 40-60 mL/kg of crystalloid solution is required to restore adequate perfusion, blood replacement must then be considered. The administration of 10 mL/kg of type specific or O negative packed red blood cells (PRBCs) should be considered in the pediatric patient presenting with hypovolemic shock.

15. **C:** The objective assessment of the burn injury itself includes estimating the burn size and depth, associated inhalation injuries, and calculation of fluid resuscitation needs. The size of the burn wound is most frequently estimated by using the rule of nines method, which divides the body into multiples of 9%. A fairly

accurate approximation can be made using the patient's entire palm size to represent 1% of the total BSA and visualizing that palm over the burned area.

BSA calculated: 9% entire face; 18% anterior torso; 9% complete left arm.

Answer: $4 \times 20 = 80$; $80 \times 36 = 2{,}880$; ½ administered in the first 8 hours = 1,440 mL. Refer table to review the rule of nines.

Rule of nines		
Body area	Adult (%)	Pediatric (%)
Head	9	18
Anterior torso	18	18
Back	18	18
Each arm	9	9
Each leg	18	14
Neck or genital area	1	0

16. **C:** Common initial symptoms for intestinal obstruction include bilious vomiting, abdominal distention, feeding intolerance, large quantities of gastric contents at delivery, absence of an anal opening, and lack of stooling in the first twenty-four hours. Presence of tenderness, metabolic acidosis, or decreasing platelets may indicate a bowel necrosis or peritonitis and should be treated as an urgent problem. *Management includes decompression of the bowel with intermittent large-bore gastric suction,* IV fluids, antibiotic therapy as indicated, and respiratory support. Severe abdominal distention may compromise respiratory status.

17. **A:** *Ethylene glycol poisoning* is caused by the ingestion of ethylene glycol (the primary ingredient in both automotive antifreeze and hydraulic brake fluid). It is a toxic, colorless, odorless, and almost nonvolatile liquid with a sweet taste and is occasionally consumed by children for its sweetness. Following ingestion, the symptoms of poisoning follow a three-step progression starting with intoxication and vomiting, before causing metabolic acidosis, cardiovascular dysfunction, and finally acute kidney failure. Treatment consists of

initially stabilizing the patient followed by the use of antidotes. *The antidotes used are either ethanol or fomepizole (Antizol)* administered by intravenous infusion. The antidotes work by blocking the enzyme responsible for metabolizing ethylene glycol and therefore halt the progression of poisoning. Hemodialysis is also used to help remove ethylene glycol and its metabolites from the blood.

Ethylene glycol toxicity stages	
Stages	Clinical manifestation
I	Stage 1 (0.5-12 hours) consists of neurological and gastrointestinal symptoms; patients may appear to be intoxicated, exhibiting symptoms such as dizziness, incoordination of muscle movements, nystagmus, headaches, slurred speech, and confusion. Irritation to the stomach may cause nausea and vomiting. Over time, the body metabolized ethylene glycol into other toxins.
II	Stage 2 (12-36 hours) is a result of accumulation of organic acids formed by the metabolism of ethylene glycol and consists of increased heart rate, high blood pressure, hyperventilation, and metabolic acidosis. Additionally low calcium levels in the blood, overactive muscle reflexes, muscle spasms, prolonged QT interval, and congestive hear failure may occur. If untreated, death most commonly occurs during this period.
III	Stage 3 (24-72 hours) of ethylene glycol poisoning is the result of kidney injury. Symptoms include acute tubular necrosis, red blood cells in the urine, excess proteins in the urine, lower back pain, decreased production of urine, anuria, hyperkalemia, and acute kidney failure. If kidney failure occurs, it is typically reversible, although weeks or months of supportive care including hemodialysis may be required before kidney function returns.

18. **D:** Meconium is normally stored in the infant's intestines until after birth, but sometimes (often in response to fetal distress) it is expelled into the amniotic fluid prior to birth, or during labor. If the baby then inhales the contaminated fluid, respiratory problems may occur. The most obvious sign that meconium has been passed during or before labor is the greenish or yellowish appearance of the amniotic fluid. After birth, rapid or labored breathing, cyanosis, slow heartbeat, a barrel-shaped chest or *low APGAR score* are all signs of the syndrome. Inhalation can be confirmed by one or more tests such as using a stethoscope to listen for abnormal lung sounds (diffuse crackles and rhonchi), performing blood gas tests to confirm a severe loss of lung function, and using chest x-rays to look for

patchy or streaked areas on the lungs. Infants who have inhaled meconium may develop RDS often requiring ventilatory support. Complications of meconium aspiration include pneumothorax and PPHN. When meconium staining of the amniotic fluid is present and the baby is born depressed, it is recommended by the newborn resuscitation guidelines that an individual trained in neonatal intubation use a laryngoscope and ETT to suction meconium from below the vocal cords. The APGAR score is determined by evaluating the newborn baby on five simple criteria on a scale from zero to two, then summing up the five values thus obtained. The resulting APGAR score ranges from zero to ten. The five criteria (*A*ppearance, *P*ulse, *G*rimace, *A*ctivity, *R*espiration) are used as a mnemonic learning aid. The test is generally done at one and five minutes after birth, and may be repeated later if the score is and remains low. Scores 3 and below are generally regarded as critically low, 4 to 6 fairly low, and 7 to 10 generally normal.

APGAR score			
Acronym	Score of 0	Score of 1	Score of 2
Appearance (skin color)	Blue or pale all over	Blue extremities, body pink	No body cyanosis, extremities pink
Pulse (heart rate)	< 60	< 100	< 100
Grimace (reflex, irritability)	No response to stimulation	Grimace, weak cry when stimulated	Crys or pulls away when stimulated
Activity (muscle tone)	None	Some flexion	Flexed arms and legs that resist
Respiratory (breathing)	Absent	Weak, irregular, gasping	Strong lusty cry

19. **B:** *Reye's syndrome* is a potentially fatal disease that causes numerous detrimental effects to many organs, especially the brain and liver, as well as causing hypoglycemia. The exact cause is unknown, and while it has been associated with aspirin consumption by children with viral illness, it also occurs in the absence of aspirin use. The disease causes fatty liver with minimal inflammation and severe encephalopathy (with swelling of the brain). The liver may become slightly enlarged and firm, and there is a change in the appearance of the kidneys. Jaundice is not usually present. Early

diagnosis is vital; while most children recover with supportive therapy, severe brain injury or death are potential complications. The *ammonia test* is primarily used to help investigate the cause of changes in behavior and consciousness. It may be ordered, along with other tests such as glucose, electrolytes, and kidney and liver function tests, to help diagnose the cause of a coma of unknown origin or to help support the diagnosis of Reye's syndrome or hepatic encephalopathy caused by various liver diseases.

Increased ammonia levels and decreased glucose levels may indicate the presence of Reye's syndrome in symptomatic children and adolescents. The following are possible reasons why this test may be done:

- hepatic encephalopathy
- inborn error of metabolism
- Reye's syndrome

The following are considered to be normal results for this test:

- adults: 10-80 µg/dL
- neonates (0-10 days): 170-341 µg/dL
- infants and toddlers (10 days to 2 years): 68-136 µg/dL
- children (older than 2 years): 19-60 µg/dL

Aspirin should not be given to those under the age of 16 years, unless specifically indicated in *Kawasaki disease* or in the prevention of blood clot formation.

20. **B:** Treatment is aimed at maintaining adequate oxygenation, maintaining the infant in an alkalemic state through hyperventilation and the use of blood buffers, sedation or neuromuscular blockade, fluid boluses, and cardiotonic drugs. *Maintenance of the systemic blood pressure discourages right-to-left shunting.*

21. **D:** *In children younger than 10 years of age,* the narrowest portion of the trachea is at the cricoid process. The vocal cords are attached lower anteriorly and the tongue (especially in infants) is proportionately larger.

22. **B:** *Hypoxia* is a major cause of bradycardia in the pediatric patient, so bradycardia during any airway procedure should be treated promptly with assuring that the airway is open, oxygenation and ventilation. Placing the child in a "sniffing position," with the midface placed superiorly and anteriorly, is the optimal alignment for airway protection. With traumatic injuries, care must be taken to maintain a neutral position of the cervical spine while opening the airway. Padding of the backboard under a child's shoulders and posterior thorax will also aid in neutral alignment of the cervical spine.

23. **B:** Sepsis is by far the most common cause of distributive shock. Goals of early resuscitation in patients with sepsis include restoration of tissue perfusion, reversal of oxygen supply dependency, and normalization of cellular metabolism. When appropriate fluid administration fails to restore adequate tissue perfusion and arterial pressure, vasopressors are usually necessary to increase mean systemic pressure, cardiac output, and oxygen delivery. Norepinephrine (Levophed) improves systemic blood pressure and does not substantially worsen end-organ ischemia in most studies of crystalloid-resuscitated septic shock patients. Norepinephrine may be preferential to other catecholamine pressors as first-line therapy for septic shock. Dosing of norepinephrine in shock patients is normally in the range of 0.01-5 µg/kg/minute and titrated to improvements in blood pressure and tissue perfusion. If sepsis is suspected, antibiotic therapy should be anticipated and discussed with both the referring and receiving physician.

24. **D:** Using the formula 16 + age in years divided by 4 equals an ET tube size of 5.0.

Methods of calculating proper ET tube size		
Age	ETT size	ETT depth (cm)
Preterm	3.0 (Preterm infants less than 28 weeks may require a smaller ET tube, 2.5)	6 + weight per kg
Full-term	3.5	6 + weight per kg
One year and above	(Age in years) + 16 divided by 4	ETT size × 3 in the orally intubated patient or 10 cm + age in years at the gums

25. **C:** The *steeple sign* is a sign on a frontal radiograph of tracheal narrowing and suggestive of the diagnosis of croup (laryngotracheobronchitis). Croup is the common term for a viral infection that affects the larynx but may extend into the trachea and bronchi. Patients generally present with a history of fever and coryza (acute inflammation of the mucous membrane of the nose, with discharge of mucus; a head cold). As the illness progresses inspiratory stridor may be present, as well as a characteristic "barking" cough. If the inflammation extends to the bronchi, rhonchi and wheezing may also be present. Care must be taken to rule out epiglottitis and retropharyngeal abscess because the presentations can be similar. Treatment is supportive and centers on treating dehydration and respiratory distress. Medications can include racemic epinephrine aerosols, dexamethasone, and prednisolone.

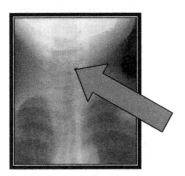

26. **B:** *Tidal volume* (V_t) is calculated in milliliters per kilogram. Traditionally 10-15 mL/kg was used but has been shown to cause barotrauma, or injury to the lung by overextension, so 6-8 mL/kg is now common practice in ICU for adults and older children. For infants and younger children without existing lung disease—a TV of 4-8 mL/kg to be delivered at a rate of 30-35 breaths/minute.

Refer to table below that describes the most commonly expected changes in pCO_2, pO_2, and MAP, which occur with increases in the ventilator parameters in the column on the left:

Changes and ventilator parameters			
Increase in	pCO_2	pO_2	MAP
FIO_2	No change	Increase	No change
Rate	Decrease	Usually no change	Increase
PIP/TV	Decrease	Increase	Increase
IT	Usually no change	Increase	Increase
PEEP	Usually no change	Increase	Increase

For example, a patient with an ABG: pH 7.28, pCO_2 50, pO_2 70, BE-3. One could improve oxygenation by increasing the FIO_2, PEEP, IT, or/and PIP or TV. One could decrease the pCO_2 and improve the pH by increasing the rate or/and PIP or TV. The best adjustment would be based on assessment of chest wall movement, aeration, expansion on chest x-ray, the patient's pulmonary problems, and the current ventilator settings. For example, if the FIO_2 is already at 95%, then it would be better to increase the PIP or IT rather than increase the FIO_2.

Consider another ABG which may be encountered when the patient is improving: pH 7.45, pCO_2 35, pO_2 130, BE +0. The pCO_2 is too low indicating that the minute ventilation is too high. The minute ventilation could be reduced by decreasing the rate and/or the PIP/TV. The pO_2 could be lowered by decreasing the FIO_2, PEEP, IT, and/or PIP or TV.

27. **B:** *Diaphragmatic hernia* is caused early in gestation when the pleuroperitoneal cavity fails to close. Abdominal contents migrate into the thoracic cavity, compressing developing lungs and causing pulmonary hyoplasia. Classic presentation by these infants includes early onset of respiratory distress with deterioration between the 1 and 5 minute APGAR scores in the delivery room. Clinical signs include dyspnea, unequal breath sounds, a shift in the PMI, and potentially scaphoid abdomen. The initial treatment efforts of preoperative stabilization are aimed at optimizing oxygenation, maintaining an adequate systemic blood pressure, and reducing the associated pulmonary hypertension. Because any distention of

the bowel further compromises respiratory function, the transport team should insert a large-bore (10 Fr) orogastric tube and initiate suction. Positive-pressure ventilation with a face mask should be avoided. When ventilation is required, immediate endotracheal intubation should be performed.

28. **B:** Newborns are susceptible to hypoglycemia because of immature glucose control mechanisms, decreased glucose stores, or both. A serum glucose of < 40 mg/dL represents hypoglycemia in the newborn. Hypoglycemia may be treated with a slow intravenous bolus of 2-4 mL/kg of 10% dextrose followed by a maintenance infusion drip of 10% dextrose in water at a rate of 80 mL/kg/24 hour. Serum glucose levels should be checked every thirty minutes to one hour until it has been demonstrated that the amount of glucose provided is adequate to maintain normal serum glucose levels. The newborn weighing less than 1,000 g should receive 5% dextrose in water because of their intolerance of the higher glucose loads resulting in hyperglycemia. Hyperglycemia, blood glucose levels greater than 125 mg/dL, is most commonly seen in the newborn weighing less than 1,000 g or in newborns whose hypoglycemia as been overcorrected.

29. **D:** *Nasal intubations* should not be performed on children less than twelve years of age because the acute angle to the glottis makes this an extremely difficult procedure while maintaining neutral cervical spine position. Needle or surgical cricothyroidotomy (dependent on age) may be necessary for airway protection for patients who cannot be successfully intubated and who cannot be ventilated and oxygenated by any other means. Children with Glasgow coma scores (GCS) of 8 or less, children with ongoing seizure activity, or those with deteriorating neurologic status should be intubated so that adequate oxygenation and airway protection is assured. Hypoxia and hypotension are the leading causes of neurologic deterioration in the head-injured patient. Preservation of stable mean arterial pressure is important to provide adequate cerebral perfusion and oxygenation. Elevation of the backboard to thirty degrees unless precluded by other injuries may assist in decreasing intracranial pressure.

30. **C:** Newborn (34-38 weeks) (2,000-3,000 g) should be intubated with a 3.5 ET tube with an estimated tube depth at approximately 9 cm at the gums.

31. **B:** *Blunt trauma* is the cause of the majority of abdominal injuries in children. Abdominal examination can be extremely difficult in the pediatric population because fear from exam or pain from distracting injuries interferes with assessment. A high index of suspicion should always be maintained with patients suffering multisystem injury. The solid organs most commonly injured in the pediatric patient are the spleen and the liver. Disruption of the vascular supply to these organs can result in massive hemorrhage. *Radiation of pain to the left shoulder (Kehr's sign) can indicate splenic injuries.*

32. **D:** The *thumbprint sign* is a finding on a lateral C-spine radiograph that suggests the diagnosis of epiglottitis. The sign is caused by a thickened free edge of the epiglottis, which causes it to appear more radiopaque than normal, resembling the distal thumb. *Epiglottitis* is a rare but life-threatening bacterial infection of the epiglottitis and surrounding airway structures. Epiglottitis is second only to croup as a cause for infectious stridor. Clinical presentation includes symptoms that often occur rapidly causing caretakers to seek medical attention in twenty-four hours of the onset of initial symptoms, fever, stridor, labored respirations, and because of supraglottic edema, often present with drooling. They are often anxious and present in a classic tripod position (sitting forward with their arms supporting them with their jaws thrusted forward), which increased air entry. Endotracheal intubation should only be undertaken by staff capable of securing the airway, surgically if necessary.

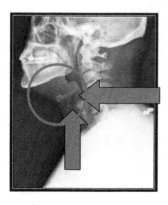

33. **B:** If a transport team suspects hypovolemia, the treatment would include careful transfusion with 10 mL/kg of an isotonic crystalloid solution such as normal saline or Ringer's lactate solution.

34. **C:** Using the formula (age in years × 2) + 8 gives an approximate weight of 16 kg for a-year-old child.

35. **A:** Preparation for endotracheal intubation is the most overlooked but often the most important part of the procedure. Being properly prepared for problems that may arise can often prevent life-threatening complications during intubation. Use of cuffed ET tubes is recommended for children over the age of eight years and adults. Use of uncuffed ET tubes is recommended for children under the age of eight years because the normal narrowing at the cricoid cartilage functions as the "natural cuff." Alternative method is using the length-based Broselow tape.

Remember that an intubated child is at risk for the displacement of the ETT, ETT plugging, pneumothorax, or an equipment failure (ventilator malfunction). Assume that any deterioration in the child's status is an airway problem until that is ruled out as a cause. "DOPE" is a useful mnemonic to remember potential causes of airway or ventilation problems in intubated patients.

Potential causes of airway or ventilation problems	
Remember "DOPE"	Clinical manifestation
D	Displaced ETT
O	Obstructed ETT
P	Pneumothorax
E	Equipment failure (such as ventilator malfunction or disconnect)

Pediatric airway pearls		
< 10 years old	< 11 years old	< 12 years old
Narrowest portion of the airway is the cricothyroid membrane or cartilage	Needle cricothyroidotomy is recommended	Nasal intubation should not be performed

Airway formulas	
Age	Estimated ET tube size (internal diameter) (mm)
Newborn < 28 weeks (< 1,000 g)	2.5
Newborn 28-34 weeks (1,000-2,000 g)	3.0
Newborn 34-38 weeks (2,000-3,000 g)	3.5
Newborn >38 weeks (>3,000 g)	3.5-4.0
Infant under 6 months	3.5-4.0
Infant (6 months to 1 year)	4.0-4.5
Child over 2 years	16 + age in years/4
Adult (female)	7.0-8.0
Adult (male)	8.0-8.5
Age or weight (kg)	Distance or depth of ET tube insertion
Newborns	"ETT tip to gum" distance = 6 + weight in kg
Weight 1 kg	Insert 7 cm depth
Weight 2 kg	Insert 8 cm depth
Weight 3 kg	Insert 9 cm depth
Weight 4 kg	Insert 10 cm depth
< 6 months	10 cm
6 months to 1 year	10-11 cm
1 year and older	10 + age in years
Adult	19-23 cm or (ET tube size × 3)
ET tube suction catheter size formula	Chest tube size formula
ET Tube size × 2	ET Tube size × 4

36. **C:** The umbilical vein remains patent and viable for cannulation until approximately one week after birth. The transport team must be able to identify the two thick-walled, constricted arteries (four o'clock and eight o'clock position) and the thinner-walled larger vein (twelve o'clock position).

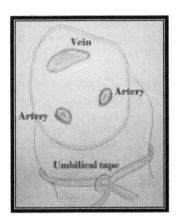

37. **D:** A pediatric patient has only 80 mL of circulating volume/kg, so small amounts of fluid or blood loss can cause serious physiologic effects. The goal in supporting cardiac output in shock is the replacement of lost circulating volume.

Circulating volume parameters		
Newborn	Pediatric	Adult
80 mL/kg	70-80 mg/kg	60 mL/kg

38. **C:** A rare occurrence in the pediatric population is the necessity for control of the airway via surgical means. *A surgical airway can be placed through the cricothyroid membrane on children older than eleven years,* but it is recommended that needle cricothyroidotomy be performed on children younger than eleven years. Indications for needle cricothyroidotomy include complete airway obstruction, severe orofacial injuries, and laryngeal transaction where there is an inability to secure the airway and/or provide adequate ventilation and oxygenation by less-invasive means. Needle cricothyroidotomy does not protect the paitent's airway from passive aspiration and is considered a temporary measure until ETT placement or removal of the obstruction can be achieved.

39. **B:** The principal indication for umbilical vein catheterization is to gain vascular access during emergency resuscitation. Umbilical vein catheterization may be a life-saving procedure in neonates who require vascular access and resuscitation. A 3.5 F catheter is used for preterm newborns, and a 5 F catheter is used for full-term newborns. In an emergency, the catheter is best advanced only 1-2 cm beyond the point at which good blood return is obtained to avoid injecting hyperosmolar fluids into the portal vessels and causing liver necrosis. This is approximately 4-5 cm in a full-term neonate. Umbilical vein catheters may be placed in the inferior vena cava above the level of the ductus venosus and below the level of the right atrium (10-12 cm). This acts as central venous access, allowing central venous pressure (CVP) monitoring, medication infusions, and the administration of hyperalimentation solutions. The position of the catheter must be confirmed radiographically. After proper placement of the umbilical line, intravenous fluids and medication may be administered to critically ill neonates.

40. **C:** The International Guidelines for Neonatal Resuscitation include recommendations for noninitiation or discontinuation of resuscitation, which include birth weight < 500 g, confirmed trisomy (13 or 18), congenital hydrocephalus, severe fetal growth restriction, and *gestational age < 24 weeks.*

41. **B:** Bronchiolitis is a lower respiratory tract infection (primarily viral), which is one of the more common causes of new-onset wheezing in children. Respiratory syncytial virus (RSV) is the causative agent in the majority of cases, but parainfluenza and *Mycoplasma pneumoniae* have also been isolated. Wheezing is the most common presenting complaint, often with an accompanying 2-5 days' history of coryaz and cough. Most cases occur in the winter months, with the majority of infections in children below one year of age. Apnea in children younger than three months is also characteristic of RSV infections.

42. **C:** Oral albuterol solutions are not indicated for patients who do not respond to aerosol therapy. Corticosteroids are not indicated for the treatment of bronchiolitis. Patients in severe distress, who are

unresponsive to therapy, may require intubation and mechanical ventilation.

43. **B:** Brown recluse spiders usually have a dark violin-shaped mark on their cephalothorax, just behind their eyes, resulting in the nicknames *fiddleback spider, brown fiddler, or violin spider.* Unlike most spiders, the brown recluse has six eyes arranged in three pairs, instead of the usual eight. The bite forms a necrotizing ulcer, "bull's-eye" in appearance, that destroys soft tissue and may take months to heal, leaving deep scars. These bites usually become painful and itchy within 2-8 hours. Pain and other local effects worsen 12-36 hours after the bite, and the necrosis develops over the next few days. Over time, the wound may grow to as large as 25 cm (10 in.) in extreme cases. The damaged tissue becomes gangrenous and eventually sloughs away.

44. **A:** The female black widow's bite is particularly harmful to humans because of their unusually large venom glands (males almost never bite humans). The black widow spider produces a protein venom that affects the victim's nervous system. This neurotoxic protein is one of the most potent venoms secreted by an animal. Some people are slightly affected by the venom, but others may have a severe response. The first symptom is acute pain at the site of the bite, although there may only be a minimal local reaction. Symptoms usually start within twenty minutes to one hour after the bite. *Local pain may be followed by localized or generalized severe muscle cramps, abdominal pain, weakness, and tremor.*

The southern black widows, as well as the closely related western and northern species, which were previously considered the same species, have a *prominent red hourglass figure on the underside of their abdomen.* A person bitten by a black widow spider, who has pain severe enough to seek treatment at an emergency department, will require narcotic pain relief. Muscle relaxants given by injection may also be of value. Although calcium gluconate given through an IV has long been advocated, it does not seem to produce much relief of symptoms.

45. **D:** The care of viper envenomation should include wound cleansing, immobilization of the affected part (decreases the circulation of venom throughout the body), *no use of compression techniques (including ice),* and transport. Included in the coagulation studies should be fibrin split products and fibrinogen levels. Treatment can include fluids, administration of steroids, medications to decrease risk of anaphylaxis, and snake antivenin. If the patient exhibits signs of severe envenomation, such as edema that has progressed 30 cm in 1 hour of the bite, shock, kidney failure, pulmonary edema, bleeding, or paralysis, administration of antivenin should be started.

46. **B:** The infant who is hypoxic in room air but demonstrates a partial pressure of oxygen (pO$_2$), greater than 150 in 100% oxygen is more likely to have *pulmonary disease* than heart disease with a fixed right-to-left shunt. Comparison of simultaneous ABGs demonstrating a PaO$_2$ at least 10 mm higher from a preductal site versus a postductul site indicates right-to-left shunting of desaturated blood at the ductal level.

47. **D:** *Gastrochisis* is a defect in the abdominal wall that has completed its development. The *defect allows for protrusion of abdominal contents and is not covered by a membrane.* Because the defect is normally very close to the umbilicus, it is frequently mistaken for an omphalocele. An omphalocele is an arrest of development of the abdominal wall, with the abdominal contents remaining externalized. The defect remains covered by a membrane in utero, although the sac may be broken during delivery.

48. **B:** Findings related to identification of esophageal atresia include inability to pass an oral gastric tube to the stomach, excessive oral secretions, and feeding intolerance. Management of these infants during transport should include the following: intermittent suction of the upper esophageal pouch, *elevation of the head of the bed to prevent gastric reflux,* and intravenous fluid therapy for fluids and glucose.

49. **C:** A high clinical index of suspicion based on the mechanism of injury should always guide one's assessment and management. The possibility of non-accidental trauma (i.e., child abuse) should always be considered under certain circumstances, which can include a discrepancy between the history that is presented by the caregivers and the actual physical examination findings; *injuries that are incompatible with a infant's neurodevelopmental capabilities;* a delay in seeking medical advice or treatment for what appears to be a serious injury; findings of multiple injuries at various chronological stages; bites marks, cigarette burns or rope/cord marks; burns with sharply demarcated margins; genital or perianal trauma (including burns to these areas); multiple subdural hematomas; retinal hemorrhages; and rib fractures involving multiple ribs and/or at various chronological stages.

50. **D:** One of the first very obvious physiologic differences between children and adults is the variation of normal pediatric vital signs based on the age of the child. A thorough understanding of pediatric vital signs is imperative in being able to detect very subtle abnormalities in a child's heart rate and RR. For example, a subtle tachycardia may be the only clue to the possibility of early hemorrhagic shock in a child who otherwise looks stable. A subtle tachypnea may be the earliest clue to possible intrathoracic injuries in a child with a normal room air oxygen saturation. Thus, anyone involved in the emergency care of children must be aware of normal vital signs based on a child's age. A simplified method to easily and quickly recall pediatric vital signs is as follows:

Vital signs	
Systolic blood pressure (SBP) (age in years × 2) + 70	Average range (mmHg)
Newborn	> 60
Infant (< 1 year old)	> 70
Child (1-8 years old)	> 80
Adult	> 90
Diastolic blood pressure (DBP)	2/3 of SBP
Heart rate	Average range (beats per minute)
Newborn	>120-160
Infant (< 1 year old)	100-120
Child (1-8 years old)	80-110
Adult	60-100
RR	Average range (breaths per minute)
Newborn	40
Infant (< 1 year old)	30
Child (1-8 years old)	20
Adult	12-18

Bibliography

2005 American Heart Association. Guidelines for cardiopulmonary resuscitation and emergency cardiovascular care. Part 10.5 Near-fatal asthma. *Circulation* 112 (Suppl. 24): 139.

Allen, JY, Charles, GM. (2005). The efficacy of ketamine in pediatric emergency department patients who present with severe acute asthma. *Annals of Emergency Medicine* 46(1): 43-50.

Apgar, V. (1953). A proposal for a new method of evaluation of the newborn infant. *Current Researches in Anesthesia & Analgesia* 32(4): 260-267.

Association of Air Medical Services. (2003). *Guidelines for Air Medical Crew Education.* Iowa, Kendall/Hunt Publishing Company

Buckley, NA, et al. (1995). Relative Pediatric benzodiazepine ingestion resulting in hospitalization. *Journal of Toxicology—Clinical Toxicology* 36 (3): 227-231.

Butler-O'Hara, M, et al. (2006). A randomized trial comparing long-term and short-term use of umbilical venous catheters in premature infants with birth weights of less than 1251 grams. *Pediatrics* 118(1): e25-35.

Casey, BM, McIntire, DD, Leveno, KJ. (2001). The continuing value of the Apgar score for the assessment of newborn infants. *The New England Journal of Medicine* 344(7): 467-471.

Chipps, BE, Murphy, KR. (2005). Assessment and treatment of acute asthma in children. *Journal of Pediatrics* 147: 288.

Denmark, TK, et al. (2006). Ketamine to avoid mechanical ventilation in severe pediatric asthma. *The Journal of Emergency Medicine* 30(2): 163-166.

Finster, M, Wood, M. (2005). The Apgar score has survived the test of time. *Anesthesiology* 102(4): 855-857.

Gosalakkal, JA, Kamoji, V. (2008). Reye syndrome and reye-like syndrome. *Pediatric Neurology* 39(3): 198-200.

Helfaer, MA, Nichols, DG, Rogers, MC. (1996). Lower airway disease: bronchiolitis and asthma. In: Rogers, MC, Nichols, DG., (Eds.), *Textbook of Pediatric Intensive Care* (3rd edition), Baltimore: Williams & Wilkins. p. 133.

Hesselvik, JF, Brodin, B. (1989). Low-dose norepinephrine in patients with septic shock and oliguria. *Critical Care Medicine* 17: 179-180.

Hills, BA. (1999). An alternative view of the role(s) of surfactant and the alveolar model. *Journal of Applied Physiology* 87(5): 1567-1583.

Holleran, R. (1996). *Flight Nursing: Principles and Practice.* (2nd edition). St. Louis, Mosby.

Holleran, R. (2003). *Air and Surface Patient Transport: Principles and Practice* (3rd edition). St. Louis: Mosby.

Holleran, R. (2009). *ASTNA Patient Transport: Principles and Practice* (4th edition). St. Louis, Mosby.

Hotchkiss, RS, Karl, IE. (2003). The pathophysiology and treatment of sepsis. *The New England Journal of Medicine* 348: 138-150.

Kattwinkel, J. (2000). *Textbook of Neonatal Resuscitation* (4th edition). Elk Grove Village, IL: American Academy of Pediatrics.

Klingner, MC, Kruse, J. (1999). Meconium aspiration syndrome: pathophysiology and prevention. *The Journal of the American Board of Family Practice/American Board of Family Practice* 12(6): 450-466.

Krishnan, JA, Brower, RG. (2000). High-frequency ventilation for acute lung injury and ARDS. *Chest* 118(3): 795-807.

Krupa, D. (1997). *Flight Nursing Core Curriculum.* Park Ridge, IL: National Flight Nurses Association.

Martin, C, et al. (2000). Effect of norepinephrine on the outcome of septic shock. *Critical Care Medicine* 28: 2758-2765.

O'Gorman, CS. (2005). Insertion of umbilical arterial and venous catheters. *Irish Medical Journal* 98(5): 151-153.

Onal, EE, et al. (2004). Cardiac tamponade in a newborn because of umbilical venous catheterization: is correct position safe? *Paediatric Anaesthesia* 14(11):953-956.

Orlowski, JP, Gillis, J, Kilham, HA. (1987). A catch in the Reye. *Pediatrics* 80(5): 638-642.

Petrillo, TM, et al. (2001). Emergency department use of ketamine in pediatric status asthmaticus. *Journal of Asthma* 38(8): 657-664.

Remington, PL, Sullivan, K, Marks, JS. (1988). A catch in "a catch in the Reye." *Pediatrics* 82(4): 676-678.

Rivers, E, et al. (2001). Early goal-directed therapy in the treatment of severe sepsis and septic shock. *The New England Journal of Medicine* 345: 1368-1377.

Rotta, AT. (2006). Asthma. In: Fuhrman, BP, Zimmerman, JJ. (Eds.), *Pediatric Critical Care* (3rd edition). Philadelphia: Mosby Elsevier, p.589.

Salour, M. (2000). The steeple sign. *Radiology* 216(2): 428-429.

Schwarz, AJ, Lubinsky, PS. (1997). Acute severe asthma. In: Levin, DL, Morriss, FC. (Eds.), *Essentials of Pediatric Intensive Care* (2nd edition). New York: Churchill Livingstone, Inc, p.130.

Short, B. L. (2008). Extracorporeal membrane oxygenation: use in meconium aspiration syndrome. *Journal of Perinatology* 28: S79.

Usta, IM, Mercer, BM, Sibai, BM. (1995). Risk factors for meconium aspiration syndrome. *Obstetrics and Gynecology* 86(2): 230-234.

Venkataraman, ST, Orr, RA. (1992). Mechanical ventilation and respiratory care. In: Fuhrman, BP, Zimmerman, JJ. (Eds.). *Pediatric Critical Care*. St. Louis: Mosby Year Book, Chap. 48, pp. 519-543.

West, JB. (1994). *Respiratory Physiology—The Essentials*. Baltimore: Williams & Wilkins.

Wiley, CC, Wiley, JF. (1998). Toxicity of benzodiazepines in overdose. *British Medical Journal* 310 (6974): 219-221.

Module 10
Flight Physiology, Safety, Survival, CAMTS

1. Initial intervention for managing a patient presenting with bariobariatrauma is?

   A. Administer high flow oxygen
   B. Decrease oxygen to 4 L/minute by NC
   C. Administer high flow oxygen by NRM 15 minutes prior to lift off
   D. Maintain cabin pressure at 2,500 feet

2. An expanding ETT cuff in flight is an indication of what gas law?

   A. Henry's law
   B. Dalton's law
   C. Boyle's law
   D. Charles' law

3. Your oxygen tank pressure reading at 1,200 hours was 1,800 psi. The pilot rechecked the unused oxygen tank in the evening and reported that the gauge reading was 1,500 psi. Which gas law best describes the decrease in pressure?

   A. Gay-Lussac's law
   B. Dalton's law
   C. Boyle's law
   D. Henry's law

4. How should your flight suit fit to provide space of insulation per CAMTS recommendations?

   A. ½ in.
   B. 1 in.
   C. Skin tight so I look really hot for the firefighters on scene
   D. ¼ in.

5. You are beginning to prepare for landing and you have news reporter riding along for the day. You see a high-rise tower at 1,100 high. Sterile cockpit applies how?

    A. The news reporter can speak anytime during the flight
    B. Flight crew members are the only one allowed to speak
    C. Say nothing about the high-rise tower
    D. Pilot is the only crew member to speak during all phases of flight

6. You have just crash landed your aircraft and your pilot has asked you to exit the aircraft. What should you take with you?

    A. Helmet
    B. Bags of normal saline
    C. Survival kit
    D. Seat cushion

7. You are transporting a non-intubated seventy-year-old man with a history of bilateral pneumonia on 2 L of oxygen by nasal cannula. You are at 10,000 feet and the patient's vital signs are BP 190/100, HR 102, RR 24, and SaO_2 86%. What is the immediate intervention for this patient?

    A. Decrease cabin pressure
    B. Increase oxygen delivery to the patient
    C. Administer fluid bolus to increase perfusion to the heart
    D. RSI and intubate the patient

8. You are transporting a thirty-year-old man who was involved in a motor vehicle crash. He has a closed femur fracture with a history of alcohol consumption of unknown amount. On the basis of the physiologic effects elicited on the body, which type of hypoxia problems may occur in flight?

    A. Histotoxic and hypemic
    B. Hypoxic and stagnant
    C. Stagnant and hypemic
    D. Hypoxic and hypemic

9. Which one of the following has been determined to be an unreliable sign of hypoxia?

    A. Cyanosis
    B. Hypertension
    C. Tachycardia
    D. Tachypnea

10. An increase in altitude produces?

    A. High humidity and high temperature
    B. Low humidity and low temperature
    C. High humidity and low temperature
    D. Low humidity and high temperature

11. After a forced aircraft landing, the pilot is incapacitated; your main priority is to?

    A. Assume crash position
    B. Turn off oxygen
    C. Turn off throttle, fuel, and then battery
    D. Turn on the emergency locator transmitter (ELT)

12. Your immediate concerns of survival after an aircraft accident include all of the following, *except*?

    A. Obtain water and go for help
    B. Building a fire
    C. Making appropriate fire signals
    D. Creating or seeking shelter

13. No pilot may takeoff or land an aircraft under visual flight rules (VFR) when the reported ceiling or visibility is less than which of the following for local day weather minimums?

    A. 1,000 feet and 1 mile
    B. 500 feet and 1 mile
    C. 500 feet and 2 miles
    D. 800 feet and 1 mile

14. The emergency transmit frequency is?

    A. 121.5
    B. 155.5
    C. 120.5
    D. 105.5

15. Average time of useful consciousness (TUC) for a non-pressurized aircraft at 45,000 feet is?

    A. 90 seconds
    B. 3-5 minutes
    C. 30-60 seconds
    D. 15 seconds or less

16. You are asked to respond to a local scene call with night vision goggles (NVG) capability involving an MVA with multiple injured patients at 2,300. You have been having bad weather off and on. The pilot-in-command (PIC) advises you that weather minimums are currently at 800 and 1. What will you do?

    A. Continue and fly to the scene
    B. Attempt to fly to the scene and see if you can get there
    C. Abort the flight due to weather
    D. Say nothing because the PIC is responsible for deciding wheather or not you continue with the mission

17. The percentage of oxygen at 25,000 MSL is

    A. 4%
    B. 21%
    C. 18%
    D. 7%

18. The altitude at which one begins to lose their night vision is

    A. 500 feet
    B. 1,000 feet
    C. 3,000 feet
    D. 5,000 feet

19. The pilot made contact upon the aircraft lifting at 1455. The second contact was at 1510 after landing. The communication center has not heard from the transport team since the last flight following transmission. The postaccident incident plan (PAIP) should be initiated at what time?

    A. 1525
    B. 1540
    C. 1555
    D. 1610

20. Gas that diffuses from an area of higher concentration to an area of lower concentration, best describes which gas law?

    A. Graham's law
    B. Charles' law
    C. Gay-Lussac's law
    D. Henry's law

21. Your patient would most likely experience barodontalgia during which phase of flight?

    A. Ascent
    B. Descent
    C. Cruise flight
    D. None of the above

22. You will be transporting a stable twenty-seven-year-old man with nontraumatic pneumocephalous secondary to gas producing necrotizing bacteria from rural hospital at 8,500 feet elevation to a local hospital at 1,200 feet sea level. What might be the best transport option? What gas law will most affect this patient negatively?

    A. Ground; Boyle's law
    B. Fixed wing transport pressurized to 9,000 AGL; Charles' law
    C. Rotor transport; Boyle's law
    D. Rotor transport; Charles' law

23. You are transporting a sixty-year-old man with a history of nonembolic stroke by rotor-wing aircraft in the middle of a sunny afternoon. When the pilot begins to turn the rotors, the flight team notices that the patient's eyes are blinking rapidly and he begins to experience a generalized tonic-clonic seizure. The monitor shows what appears to be ventricular fibrillation, but a pulse can be palpated. The seizure activity ceased when the rotor blades stopped and started again with start-up. The seizure activity is most likely due to?

A. Flicker vertigo
B. Spatial disorientation
C. Hypoxia
D. Increasing intracranial pressure

24. You are doing a night flight when you encounter bad weather. The helicopter suddenly impacts the ground and the cockpit is filled with smoke. The best action of the flight team immediately after experiencing the hard landing should be which of the following?

A. Grab the fire extinguisher and portable radio
B. Make a call for help on the emergency frequency
C. Exit the helicopter after the aircraft has come to a complete stop and meet at a predesignated position a safe distance from the aircraft
D. Stay in the helicopter as it offers the only available shelter in the area

25. Your IABP begins to purge during ascent. The triggering mechanism for this function was initiated as a result of which gas law?

A. Boyle's law
B. Gay-Lussac's law
C. Charles' law
D. Henry's law

26. Henry's law best describes which of the following patient conditions?

    A. Bends
    B. Barotrauma
    C. Shallow water blackout
    D. Arterial gas embolism (AGE)

27. On a long fixed wing flight, an option may be to place water on the ET tube cuff to counteract. Which gas law is it?

    A. Henry's law
    B. Graham's law
    C. Dalton's law
    D. Boyle's law

28. Overdue aircraft procedures during flight start after

    A. 15 minutes without contact
    B. 30 minutes without contact
    C. 45 minutes without contact
    D. 60 minutes without contact

29. The absolute minimum hours required by the Federal Aviation Regulation (FAR) Part 135 with regard to a pilot's "bottle to throttle" rule is

    A. 8
    B. 12
    C. 24
    D. 48

30. Who has the ultimate authority to initiate or complete a mission?

    A. The flight paramedic
    B. The flight nurse
    C. The PIC
    D. The communication specialist

31. The flight team should be prepared that an aircraft will capsize when it hits water because helicopters are top heavy as a result of the weight of the engines and transmission. Once in the water, the flight team can minimize heat loss by using which of the following?

A. Heat escape-lessening posture (HELP)
B. Lateral recumbent position
C. Seat cushions
D. Arms and legs should be moved quickly during ascent to the surface

32. The total pressure of a gas mixture is the sum of the partial pressures of all gases. Which gas law best describes?

A. Boyle's law
B. Graham's law
C. Dalton's law
D. Charles' law

33. Malpractice is based on a professional standard of care. The elements that must be proved for a malpractice case include all of the following, *except?*

A. Causation
B. Injury
C. Abandonment
D. Damages

34. Air medical programs that frequently fly over large bodies of water need to be familiar with emergency egress procedure in the event of a forced water landing. All of the following are correct regarding the emergency egress, *except?*

A. During surface ascent, exhalation should be done rapidly to prevent serious lung injury
B. Personal flotation devices should be worn
C. No attempt should be made to exit the aircraft until the blades have completely stopped
D. Maintain a fixed reference orientation with hands

35. Administration of the wrong medication to a patient best describes which element of malpractice?

A. Breach of duty as a result of malfeasance
B. Breach of duty as a result of nonfeasance
C. Breach of duty as a result of forseeability
D. Negligence

36. During descent, gas will

A. Expand
B. Contract
C. Equalize
D. Purge

37. The radio signal that follows the curvature of the earth and has the greatest range is?

A. Very high frequency (VHF) AM
B. VHF high-band FM
C. VHF low-band FM
D. Ultra high frequencies (UHF)

38. The ELT takes a minimum of _____ g's to activate.

A. 2
B. 4
C. 6
D. 8

39. A repeater system is a type of which of the following radio systems?

A. Simple duplex
B. Full duplex
C. Half duplex
D. Multiplex

40. In aviation, "You may fly instrument flight rules (IFR) in visual meteorological conditions (VMC), you cannot fly VFR in _____."

    A. VMC
    B. IFR
    C. Instrument meteorological conditions (IMC)
    D. DMC

41. Decompression illness is mostly attributed to which gas law?

    A. Boyle's law
    B. Charles' law
    C. Henry's law
    D. Dalton's law

42. During flight, you notice that the IV drip rate has increased. Which gas law is responsible for this to occur?

    A. Graham's law
    B. Henry's law
    C. Charles' law
    D. Boyle's law

43. The number one cause of aero-medical crashes is

    A. Pushing the weather (weather-related)
    B. Pilot fatigue
    C. Night missions
    D. Flying IFR in VMC

44. Unless it is acted on by a force, a body at rest will remain at rest and a body in motion will move at a constant speed in a straight line best describes which of the following laws?

    A. Boyle's law
    B. Newton's law
    C. Graham's law
    D. Dalton's law

45. Four basic variables that affect gas volumetric relationships include all of the following, *except?*

    A. Temperature
    B. Altitude
    C. Pressure
    D. Mass of gases

46. CAMTS requires a minimum of _____ successful live intubations during initial flight training.

    A. 1
    B. 3
    C. 5
    D. 10

47. During an in-flight emergency procedure, all of the following are correct, *except*

    A. Place patient in high-fowlers position
    B. Turn oxygen off
    C. Helmet visors in down position
    D. All equipment is secured

48. CAMTS requires that helipads must have all of the following, *except*

    A. Perimeter lighting for night operation
    B. Fence around helipad
    C. Have a device to identify wind direction and velocity
    D. Evidence of adequate security

49. Which of the following is a leading cause of death among scuba divers?

    A. AGE
    B. Bends
    C. Chokes
    D. Pulmonary decompression illness

50. All of the following are considered stressors of flight, *except?*

    A. g-forces
    B. Increased partial pressure of oxygen
    C. Barometric pressure
    D. Decreased humidity

Answer Key and Rationale

1. **C:** Nitrogen, always present in body fluids, comes out of solution and forms bubbles if the pressure on the body drops sufficiently as it does during ascent into the higher altitudes. Overweight persons (bariobariatrauma) are more susceptible to evolved gas decompression sickness (DCS) as fatty tissue contains more nitrogen.

Evolved gases	
DCS	Clinical manifestation
Bends	Characterized by pain in and around the joints and can become progressively worse, during ascent to higher altitudes.
Chokes	Are pains in the chest caused by blocking of the smaller pulmonary blood vessels by innumerable small bubbles. In severe cases, there is a sensation of suffocation.
Paresthesia or creeps	Is another DCS with symptoms of tingling, itching, and cold and warm sensations.

Henry's and Dalton's laws predict that, as the diver descends, excess nitrogen will enter the blood and all body tissues. These laws also predict that, on ascent (as ambient pressure decreases) the extra nitrogen that accumulated will diffuse out of the tissues and into the circulation. DCS arises when excess nitrogen leaving tissue forms bubbles large enough to cause symptoms. Size of bubbles is important, since small bubbles can often be found in divers with no symptoms. DCS arises when the pressure gradient for nitrogen leaving the tissues is so great that large bubbles form, probably by coalescence of many smaller bubbles. Large bubbles within tissues and the circulation cause the symptoms and signs of DCS.

Diving DCS: A diver ascends from a dive.
Altitude DCS: An aircraft flies upward (ascent).

Trapped gases	
DCS	Clinical manifestation
Bariosinusitis *(sinus block)*	The sinuses are air filled, bony cavities connected with the nose by means of one or more small openings. If these openings are obstructed by swelling of the mucous membrane lining of the sinuses (as during a cold), equalization of the pressure is difficult. Pain in the cheekbones on either side of the nose, or in the upper jaw, or above the eyes, will result.
Bariodontalgia *(toothache)*	Toothaches may occur at altitude due to abscesses, imperfect fillings, and inadequately filled root canals. Anyone who suffers from toothache at altitude should see his dentist. However, the pain caused by a sinus block can be mistaken for toothache. If air is able to enter below a filling, the filling may well be blown out as the pilot reaches higher altitude
Bariotitis media *(ear block)*	Painful ear block generally occurs, as a result of too rapid descent. If air is trapped in the middle ear, the eardrum stretches to absorb the higher pressure. The result is pain and sometimes temporary deafness.
Gastrointestinal	Gas pains are caused by the expansion of gas within the digestive tract during ascent into the reduced pressure at altitude. Relief from pain may be accomplished by descent from altitude.

2. **C:** *Boyle's law (expansion or contraction of a gas)* describes the inversely proportional relationship between the absolute pressure and volume of a gas, if the temperature is kept constant within a closed system. The air in the ETT cuff, for example, expands with altitude (ascent) and contracts during descent. Boyle's law is one of three gas laws that thoroughly describe the behavior of gases under varying temperatures, pressures, and volumes. The other two laws are Gay-Lussac's law and Graham's law.

Graham's law of effusion and diffusion states that the rates of movement of gases at the same temperature and pressure are inversely proportional to the square root of its molecular mass.

Dalton's law of partial pressures states that the total pressure of a gas mixture is the sum of the individual or partial pressures of all the gases in the mixture.

Charles's law, or the law of volumes, states that for an ideal gas at constant pressure, the volume is proportional to the absolute temperature, which describes how gases tend to expand when heated.

http://en.wikipedia.org/wiki/Boyle's_law—cite_note-0# cite_note-0

3. **A:** *Gay-Lussac's law* states that the pressure of a sample of gas at constant volume is directly proportional to its temperature. Simply, if a gas temperature decreases, then so does its pressure, if the mass and volume of the gas are held constant. The oxygen tank pressure (psi) changes are directly proportional to temperature is an example of this law.

4. **D:** The uniform should fit to allow 0.25 in. (1/4 in.) of air space between the suit and undergarments.

5. **B:** Observance of a sterile cockpit is a regulation of the Federal Aviation Administration (FAA) (FAR 135.100) that prohibits nonessential communications between the medical crew and pilot during critical phases of flight. The critical phases of flight include all ground operations that involve taxi, takeoff, and landing and all other flight operations except cruise flight. The medical crew should be aware that there are certain times when they should refrain from speaking to the pilot unless absolutely imperative. These times include the following: during takeoff, during landing, during instrument approaches, and in dense air traffic areas.

6. **C:** *Survival equipment* (kit or bag) should be standard on every air medical aircraft. Specific service area, climate, type of aircraft, and time of year are considerations when survival gear is assembled. The survival gear should be assembled and stored in a manner that affords easy access.

7. **B:** Hypoxic hypoxia is also referred to as altitude hypoxia because its primary cause is exposure to low barometric pressure. It is a deficiency in alveolar oxygen exchange, which interferes with gas exchange in two phases of respiration: ventilation and diffusion. A reduction in PO_2 in inspired air or the effective gas exchange area of the lung may cause oxygen deficiency. The result is an inadequate oxygen supply to the arterial blood, which in turn decreases the amount of oxygen available to the tissues. Decreased barometric pressure at high altitudes causes a reduction in the alveolar partial pressure of oxygen (PaO_2). The blood oxygen saturation, which is 98% at sea level, is reduced to 87% at 10,000 feet and 60% at 22,000 feet. The most effective way to prevent physiologic problems is to provide an aircraft pressurization system so that occupants of the aircraft are never exposed to pressure outside the physiologic zone. In those cases in which ascent above the physiologic zone is required, protective oxygen equipment must be provided. Treatment of hypoxia is administration of 100% oxygen.

Cabin pressurization	
Zone	Definition
Physiologic	From sea level to altitudes up to 10,000 feet
Physiologically deficient	Altitudes from 10,000-50,000 feet
Space equivalent	Altitudes from 50,000-250,000 feet
Space	Altitudes greater than 250,000 feet

8. **A:** *Histotoxic hypoxia* is the inability of cells to take up or utilize oxygen from the bloodstream, despite physiologically normal delivery of oxygen to such cells and tissues. Histotoxic hypoxia results from tissue poisoning, such as that caused by alcohol, narcotics, cyanide (which acts by inhibiting cytochrome oxidase), and certain other poisons like hydrogen sulfide (byproduct of

sewage and used in leather tanning). *Hypemic hypoxia* is where arterial oxygen pressure is normal, but total oxygen content of the blood is reduced, as from various types of anemia or from a loss of blood. *Stagnant hypoxia* occurs when conditions exist (cerebral ischemia, ischemic heart disease, intrauterine hypoxia) that result in reduced cardiac output, pooling of the blood within certain regions of the body, a decreased blood flow to the tissues, or restriction of blood.

9. **A:** *Cyanosis* has been determined to be an unreliable sign of hypoxia because the oxygen saturation must be below 75% in patients with normal hemoglobin before it is detectable. Hypotension and cyanosis are late signs of hypoxia. Providing adequate supplemental oxygen is the prime consideration in the treatment of hypoxia.

10. **B:** Humidity is the concentration of water vapor in the air; as air cools, it loses its ability to hold moisture because temperature is inversely proportional to altitude; an increase in altitude produces a decrease in temperature and, therefore, a decrease in the amount of humidity. *Increase in altitude = low temperature and low humidity.*

11. **C:** After a forced aircraft landing, the main danger is fire. If the pilot has become incapacitated, the throttle, fuel switch and master battery in sequence, should be turned off. The position of these switches varies with the aircraft, and the flight team must be familiar with the procedure for their specific aircraft.

12. **A:** Knowledge of the rule of threes when priorities are set will greatly increase the chances of survival in the outdoors. This rule states that the average person can survive three minutes without oxygen, three hours without shelter in extreme conditions, three days without water, and three weeks without food. Medical concerns and safety are important in accident, but once these are addressed, the rule of threes should guide priorities. With this rule in mind, the flight team's immediate concerns after an accident should be creating or seeking shelter, building a fire, and making appropriate fire signals.

13. **B:** One of CAMTS's standards is a recommendation for weather minimums. It seems that weather, particularly fog, which can impair pilot visualization, continues to be a cause of helicopter crashes. Flight programs need to establish weather minimums based on the terrain in which they operate and then adhere to them. The definition of weather minimums is the lowest (worst) visibility conditions under which an aircraft may legally be flown under (VFR). When visibility is less than specified minimums, an aircraft must fly under IFR or not at all. VFR "response" weather minimums must meet or exceed as outlined in FAA-A021.

VFR weather minimums *(ceiling = foot) and (visibility = miles)*		
Condition	Local	X-country
Day	500 and 1	500 and 2
Night	1,000 and 1	1,000 and 3

CAMTS 8th edition VFR weather minimums *(ceiling = foot) and (visibility = miles)*				
	Non-mountainous	Non-mountainous	Mountainous	Mountainous
Condition	Local	X-country	Local	X-country
Day	800 and 2	800 and 3	800 and 3	1,000 and 3
Night with NVGs	800 and 3	1,000 and 3	1,000 and 3	1,000 and 5
Night without NVGs	1,000 and 3	1,000 and 5	1,500 and 3	1,500 and 5

14. **A:** Airband frequencies of 121.5 MHz and 243.0 MHz are internationally designated distress signal channels.

15. **D:** TUC refers to the elapsed time from the point of exposure to an oxygen-deficient environment to the point at which deliberate function is lost. *Rapid decompression,* which occurs when a quick loss of cabin pressure occurs in a pressurized aircraft at *high altitudes,* dramatically reduces the time of useful consciousness. On decompression at altitudes above 33,000 feet, an immediate

reversal of oxygen flow in the alveoli takes place, caused by higher PO_2 within the pulmonary capillaries that depletes the blood's oxygen reserve. The causes of *hypoxia* include high altitude, hypoventilation, and pathologic condition of the lung.

Average time of useful consciousness for non-pressurized aircraft	
Altitude (feet)	Time
18,000 and lower	30 minutes
25,000	3-5 minutes
30,000	90 seconds
35,000	30-60 seconds
40,000 and higher	15 seconds or less

16. **C:** Each program must have a policy that allows any crew member to refuse or abort a flight if they feel uncomfortable. The flight is aborted because the weather minimum of 800 foot ceiling and 1 mile visibility is less than the specified minimums recommended for local-night with the use of NVG of a 800 foot ceiling and 3 mile of visibility. Refer to table in question 13 for review of weather minimums.

17. **B:** *Oxygen concentration remains at 21% regardless of altitude.* However, oxygen availability decreases with altitude because the oxygen molecules are farther apart, potentially resulting in hypoxia.

18. **D:** *Night vision loss occurs at 5,000 feet, which is part of the first stage of hypoxia which is called the indifferent stage.* Four stages of hypoxia need to be considered when examining its effect on human pathophysiology. The four stages are divided by altitude.

Stages of hypoxia by altitude	
Stage of hypoxia	Definition and clinical manifestation
First stage = indifferent	Physiologic zone for this stage begins at sea level and extends to 10,000 feet. The body reacts to the lessened availability of oxygen in the air with a slight increase in heart rate and ventilation. Night vision loss occurs at 5,000 feet.
Second stage = compensatory	Occurs from 10,000 to 15,000 feet. The body attempts to protect itself against hypoxia. An increase in blood pressure, heart rate, and depth and rate of respiration occurs. This stage is when efficiency and performance of tasks requiring mental alertness become impaired.
Third stage = disturbance	Occurs between 15,000 and 20,000 feet. It is characterized by dizziness, sleepiness, tunnel vision, and cyanosis. Thinking ability becomes slow, and muscle coordination decreases.
Fourth stage = critical	Occurs between 20,000 and 30,000 feet and features marked mental confusion and incapacitation followed by unconsciousness, usually within a few minutes.

19. **C:** The PAIP becomes the road map for the communication center staff to initiate the necessary critical steps that enhance crew survival and limit the program's liability. Priorities include verifying facts (crash location, etc.); dispatching rescue crews (civil air patrol, air medical, or ambulance response to the crash site); activating notification list according to the PAIP; and notifying security for crowd control at base of operations and/or hospitals. CAMTS recommends the following for time between each communication during flight and ground operations.

Flight following	
Air vs. ground	Time between communication
During flight and ground transport operations	Should not exceed 15 minutes while in flight unless a system of continuous automatic position tracking is utilized and 30 minutes on ground transports.
On the ground operations	Should not exceed 45 minutes.

20. **A:** *Graham's law,* also known as *Graham's law of effusion* states that the rate at which gas molecules diffuse is inversely proportional to the square root of its density (same as the square root of its molecular weight). This means that gases will flow from a higher pressure or concentration to an area of lower pressure or concentration. Simple diffusion and gas exchange at the cellular level are examples of this gas law.

21. **A:** *Barodontalgia or aerodontalgia* is a toothache that is caused by exposure to changing barometric pressure during actual or simulated flight. It is common for this to *occur during ascent,* with descent bringing relief. Barotitis media, frequently referred to as ear block, results from failure of the middle ear space to ventilate when going from low to high atmospheric pressure (descent). Barosinusitis, referred to as sinus block, usually present little problem when subjected to changes in barometric pressure. Sinus block is an acute or chronic inflammation of one or more of the paranasal sinuses produced by the development of a pressure difference, usually negative (ascent), between the air in the sinus cavity and that of the surrounding atmosphere. Patient should be monitored closely during ascent and descent.

22. **A:** The most correct answer is *ground transport; Boyle's law. Pneumocephalus* is the presence of air or gas within the cranial cavity. It is usually associated with disruption of the skull: after head and facial trauma, tumors of the skull base, after neurosurgery or otorhinolaryngology, and rarely, spontaneously. Pneumocephalus can occur in scuba diving, but is very rare in this context. Unpressurized aircraft is not recommended for this patient's condition.

23. **A:** *Flicker vertigo* can occur when transport team members and patients are exposed to lights that flicker at a rate of 4-20 cycles per second. Flicker vertigo can cause nausea and vomiting. In severe cases, it can cause seizures and unconsciousness. Even though flicker vertigo is not a common condition, sunlight flickering through rotor blades can trigger seizure activity in persons with seizure disorders or neurologic disorders. This patient had been recently diagnosed as having a stroke. Other clues to consider that flicker vertigo was

the cause of the seizure activity included; sunny afternoon and the seizure activity ceased when the rotor blades stopped and started again with start-up. Treatment can include covering the patient's eyes to prevent flicker vertigo from occurring.

24. **C:** *After the aircraft has come to a complete stop, the aircraft should be exited by normal means first,* jettison doors only if necessary, and forcible means if required. Crew members should meet at a predesignated position (usually meeting at the nose of the aircraft, which is twelve o'clock position) a safe distance from the aircraft.

25. **A:** *Boyle's law* describes the inversely proportional relationship between the absolute pressure and volume of a gas, if the temperature is kept constant within a closed system.

26. **A:** *Henry's law* states that at a constant temperature, the amount of a given gas dissolved in a given type and volume of liquid is directly proportional to the partial pressure of that gas in equilibrium with that liquid. An everyday example of Henry's law is given by carbonated soft drinks. Before the bottle or can is opened, the gas above the drink is almost pure carbon dioxide at a pressure slightly higher than atmospheric pressure. The drink itself contains dissolved carbon dioxide. When the bottle or can is opened, some of this gas escapes, giving the characteristic hiss (or "pop" in the case of a champagne bottle). Because the pressure above the liquid is now lower; some of the dissolved carbon dioxide comes out of solution as bubbles. If a glass of the drink is left in the open, the concentration of carbon dioxide in solution will come into equilibrium with the carbon dioxide in the air, and the drink will go "flat."

27. **D:** *Boyle's law (expansion or contraction of a gas)* describes the inversely proportional relationship between the absolute pressure and volume of a gas, if the temperature is kept constant within a closed system. The air in the ETT cuff, for example, expands with altitude (ascent) and contracts during descent.

28. **C:** Time between each communication should not exceed *15 minutes* while in flight unless a system of continuous automatic position tracking is utilized *or 30 minutes on ground transport.* Time between communications should not exceed 45 minutes while on the ground.

29. **A:** The *FARs* are rules prescribed by the FAA governing all aviation activities in the United States. Pilots need to be mindful that the *"eight-hour bottle-to-throttle" rule* is the absolute minimum. Some individuals may require a longer period between drinking and flying depending on the amount of alcohol consumed and their personal metabolism.

30. **C:** The PIC is accountable for nonmedical aspects of the flight and has final authority in flight-related issues. It is imperative that the PIC establishes clear leadership and command authority and appropriately applies the use of authority based on the current situation. Flight team members are in a valuable position to observe the pilot and assist in making safe decisions. Flight crew members assist in flight-related duties as outlined by the PIC. Each program must have a policy that allows any crew member to refuse or abort a flight if they feel uncomfortable.

31. **A:** *Once in the water, the flight team can minimize heat loss by using the HELP.* Flight crew members can achieve this position by bringing the knees up to the chest and putting the arms across the chest. The flotation device must be used with the HELP to stay afloat. The surviving flight team should huddle together to decrease heat loss. Protection against exposure, care of the raft, and signaling are the primary objectives in open-water survival.

32. **C:** *Dalton's law of partial pressures* states that the total pressure of a gas mixture is the sum of the individual or partial pressures of all the gases in the mixture.

33. **C:** *Elements that must be proved in a malpractice case are causation, injury, and damages.* Negligence and malpractice are often incorrectly used as interchangeable terms. *Negligence* is a deviation from accepted standards of performance. *Malpractice* is based on a professional standard of care, as well as the professional statutes of the caregiver. Other elements included in a malpractice case are presence of duty, breach of duty, and forseeability.

34. **A:** Air bubbles travel to the surface observing them may help crew members establish orientation; however, poor lighting conditions may prevent adequate visualization of bubbles. Crew members should gently use their arms to push themselves out of the aircraft and avoid kicking to prevent injury to crew members following behind. During surface descent the crew member should exhale slowly to prevent serious lung damage, should they attempt to hold their breath.

35. **A:** Once it is established that a duty exists, the second element is a breach of duty. Breach of duty may occur as a result of malfeasance (act of commission) or nonfeasance (act of omission). *Administering the wrong medication would be malfeasance,* whereas failure to follow a procedure would be nonfeasance.

36. **B:** *Boyle's law* describes the inversely proportional relationship between the absolute pressure and volume of a gas, if the temperature is kept constant within a closed system.

    Boyles law: Volume decreases and pressure increases; *pressure* increases and volume decreases.

    Charles' law: Temperature decreases and *volume* decreases; temperature increases and volume increases.

    Gay-Lussac's law: Pressure decreases and *temperature* decreases; pressure increases and temperature increases.

37. **C:** *VHF low-band FM (30-50 MHz); the VHF radio signal in this band follows the curvature of the earth and has the greatest range.*

Radio bands	
Type	Definition
VHF low-band FM (30-50 MHz)	The VHF radio signal in this band follows the curvature of the earth and has the greatest range.
VHF high-band FM (148-174 MHz)	Follows a straight line.
VHF AM (118-136 MHz)	Is typically used for aviation-related communications.
UHF (403-941 MHz)	Have a limited range and are most often used between ground units and base stations. These UHFs can be used for air-to-ground and ground-to-air communications for relatively short distances that will fluctuate with the terrain.
800 MHz	Is digital communication controlled by computers and allows multiple agencies to communicate with each other. This digital communication has higher frequency, less noise, and greater penetration outside of buildings.

38. **B:** All EMS aircraft are required by the FAA to carry an ELT, which are designed to emit a radio signal when activated that will be received by satellites and relayed to rescue personnel. The radio signal does not pinpoint the position of the aircraft but gives rescuers a general area in which to begin search. The ELT is activated by an impace exceeding 4g's (four times the force of gravity) and broadcasts on the universal distress channel 121.5. Flight team members should know the location of the ELT and ensure that it has been activated. If an impact does not automatically activate the ELT, it can be activated manually by use of the directions on the box.

39. **C:** A *radio repeater* is a combination of a radio receiver and a radio transmitter that receives a weak or low-level signal and retransmits it at a higher level or higher power, so that the signal can cover longer distances without degradation. A repeater system is a type of half duplex system that involves a base station "repeater" at an elevated site remote from the communications center. A repeater

system receives a signal on one frequency and instantly retransmits it on a second frequency to the other radios in the system, extending the communication's center's range. The process is reversed when the repeater receives signals coming into the base station.

Radio systems	
Type	Definition
Simple	Has the ability to transmit on one direction at a time by using a single frequency.
Full duplex	Has the ability to transmit and receive simultaneously by using two frequencies, typically UHF.
Half duplex	Has the ability to transmit or receive in one direction at a time by using two frequencies, typically UHF high-band.
Mulitplex	Has the ability to transmit from two or more sources over the same frequency.

40. **C:** In aviation, *VMC* is an aviation flight category in which VFR flight is permitted—that is, conditions in which pilots have sufficient visibility to fly the aircraft maintaining visual separation from terrain and other aircraft. They are the opposite of IMC. IMC, sometimes referred to as *blind flying*, is an aviation flight category that describes weather conditions that normally require pilots to fly primarily by reference to instruments, and therefore under IFR, rather than by outside visual references under VFR. Typically, this means flying in cloud, bad weather or at night. *So the rule is, you may fly IFR in VMC, but you cannot fly VFR in IMC.* It is important not to confuse IMC with IFR—"IMC" describes the actual weather conditions, while "IFR" describes the rules under which the aircraft is flying. Aircraft can (and often do) fly IFR in clear weather, for operational reasons, or when flying in airspace where flight under VFR is not permitted; indeed by far the majority of commercial flights are operated solely under IFR.

41. **C:** Henry's law has two parts: part one states that as pressure increases, solubility of gases in liquids increases; and part two

state that as temperature increases, solubility of gases in liquids decreases (colder liquids hold more gas than warmer liquids, as liquid warms up, the gas starts to come out of solution). When a diver goes underwater and subjects the body to increase pressure, the tissues are able to absorb more gases. The oxygen is used up by cellular processes, but the nitrogen is inert and just packs into the tissues. The deeper the diver goes and the longer he stays, the more nitrogen packs into the tissues.

Together, Boyle's and Henry's laws explain why, as a diver descends while breathing compressed air:

1. Inhaled PO_2 and PN_2 increase.
2. The amount of nitrogen and oxygen entering the blood and tissues also increase.

Henry's and Dalton's laws predict that, with descent, inhaled PO_2 and PN_2 will increase and cause an increased amount of nitrogen and oxygen to enter the blood and tissues. The opposite occurs on ascent: inhaled PO_2 and PN_2 decrease, and allow the excess nitrogen and oxygen to leave the blood and tissues.

The problem begins when the diver ascends and reduces the pressure the body is under, making the nitrogen less soluble in the tissues. If the diver comes up too fast (releases the pressure to fast), the nitrogen comes out in the form of bubbles, just like soda (the bottle of carbonated soda before it is opened is under pressure, when the bottle is opened, you release the pressure and the carbon dioxide becomes less soluble and comes out of solution in the form of bubbles). In order to avoid DCS, "the bends" and to prevent the bubbles from being released from the tissues, the diver must ascend slowly enough that the pressure is released slow enough to allow the nitrogen to leave the tissues without forming bubbles.

42. **D:** *Boyle's law* describes the inversely proportional relationship between the absolute pressure and volume of a gas, if the temperature is kept constant within a closed system.

Decompression sickness (DCS)		
DCS type	Bubble location	Clinical manifestation
Bends	Mostly large joints of the body (elbows, shoulders, hip, wrists, knees, and ankles)	Localized deep pain, ranging from mild to excruciating. Sometimes a dull ache, but rarely a sharp pain. Active and passive motion of the joint aggravates the pain. The pain may be reduced by bending the joint to find a more comfortable position. If caused by altitude, pain can occur at altitude, during the descent, or many hours later
Neurologic	Brain	Confusion or memory loss, headache, spots in visual field (scotoma), tunnel vision, double vision (diplopia), or blurry vision, unexplained extreme fatigue or behavior changes, seizures, dizziness, vertigo, nausea, vomiting, and unconsciousness may occur.
Neurologic	Spinal cord	Abnormal sensations such as burning, stinging, and tingling around the lower chest and back. Symptoms may spread from the feet up and may be accompanied by ascending weakness or paralysis. Girdling abdominal or chest pain.
Neurologic	Peripheral nerves	Urinary and rectal incontinence, abnormal sensations, such as numbness, burning, stinging and tingling (paresthesia), muscle weakness, and twitching.
Chokes	Lungs	Burning deep chest pain (under the sternum), pain is aggravated by breathing, shortness of breath (dyspnea), dry constant cough.
Skin bends	Skin	Itching usually around the ears, face, neck arms, and upper torso, sensation of tiny insects crawling over the skin, mottled or marbled skin usually around the shoulders, upper chest and abdomen, with itching, swelling of the skin, accompanied by tiny scar-like skin depressions (pitting edema).

Comparison of AGE and DCS		
Characteristic	**AGE**	**DCS**
Cause	Pulmonary expansion barotrauma	Excess nitrogen leaving tissues too quickly
Risks	Breath-hold ascent; noncommunicating air spaces	Exceeding prescribed limits for depth and time under water
Location and natures of bubbles	Air bubbles in arterial circulation	Nitrogen bubbles in tissues and venous circulation
Onset of symptoms	Within a few minutes of surfacing	Ranges from a few minutes to 48 hours after surfacing, but usually within 6 hours
Clinical syndrome	Unconsciousness, discrete neurological injury, or a cardiac event	Variable. Usually pain or paresthesias initially can progress to paralysis, shock. May mimic AGE
Effect of first aid, including oxygen	Symptoms may improve or go away altogether	Variable. Often no effect
Definitive treatment	Recompression in a hyperbaric chamber	Recompression in a hyperbaric chamber

43. **A:** In 1988, the National Transportation Safety Board (NTSB) released the results of an investigation of fifty-nine EMS accidents that occurred between 1978 and 1986. The study concluded that weather-related (pushing the weather) accidents were the most common and most serious type of accident experienced by EMS helicopters. In comparison with the 1980s, the 1990s saw a 10% increase in weather-related accidents.

44. **B:** *Newton's first law of motion* states unless it is acted on by a force, a body at rest will remain at rest and a body in motion will move at a constant speed in a straight line. The remaining three are gas laws.

45. **B:** *Four basic variables that affect gas volumetric relationships are temperature, pressure, volume, and the relative mass of gas or the number of molecules.* Gas laws govern the body's physiologic response to barometric pressure changes. When the transport team is taking care of the patient being transported by air, these changes become particularly important on ascent and descent.

46. **C:** Since airway management is an essential life-saving measure, and endotracheal intubation is an important aspect of airway management; *the initial education and training must include no less than five live* (animal labs are also acceptable) cadaver or dynamic human patient simulator (HPS) experience specific to age groups in program's scope of care and patient population. An experienced transport team member may show documentation that demonstrates this requirement has been previously met. Both crewmembers must be trained in airway management although license or state regulations may dictate who is allowed to intubate before and during transport.

47. **A:** During an actual flight emergency, flight team members are responsible for confirming with the pilot that an actual emergency crisis exists and assisting as necessary, shutting off the main oxygen supply, preparing patients by placing them flat and tightening the stretcher straps, and securing all equipment. As the final step in preparation, the flight team members should have their helmet visors in down position and get into the survival position by placing the arms across the chest, forming an "X" with the forearms, and grasping the shoulder harness, while placing the knees together and the feet approximately 6 in. apart.

48. **D:** Primary *and* receiving hospital helipad(s) must: be marked (with a painted "H" or similar landing designation); be identified by a strobelight or heliport beacon. A beacon may not be necessary when the location of the hospital can be readily determined by the light(s) on a prominent building or landmark near the helipad; have perimeter lighting for night operations; have a device to identify wind direction and velocity (i.e., windsock). The wind indicator should be located in an illuminated area or lighted for night

operations; have at least two approach and takeoff paths, oriented to be 90-180 degrees apart; have adequate fire retardant chemicals readily available; have documented, ongoing safety programs for those personnel responsible for loading and unloading patients or working around the helicopter on the helipad; have evidence of adequate security—a minimum of one person to prevent bystanders from approaching the helicopter as it lands or lifts off, or perimeter security such as fencing, rooftop, etc. A means must exist to monitor the primary helipad if accessible to the public, that is, through direct visual monitoring or closed circuit TV; and have at least one clear final approach and takeoff area (FATO) according to the FAA Advisory Circular entitled Heliport Design Advisory Circular, AC 150/5390-2A which also includes: takeoff and landing area length and width, or diameter, should be 1.5 times the overall length of the helicopters that utilize the helipad; surface of the helipad should be clear of objects, including parked helicopters; and parking area should be provided if more than one helicopter at a time is to be accommodated.

49. **A:** The most serious manifestation of pressure-related injuries or barotraumas is AGE. *AGE is a leading cause of death among scuba divers.* Divers need to exhale continuously when ascending, or several things may occur, which can include air pushing through the lung tissues and enters the skin in the neck, air pushing through the lung tissues and into the spaces between the lungs causing a pneumothorax, and air forced from the lungs into blood vessels and carried to vital organs. The greatest changes in pressure and volume occur at shallower depths. Pulmonary overpressurization and alveolar rupture can occur during an ascent from a depth as shallow as four feet if compressed air is held in the lungs. Breath holding results in lung overexpansion and rupture of the alveoli. Manifestations of AGE usually begin during or in minutes of ascent. Recompression in a hyperbaric chamber is the only effective treatment for this diving emergency. The immediate treatment includes administration of 100% oxygen and placing the patient in a supine position. The head-down (Trendelenburg) position and the head-down left lateral decubitus position have been recommended to minimize further passage of air emboli to the brain.

50. **B:** Multiple stressors have been identified that may be caused by transport.

Stressors of flight	
Type	Definition or clinical manifestation
Decreased partial pressure of oxygen	Hypoxia stages and types, TUC
Barometric pressure changes	Barotitis media, barosinusitis, barodontalgia, and gastrointestinal changes
Thermal changes	Increase in altitude results in decrease in ambient pressure
Decreased humidity	Increase in altitude results in decrease in ambient pressure and therefore a decrease in humidity
Noise	Can impair the ability to perform patient assessment
Vibration	Can interfere with transport equipment
Fatigue	Is always a potential threat to safety
Gravitational forces	g-forces, ELT activates on impact beginning at 4g's

Additional stressors of flight	
Type	Definition or clinical manifestation
Spatial disorientation	Inaccurate perception of position, attitude, and motion in relation to the center of the earth
Flicker vertigo	Can occur when exposed to lights that flicker at a rate of 4-20 cycles per second, which can cause nausea and vomiting. In severe cases, it can cause seizures and unconsciousness.
Fuel vapors	Jet fuel, diesel fuel, and gasoline fuel exposures can cause altered mental status, nauseas, and eye inflammation.

Bibliography

Association of Air Medical Services. (2003). *Guidelines for Air Medical Crew Education.* Iowa, Kendall/Hunt Publishing Company.

Castka, JF, Metcalfe, HC, Davis, RE, Williams, JE. (2002). *Modern Chemistry.* Austin, TX: Holt, Rinehart and Winston.

Darovic, G. (1999). *Handbook of Hemodynamic Monitoring.* 2nd edition. Philadelphia, W. B. Saunders.

Holleran, R. (1996). *Flight Nursing: Principles and Practice* (2nd edition). St. Louis, Mosby.

Holleran, R. (2003). *Air and Surface Patient Transport: Principles and Practice* (3rd edition). St. Louis: Mosby.

Holleran, R. (2009). *ASTNA Patient Transport: Principles and Practice* (4th edition). St. Louis, Mosby.

Krupa, D. (1997). *Flight Nursing Core Curriculum.* Park Ridge, IL: National Flight Nurses Association.

Reinhart, R. (2008) *Basic Flight Physiology* (3rd edition). McGraw Hill Books.

Appendix A
CCP-C Summary of Examination

I. Advanced airway management techniques (12)

A. Identify the indications for basic and advanced airway management
B. Identify the indications and contraindications for specific airway interventions
C. Perform advanced airway management techniques
D. Administer pharmacology for airway management
E. Implement a failed airway algorithm
F. React to intubation complications
G. Perform alternative airway management techniques (e.g., needle cricothyrotomy, surgical cricothyotomy, retrograde intubation, LMA)
H. Monitor airway management and ventilation during transport
I. Manage mechanical ventilation

II. Respiratory patient (12)

A. Perform an assessment of the patient
B. Identify causes and stages of respiratory failure
C. Manage patients with respiratory compromise (e.g., acute RDS, spontaneous pneumothorax, pneumonia)
D. Manage patient's status using
    1. Laboratory values (e.g., blood gas values, ISTAT)
    2. Diagnostic equipment (e.g., pulse oximetry, chest radiography, capnography)
E. Administer pharmacologic agents
F. Manage respiratory patient's complications

III. Cardiac patient (12)

A. Manage patients experiencing a cardiac event (e.g., acute coronary syndrome, heart failure, cardiogenic shock, primary arrhythmias, hemodynamic instability)
B. Use invasive hemodynamic monitoring
C. Assist in the use of cardiopulmonary support devices as part of patient management (e.g., ventricular assist devices (VADs), transvenous pacer, intra-aortic balloon pump (IABP))
D. Use cardiopulmonary support devices as part of patient management (e.g., VADs, transvenous pacer, IABP)
E. Manage patient's status using
    1. Laboratory values (e.g., blood gas values, ISTAT)
    2. Diagnostic equipment (e.g., pulse oximetry, chest radiography, capnography)
F. Administer pharmacologic agents
G. Manage cardiac patient's complications

IV. General medical patient (12)

A. Perform an assessment of the patient
B. Manage patients experiencing a medical condition (e.g., AAA, GI bleed, bowel obstruction, HHNC)
C. Use invasive monitoring for the purpose of clinical management
D. Manage patient's status using
    1. Laboratory values (e.g., blood gas values, ISTAT)
    2. Diagnostic equipment (e.g., pulse oximetry, chest radiography, capnography)
E. Administer pharmacologic agents
F. Treat patient with general medical complications

V. Trauma patient management (12)

A. Differentiate injury patterns associated with specific mechanisms of injury
B. Rate a trauma victim using the trauma score
C. Identify patients who meet trauma center criteria
D. Perform a comprehensive assessment of the trauma patient
E. Initiate the critical interventions for the management of the trauma patient

1. Manage the patient with life-threatening thoracic injuries (e.g., pneumothorax, flail chest, tamponade, myocardial rupture)
2. Manage the patient with abdominal injuries (e.g., diaphragm, liver, and spleen)
3. Manage the patient with orthopedic injuries (e.g., pelvic, femur, spinal)
4. Manage the patient with neurologic injuries (e.g., subdural, epidural, increased ICP)

F. Manage patient's status using
   1. Laboratory values (e.g., blood gas values, ISTAT)
   2. Diagnostic equipment (e.g., pulse oximetry, chest radiography, capnography)
G. Administer pharmacologic agents and blood products
H. Manage trauma patient complications

VI. Burn patients (9)

A. Perform an assessment of the patient
B. Calculate the percentage of total body surface area burned
C. Manage fluid replacement therapy
D. Manage inhalation injuries in burn injury patients
E. Manage patient's status using
   1. Laboratory values (e.g., blood gas values, ISTAT)
   2. Diagnostic equipment (e.g., pulse oximetry, chest radiography, capnography)
F. Administer pharmacologic agents
G. Provide treatment of burn complications

VII. Neurologic patient (11)

A. Perform an assessment of the patient
B. Conduct differential diagnosis of patients with coma
C. Manage patients with seizures
D. Manage patients with cerebral ischemia
E. Initiate the critical interventions for the management of a patient with a neurologic emergency
F. Provide care for a patient with a neurologic emergency
G. Assess a patient using the GCS

H. Manage patients with head injuries
I. Manage patients with spinal cord injuries
J. Manage patient's status using
     1. Laboratory values (e.g., blood gas values, ISTAT)
     2. Diagnostic equipment (e.g., pulse oximetry, chest radiography, capnography)
K. Administer pharmacologic agents
L. Manage neurologic patient complications

VIII. Obstetrical patients (9)

A. Perform an assessment of the patient
B. Manage fetal distress
C. Manage obstetrical patients
D. Assess uterine contraction pattern
E. Conduct interventions for obstetrical complications (e.g., pregnancy induced hypertension, hypertonic or tetanic contractions, cord prolapse, placental abruption)
F. Determine if transport can safely be attempted or if delivery should be accomplished at the referring facility
G. Manage patient's status using
     1. Laboratory values (e.g., blood gas values, ISTAT)
     2. Diagnostic equipment (e.g., pulse oximetry, chest radiography, capnography)
H. Administer pharmacologic agents
I. Manage emergent delivery and postpartum complications

IX. Neonatal and pediatric patient (15)

A. Neonatal patient
     1. Perform an assessment of the patient
     2. Manage the resuscitation of the neonate
     3. Manage patient's status using
         a) Diagnostic equipment (e.g., pulse oximetry, chest radiography, capnography)
     4. Administer pharmacologic agents
     5. Manage neonatal patient complications
B. Pediatric patient
     1. Perform an assessment of the patient

2. Manage the pediatric patient experiencing a medical event
   a) Respiratory
   b) Toxicity
   c) Cardiac
   d) Environmental
   e) GI
   f) Endocrine
   g) Neuro
   h) Infectious processes
3. Manage the pediatric patient experiencing a traumaticevent
   a) Single vs. multiple system
   b) Burns
   c) Non-accidental trauma
4. Manage patient's status using
   a) Laboratory values (e.g., blood gas values, ISTAT)
   b) Diagnostic equipment (e.g., pulse oximetry, chest radiography, capnography)
   c) Administer pharmacologic agents
   d) Treat patient with pediatric complications

X. Transport fundamentals—safety and survival (9)

A. Manage the safety of the work environment
B. Conduct checks to ensure transport vehicle integrity
C. Conduct checks to ensure equipment is present, functional, and stowed
D. Observe for hazards during transport vehicle operation
E. Use safety equipment while in transport
F. Secure the patient for transport
G. Practice crew resource management (CRM)
H. Participate in mission safety decisions
I. Evaluate transport mode
J. Perform immediate postaccident duties at a crash site
K. Ensure the safety of all passengers (e.g., specialty teams, family, law enforcement, observer)

L. Identify stressors related to transport (e.g., thermal, humidity, noise, vibration, or fatigue related conditions)

M. Take corrective action for patient stressors related to transport

XI. Toxic exposure and environmental patient (12)

A. Toxic exposure patient
1. Perform an assessment of the patient
2. Decontaminate toxicological patients (e.g., chemical or biological or radiological exposure)
3. Administer poison antidotes
4. Provide care for victims of envenomation (e.g., snake bite, scorpion sting, spider bite)
5. Manage patient's status using
    a) Laboratory values (e.g., blood gas values, ISTAT)
    b) Diagnostic equipment (e.g., pulse oximetry, chest radiography, capnography)
6. Administer pharmacologic agents
7. Manage toxicological patients (e.g., medication overdose, chemical or biological or radiological exposure)
8. Manage toxicological patient complications

B. Environmental patient
1. Perform an assessment of the patient
2. Manage the patient experiencing a cold-related illness (e.g., frostbite, hypothermia, cold water submersion)
3. Manage the patient experiencing a heat-related illness (e.g., heat stroke, heat exhaustion, heat cramps)
4. Manage the patient experiencing a diving-related illness (e.g., DCS, AGE, near drowning)
5. Manage the patient experiencing altitude-related illness
6. Manage patient's status using
    a) Laboratory values (e.g., blood gas values, ISTAT)
    b) Diagnostic equipment (e.g., pulse oximetry, chest radiography, capnography)
7. Administer pharmacologic agents
8. Treat patient with environmental complications

CCP-C summary of examination	
Category	**Number of questions**
Trauma emergencies	12
Transport fundamentals—safety and survival	9
Advanced airway management techniques	12
Neurological emergencies	11
Critical cardiac emergencies	12
Respiratory emergencies	12
Toxic exposures and environmental emergencies	12
Obstetrical emergencies	9
Neonatal and pediatric emergencies	15
Burn emergencies	9
General medical emergencies	12

Appendix B
FP-C Summary of Examination

I. Trauma management (9)w

A. Perform patient triage
B. Differentiate injury patterns associated with specific mechanisms of injury
C. Identify patients who meet trauma center criteria
D. Perform a comprehensive assessment of the trauma patient
E. Initiate the critical interventions for the management of the trauma patient
F. Provide care for the patient with life-threatening thoracic injuries (e.g., pneumothorax, flail chest, tamponade, myocardial rupture)
G. Provide care for the patient with abdominal injuries (e.g., diaphragm, liver, and spleen)
H. Provide care for the patient with orthopedic injuries (e.g., pelvic, femur, spinal)
I. Administer appropriate pharmacology for trauma management

II. Aircraft fundamentals—safety and survival (12)

A. Assess the safety of the scene
B. Conduct preflight checks to ensure aircraft integrity
C. Conduct preflight checks to ensure equipment is present, functional, and stowed
D. Observe for hazards during aircraft operation
E. Utilize proper safety equipment while in flight
F. Maintain a sterile cockpit during critical phases of flight
G. Approach and depart the aircraft in a safe manner
H. Ensure safety around the aircraft
I. Secure the patient for flight
J. Participate in CRM

K. Participate in flight mission safety decisions (e.g., go/no-go, abort)
L. Respond to in-flight emergencies
    1. Fire
    2. Emergency egress
    3. Emergent landing
    4. Adverse weather conditions
M. Perform immediate postaccident duties at a crash site
N. Build survival shelters
O. Initiate emergency survival procedures
P. Ensure the safety of all passengers (e.g., specialty teams, family, law enforcement, observer)
Q. Estimate weather conditions that are below weather minimums

III. Flight physiology (10)

A. Identify causes of hypoxia
B. Take corrective measures to prevent altitude related hypoxia
C. Identify signs of barometric trauma
D. Identify stressors related to transport (e.g., thermal, humidity, noise, vibration, or fatigue related conditions)
E. Take corrective action for patient stressors related to transport
F. Relate the relevant gas laws to patient condition and treatment
G. Relate the stages of hypoxia to patient condition and treatment
H. Identify immediate causes of altitude related conditions in patients
I. Identify immediate causes of altitude-related conditions as they affect the air medical crew
J. Provide appropriate interventions to prevent the adverse effects of altitude changes during patient transport

IV. Advanced airway management techniques (5)

A. Identify the indications for basic and advanced airway management

B. Identify the indications and contraindications for specific airway interventions
C. Perform advanced airway management techniques
D. Administer appropriate pharmacology for airway management
E. Implement a failed airway algorithm
F. Identify esophageal intubation
G. React to intubation complications
H. Perform alternative airway management techniques (e.g., needle cricothyrotomy, surgical cricothyotomy, Seldinger technique, retrograde intubation, LMA)
I. Monitor airway management and ventilation during transport
J. Use mechanical ventilation

V. Burn patients (5)

A. Perform an assessment of the burn patient
B. Calculate the percentage of total body surface area burned
C. Calculate appropriate fluid replacement amounts based on the patient's burn injury and physiologic condition
D. Diagnose inhalation injuries in burn injury patients
E. Administer appropriate pharmacology for burn patients
F. Provide treatment of burn emergencies

VI. Neurological emergencies (10)

A. Conduct differential diagnosis of coma patients
B. Manage patients with seizures
C. Manage patients with cerebral ischemia
D. Initiate the critical interventions for the management of a patient with a neurologic emergency
E. Provide care for a patient with a specific neurologic emergency
F. Perform a baseline neurologic assessment of a trauma patient
G. Perform an ongoing serial evaluation of a neurologic patient
H. Assess changes in intracranial pressure using patient level of consciousness
I. Perform a focused neurological assessment
J. Assess a patient using the GCS
K. Manage patients with head injuries
L. Manage patients with spinal cord injuries

M. Evaluate muscle strength and motor function
N. Administer appropriate pharmacology for neurological management

VII. Critical cardiac patient (20)

A. Perform a detailed cardiovascular assessment
B. Identify patients experiencing an acute cardiac event (e.g., acute myocardial infarction, heart failure, cardiogenic shock, primary arrhythmias, hemodynamic instability)
C. Use invasive monitoring during transport, as indicated, for the purpose of clinical management
D. Provide treatment for patients with acute cardiac events and hemodynamic abnormalities
E. Control cardiopulmonary support devices to patient condition as part of patient management (e.g., VADs, transvenous pacer, IABP)
F. Assist in the control of cardiopulmonary support devices to patient condition as part of patient management (e.g., VADs, transvenous pacer, IABP)
G. Conduct defibrillation during transport
H. Administer appropriate pharmacology for cardiac management

VIII. Respiratory patient (10)

A. Perform a detailed respiratory assessment
B. Identify patients experiencing respiratory compromise (e.g., acute RDS, spontaneous pneumothorax, pneumonia)
C. Monitor patient's respiratory status using laboratory values and diagnostic equipment (e.g., pulse oximetry, capnography, blood gas values, chest radiography)
D. Provide treatment for patients with acute respiratory events
E. Administer appropriate pharmacology for respiratory management

IX. Toxic exposures (6)

A. Conduct a physical examination of a toxicological patient
B. Decontaminate toxicological patients when indicated

C. Administer poison antidotes when indicated

D. Provide emergency care for victims of envenomation (e.g., snake bite, scorpion sting, spider bite)

E. Administer appropriate pharmacology for toxic exposures

F. Provide treatment for toxicological patients (e.g., medication overdose, chemical or biological or radiological exposure)

X. Obstetrical emergencies (4)

A. Perform an assessment of the obstetrical patient

B. Perform fetal assessment

C. React to special transport considerations of the obstetrical patient

D. Provide treatment for high-risk obstetrical patients

E. Assess uterine contractions

F. Conduct interventions for obstetrical emergencies (e.g., pregnancy induced hypertension, hypertonic or tetanic contractions, cord prolapse, placental abruption)

G. Assess whether transport can safely be attempted or whether delivery should be accomplished at the referring facility

H. Administer appropriate pharmacology for obstetrical patients

I. Manage emergent delivery

XI. Neonatal (4)

A. Perform an assessment of the neonatal patient

B. Reevaluate the clinical assessment and management of the neonate when initial emergency measures fail

C. Administer appropriate pharmacology for neonatal patients

D. Implement neonatal resuscitation according to established practice

E. Manage the isolette transport

F. Provide treatment of neonatal emergencies

XII. Pediatric (10)

A. Perform an assessment of the pediatric patient

B. Identify the pediatric patient experiencing an acute respiratory event (e.g., epiglottitis, bronchiolitis, asthma)

C. Identify the pediatric patient experiencing an acute medical event (e.g., meningitis, overdose, seizures)
D. Identify the pediatric patient experiencing an acute cardiovascular event (e.g., shock, cardiac anomaly, dysrhythmias)
E. Identify the pediatric patient experiencing an acute traumatic event (e.g., auto vs. pedestrian, falls, child abuse)
F. Administer appropriate pharmacology for pediatric patients
G. Provide treatment of pediatric emergencies

XIII. General medical patient (16)

A. Perform a focused medical assessment
B. Identify patients experiencing a medical emergency (e.g., AAA, GI bleed, bowel obstruction, HHNC)
C. Use invasive monitoring during transport, as indicated, for the purpose of clinical management
D. Provide treatment for patients with medical emergencies
E. Manage patient condition utilizing available laboratory values (e.g., blood glucose, CBC, H/H)
F. Administer appropriate pharmacology for the medical patient
G. Prevent transmissions of infectious disease
H. Provide appropriate pain management
I. Evaluate and record patient pain levels

XIV. Environmental (4)

A. Perform an assessment of the patient suffering from an environmental emergency
B. Identify the patient experiencing a cold-related emergency (e.g., frostbite, hypothermia, cold water submersion)
C. Identify the patient experiencing a heat-related emergency (e.g., heat stroke, heat exhaustion, heat cramps)
D. Identify the patient experiencing a diving-related emergency (e.g., DCS, AGE, near drowning)
E. Identify the patient experiencing an altitude related emergency (e.g., HAPE, cerebral edema)
F. Administer appropriate pharmacology for environmental emergency patients
G. Provide treatment of environmental emergencies

FP-C summary of examination	
Category	**Number of questions**
Trauma emergencies	9
Aircraft fundamentals—safety and survival	12
Flight physiology	10
Advanced airway management techniques	5
Neurological emergencies	10
Critical cardiac emergencies	20
Respiratory emergencies	10
Toxic exposures	6
Obstetrical emergencies	4
Neonatal emergencies	4
Pediatric emergencies	10
Burn emergencies	5
General medical emergencies	16
Environmental emergencies	4

Appendix C
Flashcards

Flashcards (We don't promise that every answer is entirely correct) **Original: November 2006** **Revised: May 2010** **Orchid Lopez; RN, CFRN, NREMT-P, FP-C**	*"Back to Basics"* *Critical Care Transport* 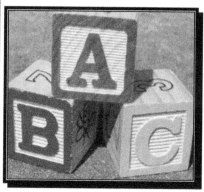
Clinical signs Kehr's Kernig's Brudzinski's Hamman's	Kehr's: referred left should pain—possible splenic injury or ectopic pregnancy Kernig's: back, leg pain on knee extension—possible bacterial meningitis Brudzinski's: back, leg pain on neck flexion—possible bacterial meningitis or subarachnoid bleed Hamman's: crunching sound heard with auscultation over the anterior chest synchronized with heartbeat—tracheobronchial injury

x-ray findings Steeple sign Thumbprint sign	**Steeple** Possible croup (laryngotracheobronchitis) A/P neck view **Thumbprint** Possible epiglottitis lateral neck view
ABG values	pCO_2 high = pH low (acidosis) pCO_2 low = pH high (alkalosis) pH low = HCO_3 low (acidosis) pH high = HCO_3 high (alkalosis) pCO_2 = 35-45 respiratory pH = 7.35-7.45 metabolic HCO_3 = 22-26 metabolic
Drugs for AAA	Nipride and beta-blockers

First adjustment on ventilator	TV first, not rate
Trauma 1. Most common dislocation 2. Most common spontaneous recurrence	1. Hip 2. Anterior shoulder
Brain natriuretic peptide (BNP)	Heart failure marker that measures BNP released by an overdistension of the heart Below 100 = normal Above 500-700 = heart failure

Rotor-wing pilot required hours	2000 hours 1000 PIC 100 hours at night
"Bottle-to-throttle" time	At least 8 hours
CVP Measures Normal parameter Which port to use	Measures: preload (right atrial pressure) Norm: 2-6 mmHg Port: proximal port Catheter placement outside line markers: RA/CVP = 25-30 cm RV = 35-45 cm PA = 50-55 cm

Spinal cord syndromes (ABC) Anterior cord Brown-Séquard Central cord syndrome **Autonomic dysreflexia**	Anterior: complete motor, pain and temperature loss below the lesion Brown: ipsilateral loss of motor, position and vibration sense; contralateral loss of pain and temperature perception Central: greater motor weakness in UE than LE with varying degrees of sensory loss Autonomic: urinary retention, massive increase in sympathetic tone which can cause HTN, treated by insertion of foley
Normal urinary output **Normal blood volume**	UO: 30-50 mL/hr (adult) UO: 1-2 mL/kg/hr (peds) Blood volume: 70 mL/kg (adult) Blood volume: 80 mL/kg (peds)

Normal temperature **Mild hypothermia** **Moderate hypothermia** **Severe hypothermia**	Normal: 37.6/98.6 Mild: 32-36 (decreasing HR) Moderate: 29-32 (loss of shivering, ALOC) Severe: 20-28 (coma, VF common)
Two major causes of heat loss? **Thermoregulation ceases at?**	Radiation, evaporation 28 degrees
Rules of flight following	Sterile cockpit during critical phase of flight 15 minutes maximum between communication center during flight 45 minutes maximum while on the ground

Rotor-wing shut-off sequence	**Remember "TFB"** Throttle Fuel Battery Take survival bag and meet at twelve o'clock position
Survival sequence	Shelter Fire Water Food
Order of how to assess the abdomen	Inspect Auscultation Palpation Percussion

Contraindications for thrombolytics	History of hemorrhagic stroke CVA last 12 months SBP over 180 Pregnancy or 1 month postpartum
FARs Local flying area determined by Cell phones prohibited	Part 91: no passengers Part 135: passengers (14 hours max for pilots) Certificate holder While airborne
PaO$_2$ SaO$_2$ Bariobariatrauma	PaO$_2$: plasma-measured as pressure SaO$_2$: hemoglobin-measured as percentage Nitrogen release in obese patients, administer high flow oxygen 15 minutes to lift off to wash out nitrogen

Normal pediatric SBP? When does it drop?	**BP last to go . . .** SBP: 90 + (2 × age) After loss of 25% DBP: 2/3 the SBP
Three killers of ventilator patients during flight	Pericardial tamponade Tension pneumothorax Hypovolemia
Death from crush injury due to? Complications of crush injury?	Death due to: renal failure Complications: DIC, compartment syndrome, renal failure, hyperkalemia

CAMTS 1. Medical director not required to: 2. Intubation requirement: 3. Live intubation required during training: 4. Specialty team response time:	1. live in same state 2. quarterly 3. five 4. 45 minutes
CAMTS 1. Pilot area orientation day/night: 2. Helipad required to have: 3. Fixed wing twin engine time: 4. Ambulance fuel requirement: 5. ELT set off at: 6. Uniform fit:	1. 5 hours day / 2 hours night 2. 2 paths, security 3. 500 hours 4. 175 miles 5. 4g's 6. ¼ in. space between body and uniform
Applied gas laws The bends, decompression, soda can, CO_2 in blood	Henry's law

Applied gas laws Tissue swelling, hypoxic hypoxia, O_2 available at altitude	Dalton's law
Applied gas laws Cellular gas exchange, diffusion	Graham's law
Applied gas laws Oxygen tank pressure in heat or cold	Gay-Lussac's law

Applied gas laws BP cuff, ETT cuff, MAST	Boyle's law IABP purges with ascent or descent
Trauma and kinematics High velocity Medium velocity Low velocity	High: above 2000 FPS Med: 1000-2000 FPS Low: under 1000 FPS
Tumbling **Yaw**	Tumbling: rotation on 360 degree axis Yaw: deviation up to 90 degrees from straight path

Normal values CVP/RAP Cardiac output Cardiac index Pulmonary artery systolic/ diastolic Wedge (PAWP/PCWP) SVR	CVP: 2-6 CO: SV x HR (4-8 L/min) CI: 2.5-4.2 PAS/PAD: 15-25/8-15 PAWP/wedge: 8-12 SVR: 800-1200 dynes/sec/cm^{-5} When assessing CVP or PA, pressures on a mechanically ventilated patient, assess pressures at the end of exhalation
Chest/ABD trauma Chest tube location? Needle thoracostomy? Suspect with fracture of first 3 ribs? Scaphoid abdomen indicates?	Fourth IC space, anterior-axillary (chest tube) Second ICS midclavicular or the fifth ICS anterior mid-axillary line (needle thoracostomy) Aortic disruption Diaphragmatic rupture
High-risk OB Abruptio placenta Placenta previa Terbutaline dose Define postpartum hemorrhage Uterine rupture	Abruptio: dark red, painful Placenta previa: red, painless Terbutaline: 0.25 SQ PP hemorrhage: over 500 mL Fetal parts can be palpated over abdomen

Effects of altitude worsen with:	Cold upper latitudes
Gay-Lussac's law Two components	Temperature increases and pressure increases Temperature decreases and pressure decreases **Example** Oxygen tank pressure at 2200 in the afternoon, pressure drops to 1800 in the evening (temperature declined in the evening, pressure decreased)
Universal law	Combines Boyle's and Charles' laws

Graham's law Definition Effects	Gas moves from high to low concentration **Examples** gas through liquid, cellular gas exchange
Henry's law	Gas in liquid proportional to gas above liquid **Examples** "the bends," CO_2 in blood, decompression
Volume of gas in GI expands thrice at what altitude? **What law affects GI the most?**	25,000 feet Boyle's law

Cardiogenic shock CVP Cardiac output Cardiac index PAS/PAD PAWP SVR Heart rate	CVP: high CO: low CI: low PAS/PAD: high PCWP: high SVR: high Heart rate initially fast, then slows down
Boyle's law Two components Effects	Increased volume = decreased pressure **Examples** Cuffs, MAST, GI, ETT, IABP
Charles' law Two Components Effects	Temperature and volume proportional (increased temperature = increased volume) Up 100 meters = down 1°C

Environmental 1. Passive rewarming? 2. Active rewarming? 3. Warm and dead? 4. Heat stroke	1. mild hypothermia only. Up 1°C/hr with blankets, heater 2. apply heat to body 3. 32°C 4. over 42°C
Clinical signs 1. Grey Turner's sign 2. Coopernail's sign 3. Halstead's sign 4. Cullen's sign 5. Murphy's sign 6. Levine's sign	1. Flank bruising (retroperitoneal bleeding) 2. Scrotum/labia (abdominal/ pelvic bleeding) 3. Marbled abdomen (bleeding) 4. Umbilical discoloration (pancreatitis) 5. RUQ pain with inspiration (gallbladder) 6. Fist to chest "clutching" (cardiac)
Types of hypoxia 1. Hypoxic hypoxia 2. Hypemic hypoxia 3. Histotoxic hypoxia 4. Stagnant hypoxia	1. altitude hypoxia, decreased alveolar oxygen, tension pneumo (e.g., altitude) 2. decreased O_2 carrying capacity in blood 3. poisoning (e.g., nitrates) 4. decreased cardiac output, poor circulation (e.g., g-forces, CHF)

High-risk OB 1. Normal FHR 2. Factors fetal well-being 3. Most important factor 4. TX for fetal distress	1. 120-160 2. FHR, fetal movement, variability 3. variability 4. LOCK: left lateral recumbent, O_2, correct contributing factors, keep reassessing
CHF considerations Preload Lab test Medications	Many CHF patients are relatively hypovolemic. Careful with diuretics and medications that can decrease preload BNP = lab test nonspecific > 500 No beta-blockers, except for carvidolol (coreg) Natracor (neseritide) = synthetic version of BNP
Primary cause of death with ventilator dependent patients	Ventilator acquired pneumonia

Digoxin Class Causes what electrolyte imbalance ECG changes	Cardiac glycoside Hypokalemia ECG—"dig dip" ST depression
ARDS Treatment CXR	PEEP CXR reveals widespread pulmonary infiltrates; glass-like appearance
PEEP Effects of PEEP Normal physiologic PEEP	PEEP Increased pulmonary vascular resistance Can cause hypotension over 15 cm H_2O Normal Range: 3-5 cm H_2O

Treat HTN when BP?	Over 220 systolic MAP over 130
Dehydration raises serum?	Sodium Normal sodium: 135-145
Objective data?	ABCs, neurological assessment Differential diagnosis for altered mental status: AEIOUTIPS

Bowel sounds in chest cavity? **Crunching sound heard over chest with auscultation, may be synchronized with heartbeat?**	**Bowel sounds heard** Diaphragmatic rupture Most common in the left chest **Crunching sounds heard** Associated with tracheobronchial injury and is called Hamman's sign
Preferred method for moving spinal injured patients	Scoop stretcher is preferred rather then performing a log roll
Differential diagnosis 1. Pulmonary contusion 2. Ruptured diaphragm 3. Tracheobronchial injury 4. Esophageal perforation 5. Fat embolus	1. low sats despite O_2, rales 2. chest/abd pain radiated to left shoulder 3. hemoptysis, sub-q air, air leak with chest tube, advance ETT below level of injury into right mainstem 4. fever, hematemesis 5. fever, rash after fracture

Blood loss Humerus Femur	Humerus: 750 mL Femur: 1500 mL
PAWP/PCWP Function Normal	Pulmonary artery wedge pressure Pulmonary capillary wedge pressure Looks at the left side of the heart, if high can indicate pulmonary congestion, CHF, and cardiogenic shock PAWP/PCWP: 8-12 mmHg Do not keep wedged for more than 15 seconds, make sure that balloon is deflated and have patient cough forcefully
ETT Depth	Adult: 3 × ETT size or average is 19-23 cm Peds: 10 + age in years Neonatal: 6 + age weight in kg

Ventilator miscellaneous
1. To change CO_2
2. To change oxygenation

1. adjust rate, TV
2. adjust PEEP, PAP

Burns
Rule of nines for adult and pediatrics
Parkland formula
Consensus formula

Know your rules of nines for both adult and pediatric patients

Parkland: 4 mL × kg × TBSA. ½ over 1st 8 hrs, rest over next 16 hours

Consensus: 2-4 mL × kg × TBSA. ½ over 1st 8 hours, rest over next 16 hours

Safety
1. ELT frequency
2. Confirm ELT working
3. Twin engine required offshore

1. 121.5
2. Tune it in and listen
3. Raft, vest

Drugs 1. Induction agent of choice with bronchospastic patients 2. Ativan: indication dose, max 3. Mannitol dose 4. Drug choice for cyclic antidepressant OD 5. Drug choice for beta-blocker OD 6. Fentanyl dose 7. Treatment for malignant hyperthermia 8. Drug for GI bleeds	1. Ketamine (ketalar) 2. Lorazepam, seizures, 1-2 mg, max 4 mg 3. 1-2 g/kg 4. Sodium bicarbonate 5. Glucagon 6. Sublimaze (3 µg/kg) 7. Dantrium (dantrolene) 8. Sandostatin (octreotide)
Neurogenic shock CVP Cardiac output Cardiac index PAWP/PCWP "Wedge" SVR Heart rate	CVP: down CO: down CI: down PCWP: down SVR: down (distributive shock) Heart rate can present as normal or slow
Arterial line Sites Purpose	Radial, femoral Monitor pressure, blood draw, ABGs Maintain pressure bag at 300 mmHg Underdampening: caused by having air in the system, loose connection, a low pressure bag, and altitude changes Overdampening: caused by kinking, increased bag pressure, and tip against the wall

ECG 1. Most common reperfusion dysrhythmia 2. Most common hypothermia dysrhythmia 3. Hypokalemia on ECG 4. Hyperkalemia on ECG	1. Reperfusion: AIVR 2. Hypothermia: VF, (osborn wave) 3. Peaked P's, flat T's 4. Flat P's, peaked T's (treat with calcium)
MAP goal with CHI CPP goal with increased ICP	MAP: 80-100 CPP: 70-90
Normal ICP Normal CPP (head) Normal MAP Normal for the other CPP (heart) (Coronary perfusion pressure)	ICP: 0-10 CPP: 70-90 MAP: 80-100 Heart CPP: 50-60 **Remember your *head* is higher than your *heart***

GCS Mild, moderate, severe	GCS or Scale Mild: 14-15 Moderate: 9-13 Severe: 3-8
CPP (head) formula **MAP formula** **CPP (heart) formula**	CPP: MAP-ICP MAP: $2 \times$ diastolic + systolic/3 Heart CPP: DBP-wedge
Rotor-wing minimums ceiling/visibility Day/local Day/cross-country Night/local Night/cross-country	Day/local: 500 foot (ceiling) and 1 mile (visibility) Day/x-country: 1000 foot (ceiling) and 1 mile (visibility) Night/local: 500 foot (ceiling) and 2 mile (visibility) Night/x-country: 1000 foot (ceiling) and 3 mile (visibility)

Number one cause of air medical crashes	Controlled flight into terrain, *pushing the weather*
Lab values 1. Normal potassium 2. Normal sodium 3. Normal chloride 4. Normal calcium 5. Metabolic acidosis elevates?	1. 3.5-5.5 2. 135-145 3. 95-105 4. 8.5-10.5 5. potassium
Time of useful consciousness with sudden decompression at: 30,000 feet 41,000 feet	30,000: 90 seconds 41,000: under 15 seconds Least amount of time is your answer on the exam

12-lead ECG Inferior Septal Anterior Lateral Posterior	"I See All Leads" = Inf/sept/ant/lat Inferior: II, III, aV_F Septal: V_1, V_2 Anterior: V_3, V_4 Lateral: I, aV_L, V_5, V = Posterior: ST segment depression or reciprocal changes noted in V_1-V_4, ST elevation V_6
Cardiac Ischemia Injury Infarct	Ischemia: ST depression (1 mm in 2 leads) Injury: ST elevation (1 mm in 2 leads) Infarct: Q wave > 25% the height of the R wave
Pediatric age guidelines ETT cuffed versus uncuffed Needle cricothyrotomy Nasal intubation	**"10, 11, 12" Rules** Uncuffed tube under 10 Needle cricothyrotomy only under 11 No nasal intubation under 12

High-risk OB 1. Primary cause of PTL 2. Terbutaline contraindications 3. PIH triad signs	1. Infection 2. IDDM, Maternal HR over 120, vaginal bleeding 3. HTN, edema, proteinuria
O_2 adjustment calculation to maintain saturation at altitude	% oxygen patient is already on X pressure at departure (mmHg) Pressure at altitude This equals percentage needed in flight **Example** Patient on FIO_2 of 0.40 Depart: 681 mmHg Altitude: 565 mmHg Answer: patient needs 48% oxygen
Ventilator modes CMV AC IMV/SIMV	CMV: preset volume or PIP at set rate. Patient can't initiate breath AC: preset volume or PIP with every breath. Can trigger breath, can't control TV IMV: preset breaths, TV, PIP. Patient breaths allowed SIMV: allows variation of support

IABP 1. Action 2. Deflates 3. Dicrotic Notch	1. Increase cardiac output, coronary perfusion 2. during ventricular systole 3. aortic valve closing, synchronized with a-line or ECG (most common trigger)
IABP 1. Signs/symptoms of balloon leak 2. Clot prevention 3. IABP increases CO by 4. Balloon rupture 5. Migration/dislodged 6. Lethal IABP timing cycles	1. blood specs in tubing, alarm 2. cycle manually every 30 minutes 3. 10-20% 4. rusty flakes in line or turn machine off 5. assess left radial and urine output 6. late deflation and early inflation
Oxyhemoglobin disassociation curve Left shift	**"L" stands for Alkalosis** Left shift = low Hemoglobin holding oxygen Alkalosis Low CO_2 Low temperature Low DPG Mxydema coma

Oxyhemoglobin disassociation curve Right shift	**"R" stands for raised** Right = raise/releases oxygen Acidosis Raised CO_2 Raised temperature Raised DPG Thyroid storm
Phlebostatic axis Where? What?	Where pressure measurements are made with invasive line Fourth intercostal space, level of atria
Boyle's law Ascent Descent	**Ascent** Barondontalgia (toothache) Barosinutis can occur on ascent Bariobariatrauma (obese) = Nitrogen in the fat cells can expand causing the "bends" administer high flow oxygen for 15 minutes prior to lift-off to remove nitrogen **Descent** Barotitis media (middle ear) can affect the patient during descent

Hypertension Mild Moderate Severe	Mild: 140-159/90-99 Moderate: 160-179/100-109 Severe: over 180/110
Volume for RBC administration **Volume for WBC**	RBC: 10 mL/kg WBC: 20 mL/kg
ABG rules 1. CO_2 and pH 2. Bicarb and pH 3. Bicarb replacement 4. PaO_2 at altitude	1. CO_2 up 10 = pH down .08 (inverse) 2. HCO_3 up 10 = pH up 15 (proportional) 3. kg/4 × base deficit = meq of bicarb needed 4. PaO_2 drops 5 for every 1000 feet elevation

Stages of hypoxia Elevation Signs or symptoms	Indifferent: (10,000 feet MSL): increased HR and RR, decreased night vision Compensatory: (10,000-15,000 feet MSL): HTN, task impairment Disturbance: (15,000-20,000 feet MSL): dizzy, sleepy, cyanosis Critical: (20,000-30,000 feet MSL): ALOC, incapacitated
Night vision lost at:	5,000' MSL
PA Catheter 1. Named? 2. Proximal port is for? 3. S/S of bad placement? 4. Procedure for bad placement? 5. Measures? 6. Which port used? 7. Pressure bag set to?	1. Swan-Ganz 2. CVP, medications 3 VT, ventricular ectopy 4. Float forward to PA or pull back to RA 5. Right heart directly, left heart indirectly 6. Distal port 7. 300 mmHg

Normal cardiac index	CI: 2.5-4.3
Stressors of flight	1. third spacing 2. fatigue 3. g-forces 4. noise 5. vibration 6. hypoxia 7. dehydration 8. temp changes 9. barometric pressure changes
Personal factors affecting stressors of flight?	DEATH Drugs Exhaustion Alcohol Tobacco Hypoglycemia

Dalton's law	Sum total of partial pressures equal to total atmospheric pressures (Dalton's gang) Examples tissue swelling, altitude hypoxia, hypoxic hypoxia This is why O_2 is needed at altitude
Cardiac Thrombolytics must be administered within	Three hours of onset of chest pain
Diving injuries ATM	1 ATM for every 33 feet descent *and* Add 1 if asking for total ATM versus water pressure

Hypovolemic shock CVP CO Cardiac Index Wedge SVR Heart rate	CVP: down CO: down CI: down PAWP: down SVR: high Heart rate: fast
Acute respiratory failure	pO_2 below 60, pCO_2 above 50
Newton's laws	*First law: an object in motion tends to stay in motion . . .* Second law: force = mass × acceleration Third law: every action has = and opposite reaction

Tetralogy of Fallot (TOF)	**Remember PROV** P = pulmonary stenosis R = right ventricular hypertrophy O = overriding aorta V = ventricular septal defect
What is a tet spell?	During a "tet" spell, blood flow across the right ventricular outflow tract is significantly decreased, resulting in shunting right-to-left through the VSD out of the aorta, thus bypassing the lungs. Causes include: spasms, sudden decrease in systemic vascular resistance secondary to hypovolemia, dehydration, hot weather, or defecation. Tet spells are usually seen in the neonatal period, and peak in incidence between two and four months of life.
Atrial waveforms	"filling pressures" Right atrial pressure (CVP) Left atrial pressure (PAWP/ PCWP)

Ventricular waveforms	Right ventricular pressure obtained upon insertion of PA catheter or if the catheter has been dislodged backward into the right ventricle resulting in a right ventricular waveform Looks like "VT," no dicrotic notch seen on the downslope of the right side of the waveform Left ventricular pressure measured during cardiac catheterization
Arterial waveforms	Arterial lines Pulmonary artery pressure (PAP) Dicrotic notch seen on the downslope of the right side of the waveform

Waves	A wave = rise in atrial pressure as a result of atrial contraction C wave = not always visible on the tracing, rise in the atrial pressure which closure of the AV valves (tricuspid and mitral) bulge upward into the atrium following valve closure V wave = rise in atrial pressure as it refills during ventricular contraction
A Wave Correlation to ECG	A wave generally coincides with the PR interval on the ECG in a right atrial pressure waveform It will be slightly delayed in a left atrial pressure waveform

C Wave Correlation to ECG	C wave generally coincides with mid to late QRS on the ECG in a right atrial pressure waveform It will be slightly delayed in a left atrial pressure waveform
V Wave Correlation to ECG	V wave is generally seen immediately after the peak of the T wave on the ECG in a right atrial pressure waveform It will be slightly delayed in a left atrial pressure waveform
Wave descents	Decline in right atrial pressure during atrial relaxation (Remember "X" in relaXation) Decline in right atrial pressure resulting from atrial emptying (Remember "Y" in emptYing)

Breathing and waveforms	**Record pressure measurements at the end of exhalation** In a spontaneously breathing patient, inspiration is the fall in pressure, expiration is the rise in pressure. End-expiration occurs just prior to the respiratory drop in pressure Positive pressure mechanical ventilated patients will cause cardiac pressure to rise upon inspiration
Measuring waveforms	The end-diastolic pressure can be estimated by identifying the "Z" point A line is drawn from the end of the QRS to the hemodynamic tracing. The point where the line intersects with the waveform is the "Z" point. The "Z" point on the PAWP tracing will be delayed by 0.08-0.12 seconds from the QRS

Cardiac output	Heart rate × stroke volume = CO
Dicrotic notch	Closure of the aortic valve
Neonatal	Maintains the PDA open = prostaglandin (PGE1) Closed the PDA = indomethacin and long-term use of high oxygen delivery 32 weeks or less in gestation = surfactant Common cause of seizures = hypoglycemia ≤ 40 mg/dL and hypoxia Scaphoid abdomen = diaphragmatic hernia managed with orogastric tube and PPV

CPK > 20,000	CPK (muscle enzyme) levels greater than 20,000 is ominous and is an indication of later DIC, acute renal failure and is potentially dangerous hyperkalemia in the heatstroke patient
Anion gap	$Na - (Cl + Bicarb/CO_2) = AG$ Normal 12 ± 4 > 16 indicates an underlying metabolic acidosis *Remember "MUDPILES"* Methanol Uremia DKA Paraldehyde Isoniazide/Iron Lactate Ethylene glycol Salicylate

Appendix D
Tips on How to Study for the Exam

Studying is only a part of getting good results on your exam. Preparation for your examination should begin several months prior; this includes studying, reviewing study materials on a regular basis, and if possible, attending a BCCTPC approved 16-hour FP-C/CCP-C review course. Students with better study methods and strategies have a better success in passing the certification examination. Everyone is different, different methods work for different people and the following are only suggestions on improving upon your current studying techniques.

Before the Exam: Tips on Improving Test Taking and Study Skills

- ✓ Budget your time; make sure you have sufficient time to study so that you are well prepared for the test.
- ✓ Go to eview sessions, pay attention to hints that the instructor may give about the test. Take notes and ask questions about items you may be confused about.
- ✓ Ask the instructor to specify the areas that will be emphasized on the examination.
- ✓ Go over any material from practice exams, review material, the textbook, class notes, and study flashcards.
- ✓ Do not try to pull an all-nighter. Get at least eight hours of sleep before the exam.
- ✓ Eat before a test. Having food in your stomach will give you energy and help you focus, but avoid heavy foods which can make you groggy.
- ✓ Do not try to do all your studying the night before the test. Instead space out your studying, review class materials at least several times a week, focusing on one topic at a time.
- ✓ Start out by studying the most important information. Learn the general concepts first; don't worry about learning the details until you have learned the main ideas.
- ✓ Take notes and write down a summary of the important ideas as you read through your study material.

✓ Take short breaks frequently. Your memory retains the information that you study at the beginning and the end better than what you study in the middle.

✓ Space out your studying, you'll learn more by studying a little every day instead of waiting to cram at the last minute. By studying every day, the material will stay in your long-term memory but if you try to study at the last moment, the material will only reside in your short-term memory that you will easily forget.

✓ Make sure that you understand the material well, don't just read through the material, and try to memorize everything.

✓ Test yourself or have someone test you on the material to find out what your weak and strong areas are. You can use the review questions and study flashcards or practice tests the instructor may give out as well as other materials.

Day of the Exam: Tips on Answering Multiple Choice Questions

✓ It is best to take the examination within 2 weeks of attending a 2-day review course, sooner if possible, the information is still fresh in your memory.

✓ Try to show up at least 15 minutes before the exam will start and make sure you have your photo ID with you.

✓ Put the main ideas or information or formulas onto a sheet that can be quickly reviewed which makes it easier to retain the key concepts that will be on the exam.

✓ Do not rush but pace yourself. Bring a watch to the testing site with you so that you can better pace yourself.

✓ *Make sure you read the last sentence first, so that you are sure of what the question is asking for, then read the whole question carefully and look for keywords before you look at the answer.* Do not make assumptions about what the question might be.

✓ Come up with the answer before looking at the possible answers, this way the choices given on the test will not throw you off or trick you.

✓ Read all the choices before choosing your answer.

✓ Eliminate answers you know are not right. There are usually two answers that can be eliminated.

✓ Do the easiest problems first. Do not stay on a problem that you are stuck on, especially when time is a factor.

✓ If you do not know an answer, skip it. Go on with the rest of the test and come back to it later. Other parts of the test may have some information that will help you out with that question.

✓ If there is no guessing penalty, always take an educated guess and select an answer.

✓ *Do not keep on changing your answer, usually your first choice is the right one, unless you misread the question.*

✓ In "All of the above" and "None of the above" choices, if you are certain one of the statements is true, do not choose "None of the above" or one of the statements are false do not choose "All of the above."

✓ In a question with an "All of the above" choice, if you see that at least two correct statements, then "All of the above" is probably the answer.

✓ A positive choice is more likely to be true than a negative one.

✓ Usually the correct answer is the choice with the most information.

✓ Keep a positive attitude throughout the whole test and try to stay relaxed. If you start to feel nervous take a few deep breaths to relax.

✓ Do not worry if others finish before you. Focus on the test in front of you.

✓ If you have time left when you are finished, look over your test. Make sure that you have answered all the questions, only change an answer if you misread or misinterpreted the question because the first answer that you put is usually the correct one.

Test anxiety is when a student excessively worries about doing well on a test. This can become a major hindrance on test performance and cause extreme nervousness and memory lapses among other symptoms. The following are tips on reducing test-taking anxiety.

✓ Being well prepared for the test is the best way to reduce test taking anxiety.

- ✓ Space out your studying over a few months and continually review class material. Do not try to learn everything the night before.
- ✓ Try to maintain a positive attitude while preparing for the test and during the test.
- ✓ Exercising for a few days before the test will help reduce stress.
- ✓ Get a good night's sleep before the test.
- ✓ Show up to the testing site early so you will not have to worry about being late.
- ✓ Stay relaxed; if you begin to get nervous, take a few deep breaths slowly to relax yourself and then get back to work.
- ✓ Read the directions slowly and carefully.
- ✓ Write down important formulas, facts, definitions, and/or keywords on a blank piece of paper, so you will not worry about forgetting them.
- ✓ Do the simple questions first to help build up your confidence for the harder questions.
- ✓ Do not worry about how fast other people finish their test; just concentrate on your own test.
- ✓ If you do not know a question skip it for the time being (come back to it later if you have time), and remember that you do not have to always get every question right to do well on the test.
- ✓ Focus on the question at hand. Do not let your mind wander on other things.

Good Luck!

About the Author

As a registered nurse for the last 28 years, my primary clinical expertise has been working in the pre-hospital environment as a flight nurse and a paramedic, as well as continuing to work in a variety of clinical areas which include the emergency department, pediatrics and endoscopy. My extensive clinical background has also given me the opportunity to work as a legal nurse consultant with one of the largest law firms in Arizona. As an EMS educator and program director of paramedic training programs for the last 20 years and most recently as the National Clinical Educator for one of the largest air medical transport companies, I truly enjoy teaching in a simple manner as to assure that students do have a strong basic understanding in making critical care decisions and that they will be providing the highest quality of patient care beginning from the least to the most invasive management of care for the patients they are transporting. My goal as a professional and as an EMS educator has always been to encourage students to have the desire to learn and grow in their profession, as well as contribute to EMS in a way that inspires positive change.

"Tell me and I'll forget;
Show me and I may remember;
Involve me and I'll understand"

Index

Made in the USA
Middletown, DE
02 September 2024

60177781R00278